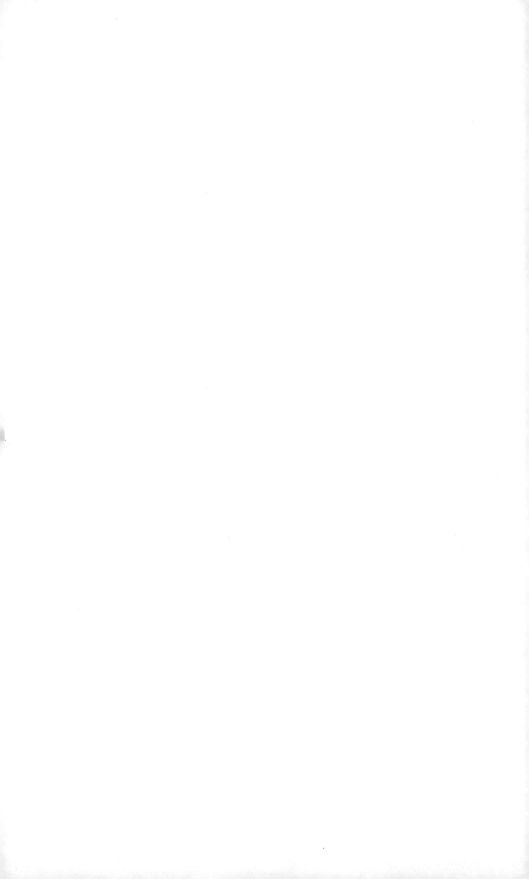

OVARIAN CANCER

Cancer Treatment and Research
Steven T. Rosen, M.D., *Series Editor*

Kurzrock, R., Talpaz, M. (eds): *Cytokines: Interleukins and Their Receptors.* 1995.
ISBN 0-7923-3636-4.
Sugarbaker, P. (ed): *Peritoneal Carcinomatosis: Drugs and Diseases.* 1995.
ISBN 0-7923-3726-3.
Sugarbaker, P. (ed): *Peritoneal Carcinomatosis: Principles of Management.* 1995.
ISBN 0-7923-3727-1.
Dickson, R.B., Lippman, M.E. (eds.): *Mammary Tumor Cell Cycle, Differentiation and Metastasis.* 1995. ISBN 0-7923-3905-3.
Freireich, E.J, Kantarjian, H. (eds.): *Molecular Genetics and Therapy of Leukemia.* 1995.
ISBN 0-7923-3912-6.
Cabanillas, F., Rodriguez, M.A. (eds.): *Advances in Lymphoma Research.* 1996.
ISBN 0-7923-3929-0.
Miller, A.B. (ed.): *Advances in Cancer Screening.* 1996. ISBN 0-7923-4019-1.
Hait , W.N. (ed.): *Drug Resistance.* 1996. ISBN 0-7923-4022-1.
Pienta, K.J. (ed.): *Diagnosis and Treatment of Genitourinary Malignancies.* 1996.
ISBN 0-7923-4164-3.
Arnold, A.J. (ed.): *Endocrine Neoplasms.* 1997. ISBN 0-7923-4354-9.
Pollock, R.E. (ed.): *Surgical Oncology.* 1997. ISBN 0-7923-9900-5.
Verweij, J., Pinedo, H.M., Suit, H.D. (eds.): *Soft Tissue Sarcomas: Present Achievements and Future Prospects.* 1997. ISBN 0-7923-9913-7.
Walterhouse, D.O., Cohn, S. L. (eds.): *Diagnostic and Therapeutic Advances in Pediatric Oncology.* 1997. ISBN 0-7923-9978-1.
Mittal, B.B., Purdy, J.A., Ang, K.K. (eds.): *Radiation Therapy.* 1998.
ISBN 0-7923-9981-1.
Foon, K.A., Muss, H.B. (eds.): *Biological and Hormonal Therapies of Cancer.* 1998.
ISBN 0-7923-9997-8.
Ozols, R.F. (ed.): *Gynecologic Oncology.* 1998. ISBN 0-7923-8070-3.
Noskin, G. A. (ed.): *Management of Infectious Complications in Cancer Patients.* 1998.
ISBN 0-7923-8150-5
Bennett, C. L. (ed.): *Cancer Policy.* 1998. ISBN 0-7923-8203-X
Benson, A. B. (ed.): *Gastrointestinal Oncology.* 1998. ISBN 0-7923-8205-6
Tallman, M.S. , Gordon, L.I. (eds.): *Diagnostic and Therapeutic Advances in Hematologic Malignancies.* 1998. ISBN 0-7923-8206-4
von Gunten, C.F. (ed.): *Palliative Care and Rehabilitation of Cancer Patients.* 1999.
ISBN 0-7923-8525-X
Burt, R.K., Brush, M.M. (eds): *Advances in Allogeneic Hematopoietic Stem Cell Transplantation.* 1999. ISBN 0-7923-7714-1
Angelos, P. (ed): *Ethical Issues in Cancer Patient Care* 2000. ISBN 0-7923-7726-5
Gradishar, W.J., Wood, W.C. (eds): *Advances in Breast Cancer Management.* 2000.
ISBN 0-7923-7890-3
Sparano, Joseph A. (ed.): *HIV & HTLV-I Associated Malignancies.* 2001.
ISBN 0-7923-7220-4.
Ettinger, David S. (ed.): *Thoracic Oncology.* 2001. ISBN 0-7923-7248-4.
Bergan, Raymond C. (ed.): *Cancer Chemoprevention.* 2001. ISBN 0-7923-7259-X.
Raza, A., Mundle, S.D. (eds): *Myelodysplastic Syndromes & Secondary Acute Myelogenous Leukemia; Directions for the new Millennium.* 2001. ISBN 0-7923-7396-0.
Talamonti, Mark S. (ed.): *Liver Directed Therapy for Primary and Metastatic Liver Tumors.* 2001 ISBN 0-7923-7523-8
Stack, M.S., Fishman, D.A. (eds.): *Ovarian Cancer.* 2001 ISBN 0-7923-7530-0

OVARIAN CANCER

edited by

M. Sharon Stack, Ph.D.
and
David A. Fishman, M.D.

*Northwestern University Medical School
Chicago, IL, U.S.A.*

KLUWER ACADEMIC PUBLISHERS
Boston / Dordrecht / London

BS

Distributors for North, Central and South America:
Kluwer Academic Publishers
101 Philip Drive
Assinippi Park
Norwell, Massachusetts 02061 USA
Telephone (781) 871-6600
Fax (781) 681-9045
E-Mail <kluwer@wkap.com>

Distributors for all other countries:
Kluwer Academic Publishers Group
Distribution Centre
Post Office Box 322
3300 AH Dordrecht, THE NETHERLANDS
Telephone 31 78 6392 392
Fax 31 78 6546 474
E-Mail <services@wkap.nl>

 Electronic Services <http://www.wkap.nl>

Library of Congress Cataloging-in-Publication Data

Ovarian cancer / edited by M. Sharon Stack and David A. Fishman.
   p. ; cm. – (Cancer treatment and research ; 107)
   Includes bibliographical references and index.
   ISBN 0-7923-7530-0
   1. Ovaries—Cancer. 2. Carcinogenesis. 3. Metastasis. I. Stack, M. Sharon, 1959- II.
Fishman, David A., 1959- III. Cancer treatment and research ; v. 107.
   [DNLM: 1. Ovarian Neoplasms—therapy. WP 322 09631 2001]
RC280.08 08832 2001
616.99'465—dc21

                                                      2001038790

*The Publisher offers discounts on this book for bulk purchases. For further
information, send email to [laura.walsh@wkap.com]*

Printed on acid-free paper. Printed in the United States of America

5/20/03

To our spouses, parents and children,

for their strength, wisdom, and love.

CONTENTS

Contributors ix

Foreword xiii

I. TREATMENT:

1. **The Scientific Basis of Early Detection of Epithelial Ovarian Cancer**
   David A. Fishman and Kenny Bozorgi...3

2. **Risk Assessment and Genetic Testing**
   Pierre O. Chappuis and William D. Foulkes....................................29

3. **Early Detection of Ovarian Cancer: Promise and Reality**
   Robert C. Bast, Jr, Nicole Urban, Viji Shirdhar, David Smith, Zhen Zhang,
   Steven Skates, Karen Lu, Jinsong Liu, David Fishman
   and Gordon Mills...61

4. **Current Diagnosis and Treatment Modalities for Ovarian Cancer**
   Peter E. Schwartz...99

5. **Ultrasound and Ovarian Cancer**
   Leeber Cohen and David A. Fishman..119

6. **Gene Therapy**
   Warner K. Huh, Mack N. Barnes, F. Joseph Kelly, and
   Ronald D. Alvarez..133

II. RESEARCH
A. Malignant Transformation

7. **Normal Ovarian Surface Epithelium**
   Alice S.T. Wong and Nelly Auersperg..161

8. **Cytopathology of the Ovary**
   D.V.S. DeFrias, A.M. Okonkwo, P.C. Keh, and R. Nayar.......................185

9. **Telomerase and Malignant Transformation**
   Jiamei Yu and Louis Dubeau...213

10. **Homeobox Gene Expression in Ovarian Cancer**
   Susan M. Pando and Hugh S. Taylor...231

B. Growth Control

11. **EGF/ErbB Receptor Family in Ovarian Cancer**
   N.J. Maihle, A.T. Baron, B.A. Barrette, C.H. Boardman, T.A.
   Christensen, E.M. Cora, J.M. Faupel-Badger, T. Greenwood, S.C. Juneja,
   J.M. Lafky, H. Lee, J.L. Reiter, and K.C. Podratz..........................247

12. **Critical Role of Lysophospholipids in the Pathophysiology, Diagnosis,
   and Management of Ovarian Cancer**
   Gordon B. Mills, Astrid Eder, Xianjun Fang, Yutaka Hasegawa, Muling
   Mao, Yiling Lu, Janos Tanyi, Fazal Haq Tabassam, Jon Wiener, Ruth
   Lapushin, Shiangxing Yu, Jeff A. Parrott, Tim Compton, Walter Tribley,
   David Fishman, M. Sharon Stack, Douglas Gaudette, Robert Jaffe,
   Tatsuro Furui, Junken Aoki, and James R. Erickson.......................259

13. **Expression of CSF-1 and Its Receptor CSF-1R in Non-Hematopoietic
   Neoplasms**
   Barry Kascinski...285

14. **Role of Inhibins and Activins in Ovarian Cancer**
   Teresa K. Woodruff..293

C. Cellular Regulation and Metastasis

15. **Adhesion Molecules**
   Amy P.N. Skubitz..305

16. **Ovarian Cancer-Associated Proteinases**
   Supurna Ghosh, Yi Wu, and M. Sharon Stack.............................331

17. **Angiogenesis and Metastasis**
   Gregory J. Sieczkiewicz, Mahrukh Hussain, and Elise C. Kohn.........353

Index 383

Contributors

Ronald D. Alvarez, Division of Gynecologic Oncology, Department of Obstetrics & Gynecology, University of Alabama, Birmingham, AL 35233

Junken Aoki, Graduate School of Pharmaceutical Sciences, University of Tokyo, 7-3-1 Hongo, Bunkyo-Ku, Tokyo 113-0033, Japan

Nelly Auersperg, Department of Obstetrics & Gynaecology, University of British Columbia, Vancouver, B.C., V6H 3V5, Canada

Mack N. Barnes, Division of Gynecologic Oncology, Department of Obstetrics & Gynecology, University of Alabama, Birmingham, AL 35233

A.T. Baron, Tumor Biology Program, Mayo Clinic, Rochester, MN 55905

B.A. Barrette, Department of Obstetrics & Gynecology, Mayo Clinic, Rochester, MN 55905

Robert C. Bast, Jr, Departments of Experimental Therapeutics, Molecular Therapeutics, Gynecologic Oncology and Anatomic Pathology, University of Texas M.D. Anderson Cancer Center, Houston, TX 77030

C.H. Boardman, Department of Obstetrics & Gynecology, Mayo Clinic, Rochester, MN 55905

Kenny Bozorgi, Section of Gynecologic Oncology, Department of Obstetrics & Gynecology, Northwestern University Medical School, Chicago, IL 60611

Pierre O. Chappuis, Division of Medical Genetics, Department of Medicine, McGill University Health Center, Montreal, QC, Canada

T.A. Christensen, Tumor Biology Program, Mayo Clinic, Rochester, MN 55905

Leeber Cohen, Division of Ultrasound, Department of Obstetrics & Gynecology, Northwestern University Medical School, Chicago, IL 60611

Tim Compton, Atairgin Technologies, 101 Theory, Irvine, CA 92612

E.M. Cora, Department of Biochemistry & Nutrition, University of Puerto Rico, School of Medicine, PO Box 365067, San Juan, PR 00936

D.V.S. DeFrias, Department of Pathology, Northwestern University Medical School, Chicago, IL 60611

Louis Dubeau, Department of Pathology, Keck School of Medicine of the University of Southern California, Norris Comprehensive Cancer Center, Los Angeles, CA 90033

Astrid Eder, Department of Molecular Therapeutics, MD Anderson Cancer Center, 1515 Holcombe Blvd., Houston, TX 77030

James R. Erickson, AGY Therapeutics, 290 Utah Ave., S. San Francisco, CA 94080

Xianjun Fang, Department of Molecular Therapeutics, MD Anderson Cancer Center, 1515 Holcombe Blvd., Houston, TX 77030

J.M. Faupel-Badger, Tumor Biology Program, Mayo Clinic, Rochester, MN 55905

David A. Fishman, Section of Gynecologic Oncology, Department of Obstetrics & Gynecology, Northwestern University Medical School, Chicago, IL 60611

William D. Foulkes, Division of Medical Genetics, Department of Medicine, McGill University Health Center, Montreal, QC, Canada

Tatsuro Furui, Department of Obstetrics & Gynecology, Gifu University School of Medicine, 40 Tsukasa-machi, Gifu, 500-8705, Japan

Douglas Gaudette, Department of Human Biology & Nutrition Science, University of Guelph, ANNU Building, Guelph, Ontario,Canada N1G2W1

Supurna Ghosh, Department of Cell & Molecular Biology, Northwestern University Medical School, Chicago, IL 60611

T. Greenwood, Tumor Biology Program, Mayo Clinic, Rochester, MN 55905

Yutaka Hasegawa, Department of Molecular Therapeutics, MD Anderson Cancer Center, 1515 Holcombe Blvd., Houston, TX 77030

Warner K. Huh, Division of Gynecologic Oncology, Department of Obstetrics & Gynecology, University of Alabama, Birmingham, AL 35233

Mahrukh Hussain, National Cancer Institute, Laboratory of Pathology, Building 10, Rm 2A33, 10 Center Drive, Bethesda, MD 20892

Robert Jaffe, Department of Obstetrics, Gynecology, & Reproductive Sciences, University of California San Francisco, 513 Parnassus Ave., San Francisco, CA 94122

S.C. Juneja, Tumor Biology Program, Mayo Clinic, Rochester, MN 55905

Barry Kascinski, Department of Therapeutic Radiology, Yale University School of Medicine, New Haven, CT 06520

P.C. Keh, Department of Pathology, Northwestern University Medical School, Chicago, IL 60611

F. Joseph Kelly, Division of Gynecologic Oncology, Department of Obstetrics & Gynecology, University of Alabama, Birmingham, AL 35233

Elise C. Kohn, National Cancer Institute, Laboratory of Pathology, Building 10, Rm 2A33, 10 Center Drive, Bethesda, MD 20892

J.M. Lafky, Tumor Biology Program, Mayo Clinic, Rochester, MN 55905

Ruth Lapushin, Department of Molecular Therapeutics, MD Anderson Cancer Center, 1515 Holcombe Blvd., Houston, TX 77030

H. Lee, Tumor Biology Program, Mayo Clinic, Rochester, MN 55905

Jinsong Liu, Departments of Experimental Therapeutics, Molecular Therapeutics, Gynecologic Oncology and Anatomic Pathology, University of Texas M.D. Anderson Cancer Center, Houston, TX 77030

Karen Lu, Departments of Experimental Therapeutics, Molecular Therapeutics, Gynecologic Oncology and Anatomic Pathology, University of Texas M.D. Anderson Cancer Center, Houston, TX 77030

N.J. Maihle, Tumor Biology Program, Mayo Clinic, Rochester, MN 55905

Muling Mao, Department of Molecular Therapeutics, MD Anderson Cancer Center, 1515 Holcombe Blvd., Houston, TX 77030

Gordon B. Mills, Department of Molecular Therapeutics, MD Anderson Cancer Center, 1515 Holcombe Blvd., Houston, TX 77030

R. Nayar, Department of Pathology, Northwestern University Medical School, Chicago, IL 60611

A.M. Okonkwo, Department of Pathology, Northwestern University Medical School, Chicago, IL 60611

Susan M. Pando, Department of Obstetrics & Gynecology, Yale University School of Medicine, New Haven, CT 06520

Jeff A. Parrott, Atairgin Technologies, 101 Theory, Irvine, CA 92612

K. C. Podratz, Department of Obstetrics & Gynecology, Mayo Clinic, Rochester, MN 55905

J.L. Reiter, Tumor Biology Program, Mayo Clinic, Rochester, MN 55905

Peter E. Schwartz, Yale University School of Medicine, Department of Obstetrics & Gynecology, 333 Cedar St., New Haven, CT 06520

Viji Shridhar, Mayo Clinic, Rochester, MN 55905

Gregory J. Sieczkiewicz, National Cancer Institute, Laboratory of Pathology, Building 10, Rm 2A33, 10 Center Drive, Bethesda, MD 20892

Steven Skates, Massachusetts General Hospital, Boston, MA 02144

Amy P.N. Skubitz, Department of Laboratory Medicine & Pathology, University of Minnesota Medical School, Minneapolis, MN 55455

David Smith, Mayo Clinic, Rochester, MN 55905

M. Sharon Stack, Department of Cell & Molecular Biology, Northwestern University Medical School, Chicago, IL 60611

Fazal Haq Tabassam, Department of Molecular Therapeutics, MD Anderson Cancer Center, 1515 Holcombe Blvd., Houston, TX 77030

Janos Tanyi, Department of Molecular Therapeutics, MD Anderson Cancer Center, 1515 Holcombe Blvd., Houston, TX 77030

Hugh S. Taylor, Department of Obstetrics & Gynecology, Yale University School of Medicine, New Haven, CT 06520

Walter Tribley, Atairgin Technologies, 101 Theory, Irvine, CA 92612

Nicole Urban, The Fred Hutchinson Cancer Center, Seattle, WA 98101

John Wiener, Department of Molecular Therapeutics, MD Anderson Cancer Center, 1515 Holcombe Blvd., Houston, TX 77030

Alice S.T. Wong, Department of Obstetrics & Gynaecology, University of British Columbia, Vancouver, B.C., V6H 3V5, Canada

Teresa K. Woodruff, Department of Neurobiology & Physiology, Northwestern University, Evanston, IL 60208

Yi Wu, Department of Cell & Molecular Biology, Northwestern University Medical School, Chicago, IL 60611

Jiamei Yu, Department of Pathology, Keck School of Medicine of the University of Southern California, Norris Comprehensive Cancer Center, Los Angeles, CA 90033

Shiangxing Yu, Department of Molecular Therapeutics, MD Anderson
Cancer Center, 1515 Holcombe Blvd., Houston, TX 77030
Zhen Shang, Medical University of South Carolina, Charleston, SC 29425

Foreword

Ovarian carcinoma continues to be responsible for more deaths than all other gynecologic malignancies combined due to our continued inability to achieve detection of early (rather than advanced) stage disease and the lack of effective tumor-specific therapeutics. Despite many diagnostic imaging, surgical, medical, and therapeutic advances, little has changed over the past 40 years, as 70-75% of women newly diagnosed with epithelial ovarian carcinoma present with disseminated carcinomatosis (stage III or IV disease) with a resultant 5-year survival of 12 %. However, if disease is identified when confined to the ovary (Stage I), surgical intervention is less morbid, chemotherapy may not be required, and the resultant 5-year survival approaches 90%. Therefore the most effective means for improving survival requires detection of early stage rather than advanced stage disease.

Ovarian carcinogenesis, invasion and metastatic dissemination require a complex cascade of interrelated genetic, molecular, and biochemical events that regulate the neoplastic transition of normal ovarian surface epithelium. Ovarian cancers accumulate genetic aberrations that alter cell cycle control, DNA repair, genomic stability, apoptosis, transmembrane signaling, adhesion, and angiogenesis. Metastatic dissemination is influenced by numerous regulatory molecules and requires diverse biologic processes including cellular adhesion, migration, extracellular matrix degradation, directed invasion into host parenchyma, proliferation, and neovascularization. Many of these genetic aberrations and/or regulatory molecules are detectable in women with ovarian cancer and may ultimately serve as both novel tumor-specific biomarkers for early detection and for unique tumor-specific therapeutics. This volume summarizes recent advances in ovarian cancer detection and treatment and provides an analysis of current research into aspects of malignant transformation, growth control, and metastasis. A more detailed understanding of these processes may ultimately translate into the development of novel approaches for the detection and control of ovarian cancer.

I. TREATMENT

Chapter 1

THE SCIENTIFIC BASIS OF EARLY DETECTION OF EPITHELIAL OVARIAN CANCER: THE NATIONAL OVARIAN CANCER EARLY DETECTION PROGRAM (NOCEDP)

David A. Fishman and Kenny Bozorgi
Section of Gynecologic Oncology, Department of Obstetrics & Gynecology, Northwestern University Medical School, Chicago, IL 60611

1. INTRODUCTION

In the United States ovarian cancer is the leading cause of death from gynecologic malignancies and is the fifth most common female malignancy. Each year approximately 24,000 women will be newly diagnosed with ovarian cancer and 14,000 will die from this disease. In industrialized countries ovarian cancer accounts for more deaths than uterine and cervical cancer combined. The incidence of ovarian cancer has been steadily increasing over the past ten years, now with an overall lifetime risk of 1.8%. Ovarian cancer rapidly increases in occurrence after age 40 with the mean age of occurrence at 60 (1). Epidemiologic factors associated with ovarian cancer include nulliparity, a personal history of colon or breast cancer, an affected first degree relative with ovarian cancer, a family history of a recognized inherited malignancy syndrome, as well as a history of prolonged use of fertility drugs (2). Due to our current inability in detecting cancer confined to the ovary (stage I disease), the majority of women (75%) are diagnosed with tumor spread throughout the abdominal cavity (stage III or IV). This extensive spread of ovarian carcinoma often is associated with subtle symptoms such as bloating, early satiety, abdominal discomfort, or changes in bowel or bladder habits; vague symptoms that may often be dismissed by patient and/or healthcare provider or simply misdiagnosed. It is the anatomic location of the ovaries that contributes to our inability to detect early stage ovarian carcinoma. Despite significant improvements in surgical techniques, critical care and new chemotherapeutic regimens, the overall 5-year survival for women with stage III/IV epithelial ovarian carcinoma has remained constant (12 – 20%) over the past 30 years. Conversely, those patients diagnosed with stage I disease usually only require surgical intervention without chemotherapy and have an overall 5-year survival approximating 90%. Therefore the early detection of early stage epithelial ovarian cancer is essential in curbing the morbidity and mortality from this disease.

For decades clinicians have sought a means of detecting early stage disease with the intention of decreasing mortality; yet, to date no screening strategy has been shown to decrease mortality. A suitable test or examination should have both high sensitivity and high specificity to be a suitable screening test for a disease (3). Unfortunately, an increase in the sensitivity of a test is associated with a reduction in specificity, and vice versa. Specificity is a major concern for ovarian cancer screening because the majority of women who test positive will require surgical intervention. For example, even a test with 98% specificity would result in 50 false positive procedures for every case of ovarian cancer detected on screening the postmenopausal population. A screening test for this population requires 99.6% specificity to yield a positive predictive value (PPV) of 10%. Lower specificity, however, may be acceptable in higher risk populations. Since the incidence of ovarian cancer in the general population is 1.8%, the specificity of any test currently available is unacceptable for screening. Less than 15% of ovarian cancers occur in women younger than 50 years and the incidence rate does not peak until the 70-74 year group. When one focuses on women that have incidences approaching 60%, as those with inherited BRCA mutations, the utility becomes practical. A test with 90% specificity would yield a PPV of 10% in BRCA carriers since the incidence of ovarian cancer in this population is so high.

The ability to detect early stage epithelial ovarian cancer by a simple blood test has long been an objective in medical screening. The advantages of such an easy to use, relatively noninvasive and operator-independent test is self-evident. At present no commercially available serum marker or combination of markers is useful for the detection of early stage epithelial ovarian cancer, and, contrary to common belief, CA125 should not be used as a screening test in either the general or high-risk population. Another objective is to develop a minimally invasive screening test that can give an assessment of the surface epithelium of the ovaries of women at risk. This is of course analogous to the cervical Pap smear that has significantly decreased the incidence and mortality from cervical cancer since its inception. Similar to the Pap smear, the goal of an "ovarian pap smear" would be to detect pre-invasive lesions as well as early stage invasive lesions of the ovary. The technology to perform an office laparoscopic "ovarian Pap smear" has been developed and the diagnostic potential of such a test is being investigated.

2. SCIENTIFIC OVERVIEW

In order to effect change in the morbidity and mortality associated with ovarian cancer it is necessary to identify those individuals at increased risk and to clinically apply our enhanced understanding of the biochemical and molecular biology of ovarian carcinogenesis. This knowledge will enable the development of ovarian cancer specific therapies that shift the current paradigm from nonspecific antiproliferative therapies to treatments to prevent invasion and metastatic dissemination. Ovarian carcinogenesis, invasion and metastatic dissemination require unique complex cascades of interrelated genetic, molecular, and biochemical events. Ovarian cancers accumulate genetic aberrations that affect cell cycle control, apoptosis, adhesion, angiogenesis, transmembrane signaling, DNA repair, and genomic stability. The metastatic processes of cellular adhesion, migration, extracellular matrix degradation, directed invasion into host parenchyma, proliferation, and neovascularization (4-8) are influenced by numerous regulatory molecules, such as epidermal growth factor (EGF) and receptors (EGFR/ErbB), urinary-type plasminogen activator (uPA) and receptor (uPAR), telomerase and lysophospholipids such as lysophosphatidic acid (LPA) (9-12).

The clinical application of the enhanced understanding of ovarian carcinogenesis and metastatic dissemination is the cornerstone of the National Cancer Institute Early Detection Research Network supported National Ovarian Cancer Early Detection Program, which is committed to the development of accurate methods to attain early detection. Using newly developed bioassays for the detection of matrix metalloproteinases (MMPs), uPA, uPAR, EGFR/ErbB1, telomerase, inhibins, and LPA, these potential biomarkers are being evaluated for the detection of early stage disease. Additionally the genetic and molecular profiles of ovarian surface epithelium will be evaluated and compared to early and advanced stage disease using newly developed high throughput techniques.

3. IDENTIFICATION OF WOMEN AT INCREASED RISK

Ovarian cancer most commonly occurs in a sporadic fashion without any antecedent history of disease in the family. Epidemiological factors associated with ovarian cancer include nulliparity, a personal history of colon or breast cancer, an affected first degree relative with ovarian cancer or a family history of a recognized inherited malignancy syndrome, as well as a history of prolonged use of fertility drugs (13-18). Approximately 5% of epithelial ovarian cancers are attributable to the inheritance of highly penetrant mutations in the breast/ovarian cancer susceptibility genes BRCA-1 and -2

(19,20). The clinical presentation of heritable cancer is similar, yet tends to occur 10-15 years younger. Over 50% of women with BRCA1 mutations develop ovarian cancer prematurely (19-21), with a 30-40% risk of cancer by age 70. Epidemiological studies and detailed analysis of familial ovarian cancer pedigrees have suggested at least three forms of inherited disease: 1) hereditary, site-specific ovarian carcinoma; 2) breast and ovarian cancer syndrome; 3) hereditary nonpolyposis colorectal carcinoma. The recognition of an unexpectedly high frequency of a specific BRCA1 mutation (185delAG) in Ashkenazi Jewish women led to the discovery that the observed carrier frequency is several times higher than the expected frequency of all BRCA1 mutations combined in the general population. Approximately 2% of the Ashkenazi Jewish population has a BRCA-1 or -2 mutation, accounting for 30-50% of early-onset breast or ovarian cancer cases. To estimate the proportion of ovarian cancers attributable to founding mutations in *BRCA1* and *BRCA2* in the Jewish population, Narod et al. interviewed 238 Jewish women with ovarian cancer in North America and Israel, and offered genetic testing for the three founder mutations. Additionally a detailed family history on all cases and on a control population of 386 Ashkenazi Jewish women without ovarian or breast cancer was performed. The cumulative incidence of ovarian cancer to age 75 was found to be 6.3% for female first-degree relatives of the ovarian cancer cases, compared to 2.0% for the female relatives of healthy controls (relative risk 3.1; 95%CI: 1.4-6.5; *P*=. 003). The relative risk to age 75 for breast cancer among the female first-degree relatives was 2.0 (95%CI: 1.4-2.9; *P*=. 0002). A BRCA-1 or -2 mutation was present in 37.8% of the cases. Overall, a greater proportion of ovarian cancers were attributable to *BRCA1* mutations (25.2%) than to the *BRCA2* mutation (12.6%). However, the cumulative incidence of ovarian cancer in the relatives of the *BRCA2* carriers (12.3% to age 75) exceeded that for the first-degree relatives of the *BRCA1* carriers (8.2% to age 75). This unexpectedly high risk is due to the high prevalence of *BRCA2* mutations among elderly Jewish patients with ovarian cancer.

A total of 87 mutations were found among the 230 patients (37.8%), including 58 in *BRCA1* and 29 in *BRCA2*. The frequency of mutations varied by age of onset (Table I); a *BRCA1* mutation was found in 37.3% of women diagnosed between the ages of 30 and 60 and in 11.1% of those diagnosed above age 60 (*P*<. 0001 for difference). A *BRCA2* mutation was found in 8.7% of women diagnosed between 30 and 60 and in 18.2% of women

Table I. Frequency of mutations in cases of ovarian cancer by age at diagnosis				
Age grouping	total	BRCA1 + (%)	BRCA2 + (%)	Either(%)
19	0	(0.0)	0 (0.0)	(0.0)
30-39	19	8 (42.1)	1 (5.3)	(47.4)
40-49	62	24 (38.7)	2 (3.2)	26 (41.9)
50-59	45	15 (33.3)	8 (17.8)	23 (51.1)
60-69	51	9 (17.6)	10 (19.6)	19 (37.3)
70-90	48	2 (4.2)	8 (16.7)	10 (20.8)
Total	230	58 (25.2)	29 (12.6)	87 (37.8)
P value (for trend)	<.001	.009	.087	

diagnosed after age 60 (*P*=. 045). Women with *BRCA1* mutations were diagnosed with ovarian cancer at a younger age than cases for which no mutation was detected (50.6 years and 57.9 years respectively; *P*=. 0004). In contrast, women with *BRCA2* mutations were older at diagnosis (62.1 years versus 57.9 years; *P*=. 08). Those women at increased risk form the cohort who might benefit from a combination of non-invasive and minimally invasive tests to detect early stage ovarian cancer.

4. CLINICAL MANAGEMENT OF WOMEN AT INCREASED RISK

Individuals with a family history suggestive of an inherited malignancy syndrome or those with a living affected relative should be considered for genetic counseling and testing. These include those with a diagnosis of breast or epithelial ovarian cancer before age 50, with a significant family history of breast or ovarian cancer, with a blood relative with a known mutation in BRCA1 or -2, and Ashkenazi women who have breast or ovarian cancer or a family history of one or both diseases. Since approximately 40% of the Jewish women with epithelial ovarian cancer treated at our institutions were found to have a BRCA-1 or BRCA-2 mutation, we now offer all affected Jewish women genetic testing. The benefits of genetic testing for the BRCA genes include the identification of those individuals at increased risk for the development of breast or ovarian cancer, individualizing surveillance measures that may enhance the early detection of cancer, offering prophylactic surgery such as mastectomy or oophorectomy as well as knowledge of the potential for passing the mutation to future generations (14,15). Genetic testing for mutations in these genes also has potential risks, adverse psychological effects, and disruption of family dynamics, insurance or employer discrimination as well as potential for revealing non-paternity.

Prior to initiation of genetic testing it is imperative to provide expert genetic counseling and obtain individual consent. The ethical, legal, and psychological considerations of genetic testing for inherited cancer syndromes are substantial and justify the need for expert counseling. The American Society of Clinical Oncology (ASCO) and the Human Genome Project emphasize the importance of expert counseling for genetic testing. In the NOCEDP, those individuals deemed at increased risk for genetic susceptibility as determined by a board certified geneticist and genetic counselor are eligible for testing. Presently several hundred Jewish women with epithelial ovarian carcinoma have received genetic testing in conjunction with Dr. Narod and 40% were found to be positive for a BRCA-1 or -2 mutation (19-21). The optimal clinical management of individuals who test positive for BRCA mutations is evolving. Therefore, ovarian cancer risk assessment and testing are most effective when performed within the context of a multidisciplinary team approach. A fundamental understanding of the genetics of ovarian cancer by all team members including the geneticists, genetic counselors, nurses, social workers, physicians and related personnel enhances the provision of services to our patients and their families. The American College of Obstetrics and Gynecology committee opinion has stated that women with a documented familial history of an inherited malignancy syndrome that increases their risk for the development of ovarian cancer who do not wish to retain fertility may be offered a prophylactic BSO after age 35 (19,20). It is our practice to offer women who have inherited BRCA mutations from affected women with documented epithelial ovarian cancer prophylactic surgery for both breast and ovarian cancer. In our experience 30% of this select group of BRCA positive women have had significant pathological changes, such as atypical hyperplasia, supporting the basis of prophylactic surgery. Unfortunately approximately 3% of women continue to develop primary peritoneal carcinoma after prophylactic BSO, yet this is a distinct entity from epithelial ovarian carcinoma. Although a prophylactic BSO significantly lowers the risk of ovarian cancer in all women, noncompliance with hormone replacement therapy may also result in significant morbidity and a significant reduction in quality of life, as well as life expectancy due to cardiovascular disease and osteoporosis in premenopausal women. Thus, primary prevention should be the focus for reducing morbidity and mortality from this disease. Women with a BRCA mutation not desirous of prophylactic surgery may be at increased risk for the development of ovarian cancer (40%) and breast cancer (60%) by age 70 and require more intensive clinical surveillance. The NIH consensus statement concluded that women at increased risk should have at least an annual comprehensive gynecological examination (pelvic and rectovaginal), serum marker CA125, and transvaginal/abdominal ultrasound annually, despite the lack of data supporting the use of these measures for ovarian cancer screening (15-18).

Upon entry into the NOCEDP, women complete multiple surveys regarding medical history, health services, quality of life, anxiety, knowledge, and cancer education. All participants undergo a comprehensive evaluation by an experienced cancer genetic counselor to determine risk assessment and are also counseled by oncology nurse practicioners. Physical examination and ultrasound are performed by a board certified gynecologic oncologist and an expert gynecologic sonologist and sonographer. Both the referring physician and patient are educated regarding the current status of ovarian cancer early detection. This program provides multidisciplinary care by combining clinical expertise in gynecologic oncology, advanced practice nursing, genetics and genetic counseling, psychiatry, psychology pathology, health services, quality of life, in conjunction with the clinical application of the scientific basis of ovarian carcinogenesis, invasion, and metastasis.

5. MOLECULAR GENETICS OF OVARIAN CANCER

Although relatively little is known about the etiology of ovarian cancer at the molecular and genetic level, progress has been made recently in identifying a spectrum of potential mechanisms in the transformation of ovarian epithelium. A variety of changes in candidate oncogenes, tumor suppressor genes, growth factors and growth factor receptors that occur in ovarian cancer have been elucidated. A better understanding of these molecular and genetic alterations will ultimately impact the clinical care of ovarian cancer patients through chemoprevention, early detection, and individualized therapy directed at specific molecular targets.

A number of oncogenes have been described in ovarian cancers. Most promising of these are the receptor and nonreceptor tyrosine kinases. Some of the earliest work focused on HER-2/neu, a transmembrane receptor tyrosine kinase whose overexpression has been reported in 20 to 30 % of ovarian cancers (23) and may be associated with a poor prognosis (24). While a ligand that binds to Her-2 alone has not been discovered, heregulin binds to heterodimers of HER-2 with HER-3 and HER-4. The relative levels of HER-2 in the heterodimers may dictate the cellular response to heregulin (25). With high levels of HER-2 expression, ligand binding leads to decreased clonogenic growth while invasiveness is enhanced (26). A recent study from M.D. Anderson showed that HER-2 might allow tumor cells to escape host immune defenses by inducing resistance to tumor necrosis factor (27). Its transmembrane location makes HER-2 an ideal target for antibody-based therapy as well as gene therapy. Herceptin, a humanized murine anti-HER-2 antibody, that has shown activity in 12-15% of HER-2 overexpressing breast cancers (28-30) is currently being investigated in ovarian cancer. Expression of another tyrosine kinase receptor, fms, along with its ligand CSF-1 is seen in over 50% over ovarian cancers and may provide potential autocrine regulation of tumor cell proliferation and function (31). Expression of fms may be associated with a poor clinical prognosis. Enhanced invasiveness and increased anchorage independent growth may result from signaling through fms via increased expression of uPA (32)

Especially relevant to ovarian cancers are two interactive nonreceptor kinase oncoproteins, phosphatidylinositol 3-kinase (PI3K) and AKT. Comparative genomic hybridization (CGH) has revealed multiple regions of recurrent, abnormal DNA sequence copy number in ovarian cancer. For example, changes in chromosome 3q26 which contains PIK3CA, the gene encoding the p110alpha catalytic subunit of PI3K occurs in 40 % of ovarian cancers (33). A number of important cancer-related functions such as proliferation, apoptosis, glucose transport, cellular adhesion, RAS signaling and oncogenic transformation have been associated with PI3K-mediated signaling. Studies using athymic mice have shown that PI3K inhibitors such as LY294002 significantly inhibit growth and ascites formation *in vivo* and ovarian cancer cell proliferation *in vitro* (34). AKT2, a member of the protein kinase B family, is activated as a downstream target of PI3K and is amplified in a significant percentage of ovarian cancers (35-37). AKT kinases can inhibit apoptosis by phosphorylating BAD to prevent binding bcl-XL and can inhibit the release of cytochrome c induced by paclitaxel (38). Since amplification of key regulators in these two kinase pathways are rarely seen in other epithelial malignancies, PI3K and AKT are especially promising areas of ovarian cancer research.

Loss of functional activity or mutation of several tumor suppressor genes has been implicated in the development and progression of ovarian cancers. Loss of p53 function is observed in over 50% of ovarian cancers as a "late event", associated with the acquisition of metastatic potential (39). Increased mutant p53 expression occurs in metastatic lesions (40-41). In keeping with the theory of incessant ovulation in the genesis of ovarian cancer, p53 mutations have been correlated with the total number of ovulatory cycles (42). Another tumor suppressor gene, PTEN/MMAC (phosphatase, tensin homologue mutated in multiple advanced cancers), appears to be mutated only in endometrioid ovarian cancers and not the other common epithelial subtypes (43,44). Inroads to understanding the molecular and genetic basis of ovarian cancer genesis and progression are being forged. With each new hypothesized mechanism come several points of opportunity for improved disease management through prevention, early detection and directed treatment.

6. BIOCHEMICAL MARKERS FOR OVARIAN CANCER
6.1 CA125

A variety of ovarian tumor markers have been studied with the most commonly utilized serum biomarker CA125, an ovarian cancer cell surface-associated protein that is expressed in 80% of nonmucinous epithelial ovarian cancers (14,15). CA125 is a cell-surface glycoprotein of high molecular weight that exists in multiple forms ranging from 220-1000 kDa. The normal physiological function of CA125 is unknown but is shed from the cell surface and has been detected in ascites and in fluids from healthy individuals. CA125 is normally present on the surface of cells that line the fallopian tube, endometrium, endocervix, peritoneum, pleura, pericardium and bronchus. Little, if any, CA125 can be detected on normal ovarian epithelium although the antigen sometimes is found in the ovary in occlusion cysts, benign papillary excresences, and when the epithelium undergoes tubal metaplasia. The CA125 antigen was defined by OC-125, a murine monoclonal antibody that was raised by immunizing a mouse with a human papillary serous ovarian carcinoma cell line. The presence of multiple identical OC-125 binding sites on each CA125 molecule has facilitated the development of a double determinant immunoradiometric assay. Using this assay, approximately 1-3% of apparently healthy non-pregnant women have CA125 levels greater than 35 units/ml, while 80-90% of clinically apparent epithelial ovarian cancers are associated with elevated serum CA125 levels. The optimal clinical application of CA125 is for surveillance of ovarian cancer after the diagnosis has been surgically confirmed. Overall, more than 80% of women with advanced ovarian cancer will have an elevated CA125 level (greater than 35 u/ml), yet the test is not useful in the detection of early stage disease (50%) (17,18). CA125 is not a specific marker for ovarian cancer. This is frequently misunderstood. Elevated serum levels have been found in the majority of patients with metastatic endometrial, fallopian tube, endo-cervical, and pancreatic carcinomas and breast, lung and colon cancers. Therefore, CA125 is not useful for determining the origin of adenocarcinomas for which the primary site is not apparent.

CA125 is even less reliable for the occult detection of ovarian cancer in premenopausal women. CA125 is also elevated in benign gynecologic conditions such as pregnancy, endometriosis, adenomyosis, benign ovarian cysts, leiomyomas, normal and ectopic pregnancy, pelvic inflammatory diseases, and normal menstruation. Non-gynecologic conditions associated with elevated CA125 include pancreatitis, cirrhosis, colitis, peritonitis, peritoneal tuberculosis, radiation therapy, intraperitoneal chemotherapy, as well as post surgical inflammation. The NIH Consensus Statement specified that CA125 should not be used as a screening test in the general or high-risk population since an elevated value accurately detects malignancy is less than 3% of women (45). However, in the postmenopausal patient the utility is sufficiently increased such that any woman presenting with a complex adnexal mass and an elevated CA125 value has ovarian cancer until proven otherwise. Despite some limitations, CA125 has been proven to be the most useful tumor marker currently developed. Its clinical applications include monitoring the status of disease in patients with metastatic gynecologic cancers, predicting the presence of residual disease at the completion of chemotherapy, detecting the presence of recurrent disease prior to clinical suspicion, and in attempting to distinguish benign from malignant adnexal masses preoperatively.

6.2. Lysophosphatidic Acid (LPA)

Recent attention has focused on phospholipids, such as LPA, lysophosphatidylserine (LPS), and sphingosylphosphorylcholine (SPC), as potential serum biomarkers for the early detection of epithelial ovarian carcinoma. These phospholipids function extracellularly to activate cells through specific receptors and induce proliferation of ovarian and breast cancer cells (46). LPA induces a rapid and transient increase in cytosolic free calcium, and stimulates tyrosine phosphorylation. Certain phospholipids appear to increase uPA and MMP expression and activation, suggesting a significant role in ovarian metastasis. The clinical application of LPA in ovarian cancer detection was recently reported by Xu wherein women with ovarian cancer had elevated plasma levels, including 9 of 10 women with stage I disease (47). Our preliminary data have also found elevated LPA levels in the plasma of women with advanced and early stage disease despite normal CA125 values. An enzymatic assay for LPA has been developed by Parrott et al. that is sensitive enough to detect LPA in plasma. Previous work on LPA testing (12) suggests that LPA may provide a sensitivity of >90% and a specificity of >89% for ovarian cancer. Xu et al. also have recently found that other closely related lysophospholipids, lysophosphatidylinositol (LPI) and lysophosphatidylcholine (LPC) may also be elevated in women with ovarian cancer.

To determine whether LPA is a diagnostic biomarker for ovarian cancer, we measured LPA levels in plasma from patients with cancer and healthy individuals (47). LPA is a normal constituent of serum, as it is produced by platelets during platelet aggregation and is not usually detectable in freshly isolated blood or plasma, where platelets are not activated (48-52). Several methods for separating and semi-quantitatively measuring LPA in biological fluids have been established based on thin layer chromatography, gas chromatography, mass spectrometry and/or nuclear magnetic resonance (53-63). Many of these approaches have limited sensitivity and are only semi-quantitative at best. Plasma was extracted by solvents and the lipid containing fractions were separated on thin layer chromatographic (TLC) plates, and analyzed by gas chromato-graphy (GC). The ovarian cancer patient group (48 patients) revealed significantly higher (p<0.0001) plasma LPA levels relative to controls. Using a cut-off of 1.3µM, elevated plasma LPA levels were detected in 9/10 patients with Stage I, 24/24 patients with Stage II, III and IV and 14/14 with recurrent ovarian cancer. The majority of patients with other gynecologic cancers also showed elevated LPA. In contrast, elevated plasma LPA was detected in a minority of healthy controls (5/48), patients with benign gynecologic diseases (4/18), and patients with breast cancer (0/11) or leukemia (0/5). CA125 data from the same group revealed a substantially lower rate of detection, especially in Stage I (Table II), suggesting that LPA may represent a promising marker for the early detection of ovarian and cervical cancers. In our preliminary studies, we have shown that the specificity and sensitivity of our current assay for LPA are 95 and 89%, respectively. Although this is a significant improvement over the CA 125 test, further improvement is necessary to make this test really useful.

Table II. CA125 and LPA levels from women with ovarian cancer

	CA125(>35U/ml)	LPA(>1.3uM)
Ovarian cancer I	2/9*	9/10
Ovarian cancer II-IV	14/24	24/24
Ovarian cancer recurrent	12/14	14/14

*CA1254 values were not available from one of the Stage I patients

6.3. Proteinases

In order to affect change in the morbidity and mortality associated with ovarian cancer a more comprehensive understanding of the biochemical and molecular biology of ovarian carcinogenesis, invasion and metastatic dissemination is required. Newly developed serum and molecular markers based on the biology of ovarian metastases may afford early detection and improve our ability to accurately detect early stage ovarian carcinoma. These novel tumor markers ultimately will be utilized to aid the clinician by detecting asymptomatic early stage disease, monitoring tumor status during treatment and early detection of disease recurrence.

Ovarian carcinogenesis, invasion and metastases require a complex cascade of interrelated events including cell exfoliation from the primary ovarian tumor, adhesion at distant sites within the abdominal cavity, cellular migration, extracellular matrix degradation, directed invasion into host parenchyma (such as diaphragm, liver, or omentum), cellular proliferation, and ultimately neovascularization. This enhanced understanding of ovarian cancer biology has led to the identification and detection of biomarkers in women with ovarian cancer that are being clinically applied in our program for asymptomatic women at increased risk for the development of this disease. Our research on ovarian metastasis has found that integrin ligation, cadherins, MMPs, and uPA play critical roles in the metastatic dissemination of ovarian cancer (64-75). The activity of ECM degrading proteinases has been correlated with invasive activity in many hematogenously metastasizing carcinomas, yet the role of proteolysis in the intraperitoneal spread of ovarian cancer continues to be elucidated (4,19,21,76,77). Predominant among the proteinases produced by invading tumor cells are enzymes in the PA and MMP families (71-75). PAs catalyze the conversion of the plasma zymogen plasminogen to the active proteinase plasmin. Plasmin is a broad-spectrum serine proteinase capable of degrading numerous extracellular matrix and matrix-associated proteins including fibrin, laminin, fibronectin and vitronectin. MMPs are a family of zinc-dependent proteinases which function in the degradation of predominantly collagen and gelatin. Expression of MMP-2 (gelatinase A, 72 kDa type IV collagenase) and MMP-9 (gelatinase B, 92 kDa type IV collagenase) has been linked to enhanced tumor invasion in numerous model systems (71-79). Clinically elevated serum levels of MMPs have been reported in women with advanced stage epithelial ovarian cancer and have been suggested as a potential new diagnostic marker. MMP-2 serum levels were measured by ELISA and were found to have a 90% sensitivity, 70% specificity, and a 75% positive predictive value, while CA125 had a 80% sensitivity, and a 73% positive predictive value. Serum MMP-2 levels were significantly increased in women with cystadenocarcinoma as compared to low malignant potential or benign tumors. To date we have evaluated serum levels of MMP-2 and -9, as well as their tissue-inhibitors (TIMP-1 and -2) from 100 women with ovarian carcinoma. The mean MMP-2 concentration for women with ovarian cancer was 9.99 ng/mg protein (SD +/-5.27) compared to control 20.15 ng/mg protein (SD+/- 9.78). The mean MMP-9 concentration for ovarian cancer patients was 11.44 ng/mg protein (+/- 9.13) and 22.89 ng/mg (+/- 16.30) for the control group. TIMP-1 mean concentration was 16.49 (+/- 9.13) in cancer patients and 24.42 ng/mg (+/-10.86) in controls. The mean TIMP-2 concentration was 1.07 ng/ml (+/-0.97) for cancer patients and 1.35 ng/ml (+/-0.87) for controls. Again our data is preliminary, yet warrant further investigation.

Short-term cell culture ovarian epithelium specimens were evaluated for proteinase and inhibitor expression (MMP, uPA, PAI, TIMP). Interestingly we found that MMP-9 levels significantly decreased in cultured cells and uPA activity was minimal in primary cultures (75,77). The MMP-2 detected in the tumor-conditioned medium was found in the active form and MMP-2 bound to the tumor cell surface increased invasiveness (72), suggesting a mechanism for amplification of cellular capacity for ECM degradation and metastatic dissemination. Similarly, we also demonstrated elevated concentration of uPA in the ascites from women with advanced stage ovarian carcinoma as well as in the ovarian cell tumor conditioned medium (76,77). Ovarian cell lines variably express uPA activity. Recently a soluble form of uPA receptor (suPAR) was detected in the blood of healthy patients and in malignant ascites of ovarian cancer patients (80). Serum from pre- and post-operative women treated for ovarian carcinoma found elevated levels in these patients as compared to healthy controls. The prognostic significance of suPAR found that high preoperative levels were associated with a poorer prognosis and survival as compared to CA125, which had no prognostic value. Although uPAR lost its significance in direct comparison to FIGO stage, its clinical implication is important since it serves as a preoperative evaluation and marker for disease. Elevated levels of suPAR, like CA125, may have prognostic implications not only for early detection in asymptomatic women but for those women with ovarian cancer in remission.

6.4. Telomerase

Telomerase, an enzyme involved in the regulation of cellular senescence, is inactive in most normal somatic cells but active in proliferative cancer cells (81). Previous studies have found that partially transformed cultured cells are telomerase negative, as are most benign hyperplasias and some early-stage malignant tumors (81-86). Presently we utilize real-time PCR (RT-PCR) for telomerase mRNA expression, which found that 100% of epithelial ovarian carcinomas and 100% of ovarian carcinoma cell lines expressed telomerase yet expression was not detected in normal ovarian epithelium (Table III). Copies of telomerase were calculated using the formula: Copy number = 10 (Ct-36.51/3.65). This formula was derived by Perkin-Elmer by averaging slope and intercept values from a representative sampling of amplification plots (unpublished data). Copies of telomerase were normalized to 10,000 GAPDH copies in order to facilitate the assessment of relative expression. There was no obvious correlation between telomerase expression and tumor grade, however, further study is warranted. These results demonstrate the utility of RT-PCR as applied for analysis of expression of telomerase. Comparable methodologies are being applied for the analysis of EGFR and its variants, MMP's and MT-MMPs, as well as uPA(R).

6.5. EGF/ErbB Receptor Family

The EGF/ErbB receptor family is comprised of 4 members: ErbB1, ErbB2, ErbB3 and ErbB4. The human EGF receptor (i.e., ErbB1) is the prototype in this family, and is distinguished by its ability to interact with a large number of polypeptide hormones with high affinity. Overexpression of ErbB1, ErbB2, and ErbB3 is common in ovarian carcinoma (87-90). Both normal and malignant cells also synthesize soluble forms of ErbB receptors (91-98). The

Table III. Telomerase expression in ovarian epithelium and malignant primary cells (OVCA).

Sample Type	GAPDH (copy #)	Ct Value	Telomerase (copy #)	Telomerase
Endometriosis (invasive)	10,000	30.9	32.5	32.5
Endometriosis (invasive)	62	31.1	30	4838
Ovarian cancer	10000	40.0	50	54.0
Ovarian cancer	2527	36.1	10	39.6
Ovarian cancer	12705	29.6	79.2	62.4
Ovarian cancer	10000	24.2	2360	2360
Normal ovary	10000	40.0	0	0
Normal ovary	4000	40.0	0	0
OVCA	1000000	28.1	201.4	12.01
OVCA	1000000	28.5	156.6	21.57
OVCA	1000000	30.0	60.81	20.61
OVCA	1000000	30.6	41.59	30.42
OVCA	1000000	40.0	53.8	22.67
OVCA	1000000	40.0	55.6	21.37

Relative copies of telomerase were normalized to expression per 10,000 copies of GAPDH

levels of sErbB2 are a good indicator of responsiveness to hormonal therapy for breast cancer patients (99). Maihle et al. have developed an acridinium-linked immunosorbent assay (ALISA) to detect sErbB1 in human body fluids (100) that detects a ~110-kDa sErbB1 protein in serum samples from healthy men and women (100). They found that serum p110 sErbB1 levels are significantly lower in women with stage III or IV disease prior to and shortly after cytoreductive staging laparotomy. For those women receiving cytoreductive surgery followed by combination chemotherapy, sErbB1 levels increased over time. These studies demonstrate that serum p110 sErbB1 levels are significantly different in women with ovarian cancer, and suggest that altered and/or changing serum p110 sErbB1 levels may provide important diagnostic and/or prognostic information useful for the patient management. Furthermore, their preliminary studies indicate that the observed decrease in serum p110 sErbB1 levels in advanced stage disease patients is also present in patients with early stage disease (n = 8; stage I/II). Maihle et al. have used this ALISA to detect and quantify sErbB1 serum levels in healthy women (median = 3,716 fmol/ml), ranging in age from 43 to 76 years (100). This median differs significantly from that of healthy men (median = 24,512 fmol/ml), ranging in age from 25 to 79 years. Serum sErbB1 levels do not appear to change with age in either healthy men or women (100). Stage III/IV ovarian cancer patients have significantly lower serum sErbB levels. We have identified serum samples collected within a period of 30 days prior to staging laparotomy and cytoreductive surgery from 21 stage III or IV EOC patients; none of these patients had received prior chemotherapy, radiation, or debulking surgery. We compared the serum sErbB1 levels in these EOC patients with the serum sErbB1 levels in a group of 21 healthy women of similar ages. The median (range) serum sErbB1 concentration of the 21 age-matched healthy women is 6,395 fmol/ml (1,846 to 23,708 fmol/ml). In contrast, the median (range) pre-operative serum sErbB1 concentration of the 21 patients with stage III or IV EOC is 284 fmol/ml (30 to 1,350 fmol/ml). These data indicate that pre-operative serum sErbB1 levels in patients with stage III or IV EOC are significantly lower than serum sErbB1 levels in healthy women of similar ages (Wilcoxon rank sum test, $P < 0.0001$). These data suggest that epithelial ovarian tumors affect circulating sErbB1 levels, and, furthermore, lead us to hypothesize that low sErbB1 levels may be useful as diagnostic biomarkers for epithelial ovarian cancer. Serum sErbB1 levels increase after cytoreductive surgery. We compared the initial post-operative (0 to 34 days) serum sErbB1 levels in these 73 EOC patients to serum sErbB1 levels in a group of 73 healthy age-matched women. The median (range) serum sErbB1 concentration of the 73 healthy women is 6,113 fmol/ml (1,292 to 51,358 fmol/ml). In contrast, the median (range) initial post-operative serum sErbB1 concentration of the 73 EOC patients is 1,799 fmol/ml (non-detectable to 11,035 fmol/ml). These data indicate that the initial post-operative sErbB1 levels in patients with stage III or IV EOC differ significantly from sErbB1 levels in an age-matched group of healthy women (Wilcoxon rank sum test, $P < 0.0001$; the one patient with a non-detectable serum sErbB1 level was excluded from this analysis). Decreasing serum sErbB1 levels may predict disease recurrence. Thirty-three patients provided a second serum sample 35 to 287 days after cytoreductive surgery. The median (range) serum sErbB1 concentration of these 33 serum samples is 6,434 fmol/ml (non-detectable to 29,666 fmol/ml). The median (range) serum sErbB1 concentration of these 33 serum samples appears similar to that seen in healthy women, with the exception of one patient who had an undetectable level of serum sErbB1. It is noteworthy that the median serum sErbB1 concentrations for both the initial and second post-operative serum samples appear higher than those seen in pre-operative serum samples of patients with stage III or IV EOC. These data have led us to hypothesize that serum p110 sErbB1 levels are significantly lower in advanced stage EOC patients than in healthy women, and that sErbB1 levels return toward normal values following tumor debulking surgery. Two of the 33 EOC patients who underwent multiple venipunctures provided five consecutive serum samples over the course of ~200 days. Interestingly, p110 sErbB1 levels in these two patients first increased and then decreased over time. Although the data presented here were generated from pre-operative and post-operative serum samples from two separate cohorts of EOC patients, these data altogether suggest that serum concentrations of p110 sErbB1 first return to the normal range of values following tumor debulking surgery, and then decline for a subset of patients. These data have led us to hypothesize that decreasing post-operative sErbB1 levels may be associated with disease recurrence and/or overall survival. While we recognize that this hypothesis is presently supported by limited preliminary data, if correct, it may prove to have significant clinical impact on the management of ovarian cancer patients.

7. THE OVARIAN PAP TEST

Histologically, epithelial ovarian carcinomas are classified as serous (60%), mucinous (10%), endometrioid (15%), clear cell (5%), Brenner (2%), mixed epithelial, and undifferentiated types (5). The heterogeneity of histological subtypes reflects the metaplastic potential of the ovarian surface Mullerian epithelium, which shares a common embryological origin with the peritoneum and urogenital system. The identification of premalignant lesions has provided a means for population-based screening and identification of patients at risk for the development of invasive cancers. This concept is easily recognized since it is the rationale behind the efficacy of the cervical Pap test. The female genital tract, due to its easy accessibility, has been well suited to noninvasive screening programs. The endometrium, although not accessible by non-invasive means, can be safely sampled in the outpatient setting with minimal morbidity in almost all women. The difficulty with ovarian screening for premalignant lesions is, in part, the result of their intraabdominal location; tissue screening of ovaries for pre-invasive disease or early stage invasive carcinoma, therefore, has not been possible. Unfortunately 75% of women continue to be diagnosed with advanced stage disease, providing ample evidence of the inadequacy of a routine pelvic examination and ultrasound. Therefore, the ability to identify a premalignant lesion or even early stage invasive ovarian carcinoma would be clinically relevant. The initial step in any screening effort is the identification of a precursor lesion and the development of a technique for diagnosing the abnormality.

The concept of ovarian cytology has become an important component of the surgical staging of ovarian carcinoma, as positive peritoneal cytology affects prognosis. The utility of peritoneal cytological analysis has become widely accepted in the surgical evaluation of gynecological malignancies (101). Subsequent studies have found that difficulties in cytological diagnosis arise from a paucity of malignant cells as well as a difficulty in distinguishing between tumor cells and reactive mesothelial cells. This difficulty could be expected in separating ovarian tumors of low malignant potential and well-differentiated epithelial ovarian cancer, as well as benign entities such as endometriosis and endosalpingiosis. Cytologic analysis of ovarian pathology can be quite difficult and therefore requires an expert cytopathologist. Poor or inappropriate cytopreparation also can prevent identification of malignant cells. Contamination with blood is expected in peritoneal cytology and requires appropriate preparation to optimize visualization of surface epithelium. The importance of specimen collection and preparation in the accurate interpretation of these samples cannot be overemphasized.

Ovarian dysplasia was initially described in 1984 by Gusberg and Deligdisch when histologic evaluation revealed significant epithelial abnormalities that did not qualify as malignancy nor low malignant potential (102). Ovarian dysplasia has been further characterized by morphometric methods revealing specific changes in the architecture and cytologic characteristics of ovarian surface epithelium (102-106). Retrospective analysis of ovarian tissues from women with stage I carcinoma assessed the presence of cellular and nuclear atypia in noncancerous tissue adjacent to the primary tumor. Atypia was more common in the cancer patients and was defined as the presence of nuclear pleomorphism or irregular chromatin distribution; cellular atypia defined as presence of stratification or loss of polarity. The presence of nuclear or cellular atypia was used to define ovarian intraepithelial neoplasia (OIN), which is believed to precede the development of ovarian cancer.

Cytological data from ovarian surface epithelium obtained by the Ovarian Pap test has been evaluated in a blinded manner by cyto- and histopathologists at Northwestern University using standardized pathological techniques. Cytological samples were individually obtained from each ovary and immediately and quickly spread onto clean glass slides. The smear was then fixed immediately to prevent cellular distortion. Immersion in 95% alcohol or use of a coating fixative by drop or spray was used. Specimens are stained using either the Papanicolaou or Geimsa technique (107). The surface of the ovary is lined by mesothelium, which yields cells with large symmetrical nuclei. The cytoplasm is abundant with well-defined cellular borders with single nucleoli. Germinal inclusion cysts can depict lining cells ranging from low cuboidal to elongated prismatic cells, and occasionally the epithelium shows ciliated metaplasia. Cells obtained by force from the ovarian surface (Ovarian Pap test) usually show the most commonly found epithelium, which is the low cuboidal type. The clusters are small, formed by uniform, small round cuboidal cells. The nuclei are round with dense granular chromatin with scanty cytoplasm. Mostly, cells are single surrounding clusters of small cells. Less commonly when metaplastic changes are retrieved, the lining cells acquire a prismatic form, resembling endosalpingeal cells. Cells obtained from the metaplastic epithelium are slightly elongated with distinct chromatin and inconspicuous nucleoli. The cytoplasm is elongated and follows the shape of the nuclei. The cells are arranged in palisades and are well organized side by side without overlapping. Cells from ciliated metaplasia are less commonly seen and they are organized in small loose groups of cells with rounded nuclei, slightly enlarged nucleoli and abundant cytoplasm. Within the cluster there are intercalated, elongated, contracted cells and rare cells with ill-defined perinuclear halos, which represent precursors of ciliated cells. Hyperplastic surface epithelium demonstrate exuberant arborization of tubules and papillae, some, of which show peripheral palisading. Very large monolayer of rounded cells are also frequently observed. The cells are larger than the non-hyperplastic surface epithelium, the chromatin is open, and small nucleoli are seen. There are irregularities of some nuclei outlines such as longitudinal infoldings and delicate nuclear protrusions, loss of polarity, and some degree of pleomorphism. The elongated hyperplastic cells are larger than the prismatic cells in non-hyperplastic surface cells, with open chromatin and small nucleoli. The hallmark of a mucinous ovarian tumor in cytological smear preparations is a background of mucinous material that is more easily recognized in Giemsa stained material. The cells are distributed in cellular groups of variable sizes. Cells from mucinous cystadenoma are rounded or oval with inconspicuous nucleoli and granular chromatin. The nuclear polarity is maintained, and the nuclei are symmetrical. Cells from malignant epithelial processes are larger, show granular chromatin and some degree of pleomorphism. The size of nucleoli, irregularity of nuclear outlines, and irregularity of chromatin distribution varies with the degree of differentiation. There is loss of polarity within cellular groups, and papillary fronds and tubular structures lined by abnormal cells are frequently encountered. The smears of malignant lesions are usually highly cellular, far more than in benign processes. Recently we have evaluated 60 women undergoing surgical exploration because of gynecologic manifestations. A total of 120 ovaries were removed, 90 ovaries were benign and 30 were malignant. All specimens were independently reviewed by an expert gynecologic pathologist and an expert gynecologic cytopathologist (Table IV). All permanent sections were correlated with cytopathologic diagnosis in a blinded manner. All malignancies as diagnosed by the pathologist were accurately identified by cytopathologic analysis. Our preliminary data demonstrate that ovarian cytology can discern malignant ovarian epithelium from normal.

Table IV. Comparison of ovarian cytology to permanent histological diagnosis.	Permanent Histology	Cytopathology
Specimen Total	120	120
Benign	90	90
Endometriosis	30	30
Malignant	30	30
Stage I	5	5
Stage III/IV	25	25
Papillary Serous	18	18
Endometrioid	5	5
Mucinous	7	7
Diagnostic Accuracy	100%	100%

8. FUTURE DIRECTIONS

The future of ovarian cancer detection lies in our ability to utilize technologic advances in scientific technique and integrate information gained from the study of other solid tumors to further elucidate the specific mechanisms of ovarian carcinogenesis. Newer, more efficient molecular techniques allow higher volume, time-efficient testing than ever before. While many mechanisms responsible for carcinogenesis of other tumors are not applicable to ovarian cancer, many of the underlying concepts and the techniques to study these concepts can be used to clarify the alterations unique to the events which occur in ovarian carcinogenesis.

Recent studies in colorectal (108), gastric (109), breast (110) and head and neck cancers (111) have detected mitochondrial mutations in tumor specimens. These mutations were found to be homoplasmic, most or all of the mitochondrial genome copies in the tumor were mutant, and such mutations may confer a replicative advantage. These mutations can be detected readily in blood or other bodily fluids and may serve as biomarkers in noninvasive screening for the presence of a malignancy (112). Currently, matched tumor and blood samples from patients with epithelial ovarian cancers are being tested for mitochondral DNA mutations. Since these mutations, if present, can occur at many positions throughout the mitochondrial genome, sequencing of the entire 16.5 kB might be necessary. With conventional screening techniques, this would not be feasible. However, utilizing high-density oligonucleotide arrays, rapid and high-throughput screening of large sequences is now possible.

Another powerful technique now being used to study the molecular genetics of ovarian cancer is comparative genomic hybridization, which allows quantitative detection of changes in chromosome copy number (113-115). It is sensitive to twofold differences in chromosome copy number and can detect deletions and amplifications as small as 2Mb. Identification of regions of amplifications and deletions by CGH analyses of ovarian cancer have contributed to the detection of the putative oncogene PIK3CA(33) as detailed earlier in the chapter. Evidence for the existence of important genes in ovarian cancers have come from studies using comparative genomic hybridization

(CGH) (113,116-121) and from analyses of allelic imbalance. The CGH analyses have revealed regions of recurrent increased copy number involving chromosomes 1p, 2p, 3q, 5p, 6p, 8q, 10p. 11q, 12p, 17q, 19, and 20q, and decreased relative DNA sequence copy number involving 4q, 5q, 6q, 8p, 13q, 16q, 18q and X. Studies of allelic imbalance have demonstrated frequent imbalances involving multiple chromosomes (122, 123). Identification of the affected genes in these regions and elucidation of their functions is essential to fully understand tumor progression.

8. CONCLUSION

The clinical application of the basic research on the mechanisms of ovarian carcinogenesis, invasion and metastasis will form the foundation for the detection of early rather than advanced stage ovarian cancer. This enhanced understanding of the disease process continues to lead to the development of clinical tests for the detection of novel lipids, gene mutations and aberrant gene methylation, as well as proteins in the blood (serum and plasma) that may serve as biological markers and aid in the diagnosis of early stage disease in asymptomatic women. Similarly based on the science of ovarian carcinogenesis, we now have the ability to offer women an innovative "ovarian Pap test" using office laparoscopy. This minimally invasive test will allow for the pathologic, molecular, and genetic evaluation of ovarian epithelial cells in women with normal gynecologic examinations. It is our belief that the combination of newly developed blood detection tests and the ability to apply molecular techniques to ovarian cytology will allow for the accurate identification of disease confined to the ovary.

REFERENCES

1. Landis, SH, Murray T, Bolden S, Wingo PA. Cancer Statistics. CA-A Cancer J Clin 1998; 48: 6-30.
2. Friedlander ML. Prognostic Factors in Ovarian Cancer. Seminars in Oncology 1998; 25:305 314.
3. Cronin KA, Weed DL, Connor RJ, Prorok PC. Case-Control Studies of Cancer Screening: Theory and Practice. J Natl Can Inst 1998; 90:498-504.
4. Kohn E, Liotta L. Molecular Insights into Cancer Invasion: Strategies for Prevention and Intervention Perspectives. Cancer Research 1995; 55: 1856-1862.
5. Link, Jr CJ, Kohn E, Reed E. The Relationship between Borderline Ovarian Tumors and Epithelial Ovarian Carcinoma: Epidemiologic, Pathologic, and Molecular Aspects-Review. Gyne Onc 1996; 60:347-354.
6. Katso RMT, Manek S, O'Bryne K, Playford MP, LeMeuth V, Ganesan TS Molecular approaches to diagnosis and management of ovarian cancer. Cancer and Metastasis Reviews 16: 81-107, 1997.
7. Fishman DA, Kearns A, Chilukuri K, Bafetti LM, O'Toole, EA, Georgacopoulos J, Ravosa MJ, and Stack MS. Metastatic dissemination of human ovarian epithelial carcinoma is promoted by a2b1-integrin mediated interaction with type I collagen. Inv Mets 1998; 18:15-26.
8. Fishman DA and Stack MS. The role of tumor cell adhesion in ovarian metastasis. CME Gynecol Oncol 1999; 4:201-204.
9. McCawley LJ, O'Brien P, Hudson LG. Epidermal Growth Factor (EGF) -and Scatter Factor/Hepatocyte Growth Factor (SF/HCF)- Mediated Keratinocyte Migration Is Coincident With Induction of Matrix Metalloproteinase (MMP)-9. J of Cellular Physiology 1998; 176:255-265.
10. Wikstrand CJ, Bigner DD Prognostic Applications of the Epidermal Growth Factor Receptor and Its Ligand, Transforming Growth Factor-$\propto$. J Natl Can Inst 1998; 90: 11-13.

11. Niikura H, Sasano H, Sato S. Yajima A. Expression of Epidermal Growth Factor-Related Proteins and Epidermal Growth Factor Receptor in Common Epithelial Ovarian Tumors. Int J Gyne Pathol 1997;16:60-68.

12. Xu Y, Fang XJ, Furui T, Sasagawa T, Pustilnik T, Lu Y, Shen Z, Wiener JR, Shayesteh L, Gray JW, Bast RC, Mills GB. "Regulation of growth of ovarian cancer cells by phospholipid growth factors". In Ovarian Cancer 5, Sharp, F., Blackett, T., Berek, J. and Bast, R.C., eds. Oxford UK., ISIS Medical Media, 1998.

13. Friedlander ML. Prognostic Factors. Ovarian Cancer Seminars in Oncology 1998; 25:305-314.

14. Berchuck A. Biomarkers in the Ovary. J Cellular Biochem 1995; 23:223-226.

15. Berek JS, Bast, Jr RC. Ovarian Cancer Screening. Cancer 1995; 76: 2092-2096.

16. Cronin KA, Weed DL, Connor RJ, Prorok PC. Case-Control Studies of Cancer Screening: Theory and Practice. J Natl Can Inst 1998; 90:7498-504.

17. Schwartz PE, Chambers JT, Taylor KJ. Early Detection and Screening for Ovarian Cancer. J Cellular Biochem 1995; 23:233-237.

18. Rosenthal A, Jacobs I. Ovarian Cancer Screening. Seminars in Oncology 1998; 25:315-325.

19. Abrahamson JA, Moslehi R, Vesprini D, Karlan B, Fishman D, Smotkin D, Ben David Y, Biran H, Fields A, Brunet JS, Narod S. No Association of the 11307K APC Allele with Ovarian Cancer Risk in Ashkenazi Jews. Cancer Research 1998; 58:2919-2922.

20. Randall TC, Rubin SC Assessing A Patient's Risk For Hereditray Ovarian Cancer. OBG Management 1998; 37-46.

21. Fishman DA. The present and future of biomarkers for the early detection of epithelial ovarian cancer. CME Gynecol Oncol 1999; 4:33-36.

22. Bast, R.C. Jr. and Mills, G.B. "Alterations in Oncogenes, Tumor Suppressor genes, and Growth Factors Associated with Epithelial Ovarian Cancers." In Ovarian Cancer Methods and Protocols, J.M.S. Bartlett, ed., Humana Press, 2000.

23. Slamon, D.J., Godolphin, W., Jones, L.A., Studies of the Her-2/neu protooncogene in human breast and ovarian cancer. Science 1989; 244:707-712.

24. Berchuck, A., Kamel, A., Whitaker, R., et al. Overexpression of HER-2/neu is associated with poor survival in advanced epithelial ovarian cancer. Cancer Res 1990; 50:4087-4091.

25. Xu F.J., Yu, Y.H., Boyer, C.M., et al. Stimulation or inhibition of ovarian cancer cell cell proliferation by heregulin is dependent on the ratio of HER2 to HER3 or HER4 expression. Proc Amer. Assoc. Cancer Res. 1996; 37:191.

26. Xu, F.J., Stack, S., Boyer, C., et al. Heregulin and agonistic anti-p185c-erbB2 antibodies inhibit proliferation but increase invasiveness of breast cancer cells that overexpress anti-p185c-erbB2: Increased invasiveness may contribute to poor prognosis. Clin Cancer Res 1997; 3:1629-1634.

27. Zhou, B.P., Hu, M.C., Miller, S.A., et al. HER-2/neu blocks tumor necrosis factor-induced apoptosis via the Akt/NF-kappaB pathway. J Biol Chem 2000; 275:8027-8031.

28. Baselga, J., Tripathy, D., Mendelsohn., et al. Phase II study of weekly intravenous recombinant humanized ant-p185 HER2 monoclonal antibody in patients with HER2/neu-overexpressing metastatic breast cancer. J Clin Oncol.1996; 14:737-744.

29. Slamon, D., Leyland-Jones, B., Shak, S., et al. Addition of herceptin (humanized anti-Her2 antibody) to first line chemotherapy for HER2 overexpressing metastatic breast cancer markedly increases anticancer activity: A randomized multinational controlled phase II trial. Proc Amer Soc Clin Oncol 1998; 17:98.

30. Ueno, N.T., Hung, M.C., and Zhang, S. Phase I E1A gene therapy in patients with advanced breast and ovarian cancers. Proc Amer Soc Clin Oncol 1998; 17:432a.

31. Kacinski B.M., Carter D, Mittal K, et al. Ovarian adenocarcinomas express fms-complementary transcripts and fms antigen, often with coexpression of CSF-1. Am J Pathol 1990; 137:135-147.

32. Chambers S.K., Ivins C.M., and Carcangiu M.L. Expression of plasminogen activator inhibitor-2 in epithelial ovarian cancer: a favorable prognostic factor related to the actions of CSF-1. Int J Cancer 1997; 74:571-575.

33. Shayesteh L, Lu Y, Kuo W.L., Baldocchi R, Godfrey T, Collins C, Pinkel D, Powell B, Mills G.B., Gray J.W. PIK3CA is implicated as an oncogene in ovarian cancer. Nat Genet 1999; 21:99-102.

34. Hu L, Zaloudek, Mills G.B., Gray J, and Jaffe R.B. In vivo and in vitro carcinoma growth inhibition by a phosphatidylinositol 3-kinase inhibitor (LY294002). Clin. Cancer Res 2000; 6:880-886.

35. Liu A.X., Testa J.R., Hamilton T.C., Jove R, Nicosia S.V, and Cheng J.Q. AKT2, a member of the protein kinase B family, is activated by growth factors, v-Ha-ras, and v-src through phosphatidylinositol 3-kinase in human ovarian epithelial cancer cells. Cancer Res 1998; 58:2973-2977.

36. Bellacosa A, de Feo D, Godwin A.K., et al. Molecular alterations of the AKT2 oncogene in ovarian and breast carcinomas. Int J Cancer 1995; 64: 280-285.

37. Yuan Z.Q., Sun M,Feldman R.I., Wang G, Ma X, Jiang C, coppola D, Nicosia S.V., and Cheng J.Q. Frequent activation of AKT2 and induction of apoptosis by inhibition of phosphoinositide-3-OH kinase/Akt pathway in human ovarian cancer. Oncogene 2000; 19:2324-2330.

38. Page C, Lin H.J, Jin Y, Castle VP, Nunez G, Huang M, and Lin J. Overexpression of Akt/AKT can modulate chemotherapy-induced apoptosis. Anticancer Res 2000; 20:407-416.

39. Marks J.R., Davidoff A.M., Kerns B.J.M, et al. Overexpression and mutation of p53in epithelial ovarian cancer. Cancer Res 1991; 5:2979-2984.

40. Sakai K, Kaku T, Kamura T, Kinukawa N, Amada S, Shigematsu T, Kobayashi H, Ariyoshi K, and Nakano H. Comparison of p53, Ki-67, and CD44v6 expression between primary and matched metastatic lesions in ovarian cancer. Gyn Oncol 1999; 72:360-366.

41. Sood A.K., Sorosky J.I., Dolan M, Anderson, and Buller R.E. Distant metastases in ovarian cancr: association with p53 mutations. Clin Cancer Res 1999; 5:2485-2490.

42. Schildkraut J, Bastos E, and Berchuck A. Relationship between lifetime ovulatory cycles and overexpression of mutant p53 in epithelial ovarian cancer. J Nat Cancer Inst 1997; 89:932-938.

43. Obata K, Morland S.J., Watson R.H., Hitchcock A, Chenevix-Trench G, Thomas E.J., and Campbell I.G. Frequent PTEN/MMAC mutations in endometrioid but not serous or mucinous epithelial ovarian tumors. Cancer Res 1998; 58:2095-2097.

44. Minaguchi T, Mori T, Kanamori Y, Matsushima M, Yoshikawa H, Taketani Y and Nakamura Y. Growth suppression of human ovarian cancer cells by adenovirus-mediated transfer of the PTEN gene. Cancer Res 1999; 59:6063-6067.

45. Gallion, HH and Bast, RC, Jr. National Cancer Institute Conference on Investigational Strategies for Detection and Intervention in Early Ovarian Cancer. Cancer Res 1993; 53:3839-3842.

46. Xu Y, Fang XJ, Casey G, and Mills GB. Lysophospholipids activate ovarian and breast cancer cells. Biochem J 1995; 309:933-940.

47. Xu Y, Shen Z, Wiper D, Wu M, Morton R, Elson P, Kennedy AW, Belinson J, Markman M, and Casey G. Lysophosphatidic Acid as a Potential Biomarker for Ovarian and Other Gynecologic Cancers. JAMA 1998; 280:719-723.

48. Watson SP, McConnell RT, Lapetina EG. Decanoyl lysophosphatidic acid induces platelet aggregation through an extracellular action. Evidence against a second messenger role of lysophosphatidic acid. Biochem. J 1985; 232:61-66.

49. Tigyi G, Henschen A, Miledi R. A factor that activates oscillatory chloride currents in Xenopus oocytes copurifies with a subfraction of serum albumin. J Biol Chem 1991; 266:20602-20609.

50. Tigyi G, Miledi R. Lysophosphatidates bound to serum albumin activates membrane currents in Xenopus oocytes and neurite retraction in PC12 pheochromocytoma cells. J Biol Chem 1992; 267:21360-21367.

51. Eichholtz T, Jalink K, Fahrenfort I, Moolenaar WH. The bioactive phospholipid lysophosphatidic acid is released from activated platelets. Biochem J 1993; 291:677-680.

52. Tokumura A, Iimori M, Niishioka Y, kitahara M, Sakashita M, Tanaka S. Lysophosphatidic acids induce proliferation of cultured vascular smooth muscle cells from rat aorta. Am J Physiol 1994; 267:C204-210.

53. Siuzdak G. in Mass Spectrometry for Biotechnology, San Diego, Academic Press, 1996

54. Weintraub ST, Pinckard RN, Hail M, Electrospray ionization for analysis of platelet-activating factor. Rapid Commun Mass Spectrom 1991; 5:309-11.

55. Kerwin JL, Tuininga AR, Ericsson LH. Identification of molecular species of glycerophospholipids and sphingomyelin using electrospray mass spectrometry. J Lipid Res 1994; 35:1102-1114.

56. Han X, Gubitosi-Klug RA, Collins BJ, Gross RW. Alterations in individual molecular species of human platelet phospholipids during thrombin stimulation: electrospray ionization mass spectrometry-facilitated identification of the boundary conditions for the magnitude and selectivity of thrombin-induced platelet phospholipid   hydrolysis. Biochemistry 1996; 35:5822-5832.

57. Hoischen C, Ihn W, Gura K, Gumpert J. Structural characterization of molecular phospholipid species in cytoplasmic membranes of the cell wall-less Streptomyces hygroscopicus L form by use of electrospray ionization coupled with collision-induced dissociation mass spectrometry. J Bacteriol 1997; 179:3437-3442.

58. Watson AD, Leitinger N, Navab M, Faull KF, Horkko S, Witztum JL, Palinski W, Schwenke D, Salomon RG, Sha W, Subbanagounder G, Fogelman AM, Berliner JA, Structural identification by mass spectrometry of oxidized phospholipids in minimally oxidized low density lipoprotein that induce monocyte/endothelial interactions and evidence for their presence in vivo. J Biol Chem 1997; 272:13597-13607.

59. Ramanadham S, Hsu FF, Bohrer A, Nowatzke W, Ma Z, Turk J. Electrospray ionization mass spectrometric analyses of phospholipids from rat and human pancreatic islets and subcellular membranes: comparison to other tissues and implications for membrane fusion in insulin exocytosis. Biochemistry 1998; 37:4553-4567.

60. Karlsson AA, Michelsen P, Odham G, Molecular species of sphingomyelin: determination by high-performance liquid chromatography mass spectrometry with electrospray and high-performance liquid chromatography/tandem mass spectrometry with atmospheric pressure chemical ionization. J Mass Spectrom 1998; 33:1192-1198.

61. Byrdwell WC, Dual parallel mass spectrometers for analysis of sphingolipid, glycerophospholipid and plasmalogen molecular species. Rapid Commun Mass Spectrom 1998; 12:256-272.

62. Hsu FF, Bohrer A, Turk J, Formation of lithiated adducts of glycerophosphocholine lipids facilitates their identification by electrospray ionization tandem mass spectrometry. J Am Soc Mass Spectrom 1998; 9:516-526.

63. Xu Y, Gaudette DC, Boynton J, Frankel A, Fang X-J, Sharma A, Hurteau J, Casey G, Goodbody AE, Mellors A, Holub BJ, Mills G. Characterization of an ovarian cancer activating factor(OCAF) in ascites from ovarian cancer patients. Clinical Cancer Res. 1995; 1:1223-1232.

64. Katso RMT, Manek S, O Bryne K, Playford MP, LeMeuth V, Ganesan TS. Molecular approaches to diagnosis and management of ovarian cancer, Cancer and Metastasis Reviews 1997; 16: 81-107.

65. Liotta, L.A., Rao, C.N., and Wewer, U.M. Biochemical interactions of tumor cells with the basement membrane. Ann. Rev. Biochem. 1986; 55:1037-1057.

66. Sawada, M., Shii, J., Akedo, H., and Tanizawa, O. An experimental model for ovarian tumor invasion of cultured mesothelial cell monolayer. Lab Invest 1994; 70:333-338.

67. Niedbala, M.J., Crickard, K, and Bernacki, R.J. Interactions of human ovarian tumor cells with human mesothelial cells grown on extracellular matrix. Exp Cell Res 1985; 160:499-513.

68. Auersperg, N., Maclaren, I.A., and Kruk, P.A. Ovarian surface epithelium: autonomous production of connective tissue-type extracellular matrix. Biol Reprod 1991; 44: 717-724.

69. Cannistra, S.A., Ottensmeier, C., Niloff, J., Orta, B., and DiCarlo, J. Expression and function of alpha1 and alphavbeta3 integrins in ovarian cancer. Gyn Oncol 1997; 58:216-225.

70. Hynes, R.O. Integrins: versatility, modulation and signaling in cell adhesion. Cell 1992; 69:11-25.

71. Huttenlocher, A., Sandborg, R.R., and Horwitz, A.F. Adhesion in cell migration. Current Opinion Cell Biol 1995; 7:697-706.

72. Fishman, D.A., Bafetti., L.M., and Stack, M.S. Membrane-type matrix metalloproteinase expression and matrix metalloproteinase-2 activation in primary human ovarian epithelial carcinoma cells. Invasion Metastasis 1997; 16:150-159.

73. Moser, T.L., Pizzo, S.V., Bafetti, L.M., Fishman, D.A., and Stack, M.S. Evidence for preferential adhesion of ovarian epithelial carcinoma cells to type I collagen mediated by the alpha2 beta1 integrin. Int J Cancer 1996; 67:695-701.

74. Fishman, D.A., Chilukuri, K., and Stack, M.S. Biochemical characterization of primary peritoneal carcinoma cell adhesion, migration, and proteinase activity. Gyn Oncol 1997; 67: 193-199.

26

75. Fishman, D.A., Bafetti, L.M., Banionis, S., Kearns, A.S., Chilukuri, K., and Stack, M.S. Production of extracellular matrix-degrading proteinases by primary cultures of human epithelial ovarian carcinoma cells. Cancer 1997; 80:1457-1463

76. Stack MS, Ellerbroek SM, Fishman DA. The role of proteolytic enzymes in the pathology of epithelial ovarian cancer. Int J Oncol 1998; 12:569-76.

77. Fishman DA, Bafetti LM, Banionis S, Kearns AS, Chilukuri K, and Stack MS. Production of extracellular matrix-degrading proteinases by primary cultures of human epithelial ovarian carcinoma cells. Cancer; 80:1457-63, 1997.

78. Gilles, C., Polette, M., Seiki, M., Birembaut, P., and Thompson, E.W. Implication of collagen type I-induced membrane-type 1-matrix metalloproteinase expression and matrix metalloproteinase-2 activation in the metastatic progression of breast carcinoma. Lab Invest 1997; 76:651-660.

79. Stack, M.S., Gray, R.D., and Pizzo, S.V. Modulation of murine B16F10 melanoma plasminogen activator production by a synthetic peptide derived from the laminin A chain. Cancer Res 1993; 53:1998-2004.

80. Sier CFM, Stephens R, Bizik J, Mariani A, Bassan M, Pedersen N, Frigerio L, Ferrari A, Dano K, Brunner N, and Blasi F. The level of urokinase-type plasminogen activator receptor is increased in serum of ovarian cancer patients. Cancer Res 1998; 58:1843-49.

81. Duggan BD, Minghong W, Yu MC, Roman LD, Muderspach LI, Delgadillo E, Wei-Zhi L, Martin SE, Dubeau L. Detection of Ovarian Cancer Cells: Comparison of a Telomerase Assay and Cytologic Examination J Nat Can Inst 1998; 90:238-242.

82. Kim NW, Wu F Advances in quantification and characterization of telomerase activity by telomeric repeat amplification protocol (TRAP), Nucleic Acids Research 1997; 25:2595-2597.

83. Yashima K, Litzky LA, Kaiser L, Rogers T, Lam S, Wistuba II, Milchgrub S, Srivastava S, Piatyszek MA, Shay JW, Gazdar AF. Telomerase Expression in Respiratory Epithelium during the Multistage Pathogenesis of Lung Carcinomas, Cancer Res 1997; 57:2373-2377.

84. Hirano Y, Fujita K, Suzuki K, Ushiyama T, Ohtawara Y, Tsuda F. Telomerase Activity as an Indicator of Potentially Malignant Adrenal Tumors, Cancer 1998; 83:772-776.

85. Bryan TM, Englezou A, Dalla-Pozza L, Dunham M, Reddel RR. Evidence for an alternative mechanism for maintaining telomere length in human tumors and tumor-derived cell tumors. Nature Medicine 1007; 3:11.

86. Mao L, Lee DJ, Tockman MS, Erozan YS, Askin F, Sidransky D. Microsatellite alterations as clonal markers for the detection of human cancer Proc Natl Acad Sci 1994; 91:9871-9875.

87. Berchuck A, Rodriguez GC, Kamel A, Dodge RK, Soper JT, Clarke-Pearson DL and Bast RCJ. Epidermal growth factor receptor expression in normal ovarian epithelium and ovarian cancer. Am J Obstet Gynecol 1991; 164:669-674.

88. Gullick WJ. Prevalence of aberrant expression of the epidermal growth factor receptor in human cancers. Br. Med. Bull 1991; 47:87-98.

89. Salomon DS, Brandt R, Ciardiello F and Normanno N Epidermal growth factor-related peptides and their receptors in human malignancies. Critical Rev. Oncol/Hematol 1995; 19:183-232.

90. Scambia, G., Panici P.B., Battaglia F., Ferrandina G., Baiocchi G., Greggi S., Vincenzo R.D. and Mancuso S. Significance of epidermal growth factor receptor in advanced ovarian cancer. J Clin Oncol 1992; 10:529-535.

91. Baron AT, Lafky JM, Boardman CH, Balasubramaniam S, Suman VJ, Podratz KC and Maihle NJ. Serum sErbB1 and EGF levels as tumor biomarkers in women with stage III or IV epithelial ovarian cancer. Cancer Epidemiol Biomarkers Prev 1998.

92. Haley J, Whittle N, Bennett P, Kinchington D, Ullrich A and Waterfield M. The human EGF receptor gene: structure of the 110 kb locus and identification of sequences regulating its transcription. Oncogene Res 1987; 1: 375-396.

93. Lin CR, Chen WS, Kruiger W, Stolarsky LS, Weber W, Evans RM, Verma IM, Gill GN and Rosenfeld MG Expression cloning of human EGF receptor complementary DNA: gene amplification and three related messenger RNA products in A431 cells. Science 1984; 224:843-848.

94. Yarden Y and Schlessinger J. Epidermal growth factor induces rapid, reversible aggregation of the purified epidermal growth factor receptor. Biochemistry1987; 26:1443-1551.

95. Spaargaren, M., Defize L.H., Boonstra J. and de Laat S.W. Antibody-induced dimerization activates the epidermal growth factor receptor tyrosine kinase. J Biol Chem 1991; 266:1733-1739.

96. Spivak-Kroizman, T., Rotin D., Pinchasi D., Ullrich A., Schlessinger J. and Lax I. Heterodimerization of c-erbB2 with different epidermal growth factor receptor mutants elicits stimulatory or inhibitory respnses. J Biol Chem 1992; 267:8056-8063.

97. Lax, I., Johnson A., Howk R., Sap J., Bellot F., Winkler M., Ullrich A., Vennstrom B., Schlessinger J. and Givol D. Chicken epidermal growth factor (EGF) receptor: cDNA cloning, expression in mouse cells, and differential binding of EGF and transforming growth factor-alpha. Mol Cell Biol 1988; 8: 1970-1978.

98. Di Fiore, P.P., Pierce J.H., Fleming T.P., Hazan R., Ullrich A., King C.R., Schlessinger J. and Aaronson S.A. Overexpression of the human EGF receptor confers an EGF-dependent transformed phenotype to NIH 3T3 cells. Cell 1987; 51:1063-1070.

99. Leitzel, K., Teramoto Y., Konrad K., Chinchilli V.M., Volas G., Grossberg H., Harvey H., Demers L. and Lipton A. Elevated serum c-erbB-2 antigen levels and decreased response to hormone therapy of breast cancer. J Clin Oncol 1995; 13:1129-1135.

100. Baron, A.T., Lafky J.M., Connolly D.C., Peoples J.J., O'Kane D.J., Suman V.J., Boardman C.H., Podratz K.C. and Maihle N.J. A sandwich type acridinium-linked immunosorbent assay (ALISA) detects soluble ErbB1 (sErbB1) in normal human sera. J. Immunol. Methods 1998.

101. Ozols RF, Rubin SC, Dembo Al, and Robboy SJ. "Epithelial Ovarian Cancer." in Principles and Practice of Gynecologic Oncology, Hoskins WJ, Perez CA, and Young RC, eds, Lippincott Co, 1997.

102. Gusberg SB, Deligdisch L. Ovarian Dysplasia- A Study of Identical Twins. Cancer 1984; 54:1-4.

103. Deligdisch L, Gil J. Characterization of Ovarian Dysplasia by Interactive Morphometry. Cancer 1989; 63:748-755.

104. Deligdisch L, Gil J. Interactive Morphometric Procedures and Statistical Analysis in the Diagnosis of Ovarian Dysplasia and Carcinoma. Path Res Pract 1989; 185:680-685.

105. Plaxe SC, Deligdisch L, Dotting PR, Cohen CJ. Ovarian Intraepithelial Neoplasia Demonstrated in Patients with Stage I Ovarian Carcinoma, Gyn Oncol 1990; 38:367-372.

106. Deligdisch L, Einstein AJ, Guera D, Gil J. Ovarian Dysplasia in Epithelial Inclusion Cysts. Cancer 1995; 76:1027-1034.

107. Koss LG, Diagnostic Cytology and its Histopathologic Basis, 3rd ed. Philadelphia, J.B. Lippincott, 1979.

108. Polyak K, Li Y, Zhu H, Lengauer C, Wilson J.K., Markowitz S.D., Trush M.A., Kinzler K.W., and Vogelstein B. Somatic mutations of the mitochondrial genome in human colorectal tumours. Nat Genet 1998; 20:291 – 293.

109. Burgart L.J., Zheng J, Shu Q, Strickler J.G., Shibata D. Somatic mitochondrial mutation in gastric cancer. Am J Pathol 1995; 147:1105– 1111.

110. Richard S.M., Bailliet G, Paez G.L., Bianchi M.S., Peltomaki P, and Bianchi N.O. Nuclear and mitochondrial genome instability in human breast cancer. Cancer Res 2000; 60:4231– 4237.

111. Yeh J.J., Lunetts K.L., van Orsouw N.J., Moore F.D., Mutter G.L., Vijg J, Dahia P.L., and Eng C. Somatic mitochondrial DNA(mtDNA) mutations in papillary thyroid carcinomas and differential mtDNA sequence variants in cases with thyroid tumours. Oncogene 2000; 19:2060–2066.

112. Fliss M.S., Usadel H, Caballero O.L., Wu L, Buta M.R., Eleff S.M., Jen J, and Sidransky D. Facile detection of mitochonddrial in tumors and bodily fluids. Science 2000; 287:2017– 2019.

113. Kallionemi A, Kallionemi O, Sudar D, Gray J.W., Waldman F, and Pinkel D. Comparative genomic hybridization for molecular cytogenetic analysis of solid tumors. Science 1992; 258:818–821.

114. Kallionemi O.P, Kallionemi A, Piper J, Isola J, Waldman F.M., Gray J.W., and Pinkel D. Optimizing comparative genomic hybridization for analysis of DNA sequence copy number changes in solid tumors. Genes Chromosom. Cancer 1994; 10:231–243.

115. Du Manoir S, Speicher M.R., Joos S, Schrock E., Popp S, Dohner H et al. Detection of complete and partial chromosome gains and losses by comparative genomic in situ hybridiization. Human Genet 1993; 90:590– 610.

116. Yu LC, Moore DH 2nd, Magrane G, Cronin J, Pinkel D, Lebo RV, Gray JW. Objective aneuploidy detection for fetal and neonatal screening using comparative genomic hybridization (CGH) Cytometry 1997; 28:191-197.

117. Yu Y, Xu F, Peng H, Fang X, Zhao S, Li Y, Cuevas B, Kuo WL, Gray JW, Siciliano M, Mills GB, Bast RC Jr NOEY2 (ARHI), an imprinted putative tumor suppressor gene in ovarian and breast carcinomas Proceedings of the National Academy of Sciences of the United States of America 1999; 96:214-219.

118. Pinkel D, Segraves R, Sudar D, Clark S, Poole I, Kowbel D, Collins C, Kuo WL, Chen C, Zhai Y, Dairkee SH, Ljung BM, Gray JW, Albertson DG High resolution analysis of DNA copy number variation using comparative genomic hybridization to microarrays Nature Genetics 1998; 20:207-11.

119. Lucito R, Nakimura M, West JA, Han Y, Chin K, Jensen K, McCombie R, Gray JW, Wigler M Genetic analysis using genomic representations Proceedings of the National Academy of Sciences of the United States of America 1998; 95:4487-92.

120. Moore DH 2nd, Pallavicini M, Cher ML, Gray JW A t-statistic for objective interpretation of comparative genomic hybridization (CGH) profiles. Cytometry 1997; 28:183-90.

121. Thompson CT, Gray JW Cytogenic profiling using fluorescence in situ hybridization (FISH) and comparative genomic hybridization (CGH) (Review and 23 refs) J Cellular Biochemistry-Supplement 1993; 17G:139-43.

122. Umayahara K, Cheneviex-Trench G, Daneshvar, L, Yang-feng, T, Collins C and Gray JW. :Molecular cytogenetic studies." In Ovarian Cancer 5, Sharp, F, Blackett, T, Berek, J and Bast, RC, eds., Oxford UK, ISIS Medical Media, 1998.

123. Gray JW, Chin K, Waldman F, "A Molecular cytogenetic view of chromosomal heterogeneity in solid tumors". In Proceedings of the Eight Pezcoller Symposium: Genomic Instability and Immortality in Cancer, E Mihich and L Hartwell, eds. New York, Plenum Press, 1996.

Chapter 2

RISK ASSESSMENT & GENETIC TESTING

Pierre O. Chappuis and William D. Foulkes
Division of Medical Genetics, Department of Medicine,
McGill University Health Center, Montreal, QC, Canada

Abstract: Ovarian cancer is the fifth most common cause of cancer death in women in Western countries and family history is one of the strongest known risk factors. Approximately 5 to 13% of all ovarian cancer cases are caused by the inheritance of cancer predisposing genes with an autosomal pattern of transmission. The inherited fraction of ovarian cancer may differ between populations. Based on analysis of familial ovarian cancer pedigrees and other epidemiological studies, three hereditary ovarian cancer syndromes have been defined. The identification of the genes responsible for most hereditary ovarian cancers has open a new area of early detection methods and preventive procedures specifically dedicated to women identified as carrying ovarian cancer predisposing genes. Predictive oncology is best performed by a dedicated unit with professionals aware of all the issues surrounding genetic testing.

1. INTRODUCTION

Ovarian cancer is the fifth most common malignancy and the fifth leading cause of cancer deaths among North American women. More women will die of ovarian cancer than from cancer arising in all other female reproductive organs combined. Ovarian cancer is mostly a disease of perimenopausal and postmenopausal women. Like breast cancer, there is a steady increase in ovarian cancer incidence with age and ovarian cancer before the age of 40 is rare. Besides age, the other risk factors associated with the disease are a family history of ovarian or breast cancer, infertility, nulliparity, early menarche and late menopause[1-5]. Other factors, including dietary intake of calcium, lactose, fiber, alcohol and coffee, have been associated less consistently with an increase risk of the disease[5-9]. High parity, oral contraceptive use, tubal ligation and hysterectomy have been associated with a reduction in risk[1,3,10-17]. After controlling for age, the factor most strongly associated with ovarian cancer risk is a family history of ovarian cancer[3,4]. The excess of ovarian cancer in women with a family history of the disease has lead to a search for inherited genetic causes of ovarian cancer. From epidemiological studies and mutation surveys, it is now estimated that between 5% and 13% of all epithelial ovarian cancers result from the autosomal dominantly inheritance of germ-line mutations in a cancer predisposing genes[5,18-22]. This estimate varies substantially by ethnicity, being approximately 5% in non-Ashkenazi Jewish populations and roughly 20% in Ashkenazim[23-26]. Among common adult malignancies, ovarian cancer was predicted to have the highest proportions attributable to susceptibility genes[16]. Nevertheless, less than 5 in 10,000 women in the United States were estimated to be at increased risk of developing ovarian cancer due to a strong genetic predisposition[27].

2. RISK ASSESSMENT
2.1. Population Risk

Approximately 140,000 new cases of ovarian cancer occur worldwide yearly[2]. This number represents 4% of all female cancers, and the disease is more prevalent in developed countries. The highest age-adjusted incidence rates are observed in Eastern and Northern Europe, North America and among Jews born in America or Europe (range 7.0-15.1 per 100,000)[28]. The lowest age-adjusted incidence rates are seen in Northern and Western Africa, and Asia, including Japan (range 0.7-6.7 per 100,000). Worldwide, one of the highest rates of ovarian cancer in the world is seen in Israeli Jews born in North America or Europe (age standardized incidence rate, 13.5 per 100,000). Some of these differences may be attributed to reporting bias, but they are probably too large to be due to biases alone. There are clearly ethnic-specific variations in incidence. For example, the prevalence of mutations in the major breast/ovarian cancer susceptibility genes *BRCA1* and *BRCA2* is extremely high in the Ashkenazi Jewish population.

In United States, the American Cancer Society estimates that 23,100 women will develop new ovarian cancer cases and 14,000 will die of the disease in 2000[29]. The lifetime probability of developing ovarian cancer in the North American population is approximately 1.4%[29]. Of note, even in the absence of a family history of ovarian cancer, this estimation is substantially influenced by the other risk factors. Based on pooled data from 7 case-control studies and the SEER incidence data, the lifetime risk of developing ovarian cancer ranges from 0.6% for women with 3 or more term pregnancies and 4 or more years of oral contraceptive use to 3.4% among nulliparous women with no oral contraceptive use[30].

2.2. Familial Ovarian Cancer

Familial aggregation of ovarian cancer has been variably defined as occurring when 1) two first-degree relatives have ovarian cancer, or 2) the proband has ovarian cancer as well as one or more of her first- or second-degree relatives[31]. Case-control studies designed to estimate the relative risk of developing ovarian cancer with a family history of the disease are summarized in Table 1. A meta-analysis of case-control and cohort studies on family history and risk of ovarian cancer has been published in 1998[32]. The relative risk to all first-degree relatives was 3.1 (95% CI, 2.6-3.7), 1.1 (95% CI, 0.8-1.6) for mothers of cases, 3.8 (95% CI, 2.9-5.1) for sisters and 6.0 (95% CI, 3.0-11.9) for daughters, respectively. The risk increased with the number of first-degree relatives affected[16].

Table 1. Relative risk of ovarian cancer associated with a family history of the disease in epidemiological studies.

Relatives studied	Country	Age group (y)	Cases	Controls	Odds ratio (95% CI)	Reference
Any	USA	All	150	300	"no positive association"	Wynder et al., 1969[33]
First- + second-degree	USA	< 50	150	150	15.7 (0.9-278)	Casagrande et al., 1979[10]
First-degree	USA	45-74	62	1068	18.2 (4.8-69)	Hildreth et al., 1981[1]
First-degree	USA	18-80	215	215	11.3 (0.6-211)	Cramer et al., 1983[11]
First-degree	Greece	All	146	243	∞ (3.4-∞)	Tzonou et al., 1984[34]
First-degree	Japan	N/A	110	220	∞ (0.1-∞)	Mori et al., 1988[8]
First-degree Second-degree	USA	20-54	493	2465	3.6 (1.8-7.1) 2.9 (1.6-5.3)	Schildkraut et al., 1988[35]
First-degree	USA	20-79	296	343	3.3 (1.1-9.4)	Hartge et al., 1989[36]
First-degree + aunts	Canada	All	197	210	2.5 (0.7-11.1)	Koch et al., 1989[37]
First-degree	Italy	25-74	755	2023	1.9 (1.1-3.6)	Parazzini et al., 1992[9]

Table 1 continued.

Relatives studied	Country	Age group (y)	Cases	Controls	Odds ratio (95% CI)	Reference
First-degree	USA	N/A	883	Population database	2.1 (1.0-3.4)	Goldgar et al., 1994[38]
First-degree	USA	< 65	441	2065	8.2 (3.0-23)	Rosenberg et al., 1994[15]
First-degree Second-degree Third-degree	USA	All	662	2647	4.3 (2.4-7.9) 2.1 (1.2-3.8) 1.5 (1.0-2.2)	Kerber et al., 1995[16]
First-degree	Australia	18-79	824	860	3.9 (1.6-9.7)	Purdie et al., 1995[17]
First-degree	Finland	< 76	559	Pop. incidence rate	2.8 (1.8-4.2)	Auranen et al., 1996[39]
First-degree	UK	< 60	1188	Population incidence rate	SMR=223 (155-310)	Easton et al., 1996[40]
Any	Canada	20-84	170	170	1.9 (0.8-4.4)	Godard et al., 1998[5]
Daughters (≤ 53y)	Sweden	n/s	n/s	Population incidence rate	2.7 (1.9-3.7)	Hemminki et al., 1998[41]
First degree	USA Israel	All	213	386	3.2 (1.5-6.8)	Mosheli et al., 2000[26]
First-degree	UK		≥ 2 OC in 316 families	Population incidence rate	7.2 (3.8-12.3)	Sutcliffe et al., 2000[42]

Three studies[39,40,42] have a population-based cohort design, the others are case-control studies. Abbreviation: CI, confidence intervals; N/A, not available; SMR, standardized mortality ratio; OC, ovarian cancer.

Initial work suggested that women who have one first-degree relative affected by or who died of ovarian cancer were at greater risk for ovarian cancer, but not at an age earlier than the general population[35,40,43-45]. However, an inverse relationship between age of onset of the ovarian cancer and risk for close relatives has been reported in some studies[26,41,46-48]. Houlston et al. analyzed 391 ovarian cancer pedigrees and found that the risk of developing ovarian cancer among the relatives of ovarian cancer case patients diagnosed before age 45, between 45 and 54 years, and after 55 years were 14.2, 5.2 and 3.7, respectively[46]. In a Swedish population-based study, the familial hazard ratios of ovarian cancer in daughters, adjusted for age and decade of birth, was 4.2 (95% CI, 2.2-8.2) when mothers were younger than 50 years at diagnosis compared to 2.3 (95% CI, 1.6-3.4) for mothers with ovarian cancer diagnosed at or after 50 years[41]. A higher risk of early onset of ovarian cancer is also recognized in the small proportion of women who have several affected relatives[45].

Besides ovarian cancer, case-control studies have also shown that breast[8,9,26,43,49], colon[5,11], pancreatic[16,26,38], prostate[11,26,49], uterine[49] cancers and leukemia[5] were all in significantly excess risk among relatives of women with ovarian cancer. The significantly elevated risk for breast and ovarian cancer noted among relatives of ovarian cancer patients is usually greater for ovarian cancer than for breast cancer[43,48]. Interestingly, an excess risk of ovarian cancers in the family members of women with borderline ovarian cancers was not reported[35,50]. Nevertheless, one study did not show a difference in ovarian cancer risk among first degree relatives of 254 patients with invasive ovarian cancer and 61 patients with borderline ovarian tumors[51]. The inverse relationship has also been reported, i.e. an increased risk of developing ovarian cancer that has been associated with family histories of breast, uterine, colon and pancreatic cancer[9,16,52-55].

Several investigators have evaluated the risks associated with more than one affected relative and showed a substantial increased risk for the relatives, but with wide confidence intervals[35,40,45]. A combined analysis of these data estimated the relative risk of developing ovarian cancer to be 11.7 (95% CI, 5.3-25.9) for these women[32]. The results of the prospective cohort from the UKCCCR Familial Ovarian Cancer Study Group has been recently published[42]. Based on 316 families with 2 or more confirmed cases of epithelial ovarian cancer in first-degree relatives, ovarian and breast cancer relative risks were estimated. Surprisingly, when the analyses were restricted to families that were not carrying a *BRCA1/2* germ-line mutation, the ovarian cancer risk was 11.6 (95% CI, 3.1-29.7), similar to the risk estimated for the *BRCA1/2*-related ovarian cancer families (11.9, 95% CI, 3.8-27.7). It is important to recognize that there is possibility that at least some of these "*BRCA1/BRCA2* negative" families do indeed carry mutation in *BRCA1/BRCA2* that were not detected by the screening methods used (see section 3.1).

2.3. Ovarian Cancer As A Feature Of Inherited Genetic Syndromes

Some characteristics of the autosomal dominantly inherited syndromes associated with an increased risk of developing ovarian cancer are summarized in Table 2. In a population-based series of 450 unselected epithelial ovarian cancers studied in Southern Ontario, Canada, Narod *et al.* estimated the proportion of hereditary ovarian cancer in the Ontario population to be between 2.9 to 6.9% of cases of ovarian cancer[19]. From other population-based studies, the fraction of hereditary ovarian cancer cases has been estimated between 5 and 13%[18,21,56]. The hallmark feature of hereditary ovarian cancer is the vertical transmission of cancer susceptibility consistent with an autosomal dominantly inherited factor[31].

Table 2. Ovarian cancer as a feature of hereditary genetic syndromes (adapted from Kasprzak et al.[57]).

Syndrome	Gene	% hereditary OC	Risk of OC by age 70	Other clinical features
Hereditary breast ovarian cancer	BRCA1	65%	20-50%	Breast, fallopian tube cancer
	BRCA2	10%	10-30%	Breast, prostate, pancreas, head and neck cancer
Site-specific ovarian cancer	BRCA1	10-15%	20-50%	
Hereditary nonpolyposis colorectal cancer	MLH1 MSH2 MSH6 PMS1 PMS2	5-10%	≤ 10%	Colorectal, endometrial, stomach, urinary tract, small bowel cancer
Peutz-Jeghers syndrome	STK11	< 1%	< 2%	Mucocutaneous melanin spots; GI hamartomatous polyps; adenoma malignum of uterine cervix; breast, GI, pancreas cancer
Cowden disease	PTEN	< 1%	< 1%	Multiples hamartomas; neurological signs; breast, renal cancer
Nevoid basal cell carcinoma (Gorlin) syndrome	PTCH	< 1%	< 1%	Basal cell nevi/carcinoma; palmar/plantar pits; skeletal abnormalities; odontogenic keratocysts; medulloblastoma
Multiple enchondromatosis (Ollier's disease)	?	<< 1%	<< 1%	Osteochondromatosis; hemangiomata
Epidermolytic palmoplantar keratoderma	KRT9	<< 1%	<< 1%	Epidermolytic hyperkeratosis

Abbreviation: AD, autosomal dominant; GI, gastrointestinal; OC, ovarian cancer.

2.3.1. Hereditary Breast Ovarian Cancer

The association between breast and ovarian cancer is well known. Since 1950[58], there have been numerous reports of familial aggregation of ovarian cancer. In most cases, breast cancer was also present in these pedigrees. Segregation analysis performed on breast/ovarian cancer families identified by Lynch *et al.* led them to conclude that the clustering of breast and of a single dominant gene[59]. In 1990, evidence was found for linkage of 15 early onset breast cancer pedigrees to a single locus on the chromosome 17q21[60]. It was subsequently confirmed in a series of 5 breast/ovarian cancer families, where 3 were linked to the same locus[61]. After intensive search, the *BRCA1* gene was finally identified in 1994[62]. The same year, a second breast/ovarian cancer susceptibility locus was located on chromosome 13q[63]. The *BRCA2* gene was characterized in 1995[64]. Most early-onset breast and ovarian cancer families are linked to *BRCA1*[20,65-67]. In fact, the presence of ovarian cancer is strongly predictive of *BRCA1* germ-line mutation, even in small breast/ovarian cancer families[68,69]. Stratton *et al.* estimated that *BRCA1* is responsible for 55% (95% CI, 29-83%) of the excess risk of ovarian cancer among first-degree relatives of ovarian cancer patients[70]. A similar estimation was previously reported[71]. The contribution of *BRCA2* is likely to be smaller, although certain mutations in the central part of *BRCA2* confer a higher risk of ovarian cancer than mutations located in the two extremities of the gene[72]. Based on various genetic linkage- or population-based studies, estimation of the cumulative risk of developing ovarian cancer for a woman carrying a *BRCA1* or a *BRCA2* mutation is summarized in Table 3. The incidence of primary serous carcinoma of the peritoneum, before or after oophorectomy, is not known among *BRCA1/2* carriers, but is likely to be substantially higher than in the general population[73].

In summary, the point estimate for risk of ovarian cancer conferred by mutations in *BRCA1* varies between 12% and 68% to age 70 and the confidence interval for all studies are wide. In virtually all studies, the incidence of ovarian cancer increases strikingly only after age 40[74]. Compared with *BRCA1*, mutations in *BRCA2* may confer a lower risk of ovarian cancer than mutations in *BRCA1* (11%-27%). Whether the differences in the estimated penetrance that have been reported for each gene are real or due to different mutation types, modifying genetic and environmental factors, ascertainment bias or simply result of chance, is unclear[75].

2.3.2. The Site-Specific Ovarian Cancer Syndrome

A woman with two affected first-degree relatives has a risk of developing ovarian cancer substantially higher than having one affected first degree relative[32,35,40,42,45]. Thus, the occurrence of ovarian cancer in a family with two or more first -degree relatives is likely to be explained by the inheritance of a mutated gene[40,76]. A family with 3 or more cases of invasive epithelial ovarian cancer at any age and no case of breast cancer diagnosed before age 50

36

Table 3. BRCA1/2 mutation and ovarian cancer penetrance.

Population studied	BRCA1/2 screening	Penetrance (age 70-75)	Reference
33 early-onset BC (< 60y) and OC families	BRCA1 linkage	BRCA1: 44% (28-56%)	Ford et al., 1994[74]
33 early-onset BC (< 60y) and OC families	BRCA1 linkage	BRCA1: 63%	Easton et al., 1995[77]
237 early-onset BOC families	Linkage or sequencing	BRCA1: 42% BRCA2: 27% (0-47%)	Narod et al., 1995[20] Ford et al., 1998[66]
14 AJ BOC families	Risk estimate for mutation carriers relatives	BRCA1 185delAG: 41% 5382insC: - BRCA2 6174delT: 30%	Abeliovich et al., 1997[78]
2 BOC families	BRCA2 linkage	BRCA2: 10% (at age 60)	Easton et al., 1997[79]
25 AJ BOC families	AJ founder mutations[#]	BRCA1 (185delAG + 5382insC): 57% BRCA2 6174delT: 49%	Levy-Lahad et al., 1997[80]
922 incident OC (population-based study)	Segregation analysis	BRCA1: 22% (5-60%)	Whittemore et al., 1997[22]
5318 Jews (population-based)	3 AJ founder mutations[#]	16% (6-28%)	Struewing et al., 1997[81]
412 AJ BC patients	3 AJ founder mutations[#]	12%	Warner et al., 1999[82]
a) 112 families with ≥ 2 relatives with OC, +/- BC < 60y b) 374 OC < 70y	PTT, SSCA, sequencing	BRCA1: 53% BRCA2: 31% BRCA1/2: 68% (36-94%)	Antoniou et al., 2000[75]
191 AJ patients, OC < 75y	3 AJ founder mutations[#]	BRCA1 185delAG: 37% BRCA1 5382insC: 21% BRCA2 6174delT: 14%	Mosheli et al., 2000[26]

[#]*AJ founder mutations: BRCA1: 185delAG, 5382insC; BRCA2: 6174delT.*
Abbreviation: AJ, Ashkenazi Jewish; BC, breast cancer; BOC, breast-ovarian cancer; OC, ovarian cancer, PTT, protein truncation test; SSCA, single strand conformation analysis; RR, relative risk.

qualifies as a site-specific ovarian cancer family[31,83]. Nearly all site-specific hereditary ovarian cancer is a result of BRCA1, or less frequently of BRCA2 mutations[75,83-88]. Gayther et al. studied 112 families identified through the Familial Ovarian Cancer Register of the UKCCCR characterized by the presence of at least two first- or second-degree relatives with epithelial ovarian cancer[87]. BRCA1 germ-line mutations were identified in 40 (36%) families and 8 (7%) BRCA2 mutations were identified. Antoniou et al. modeled ovarian cancer using the same set of families[75]. When a third high-risk ovarian cancer susceptibility gene was allowed for in the genetic models, none of the models fitted gave significant evidence for a third gene.

The authors concluded that the majority of familial ovarian cancer may be explained by mutations in *BRCA1* or *BRCA2*, and families without mutations can be explained by insensitivity of mutation testing and chance clustering of sporadic cases. The possibility of either rare or low risk susceptibility alleles is an alternative.

In summary, hereditary site specific ovarian cancer syndrome should be considered as a variant of the hereditary breast/ovarian cancer syndrome, in which early onset breast cancer has not yet appeared[83]. Thus, it is currently prudent to counsel women belonging to families with 3 or more cases of ovarian cancer that they are at increased risk of developing breast cancer[86].

2.3.3. The Hereditary Nonpolyposis Colorectal Cancer Syndrome

The hereditary nonpolyposis colorectal cancer (HNPCC) or Lynch syndrome has recently been extensively reviewed[89]. HNPCC is one of the most common autosomal conditions predisposing to cancer, accounts for 5 to 8% of all colorectal cancers. The genetic susceptibility to the disease is transmitted in a dominant fashion, generally with high penetrance. The diagnosis of HNPCC relies on the observation of familial clustering of colorectal cancers, meeting a set of obligate criteria referred to as the Amsterdam criteria, defined in 1991[90]. In fact, this syndrome is associated with an increased risk of developing cancers in several other sites. Colorectal cancers represent about two thirds of the malignancies in HNPCC families, whereas up to 40% of the malignancies are extracolonic cancers of epithelial origin. The second most frequently affected organ is the endometrium, thereafter a higher frequency of other target organs has been reported, including the stomach, the small intestine, the upper renal tract and the ovary. The Amsterdam criteria have been recently revised to better consider the spectrum of malignant diseases of this syndrome[91].

Greater than 90% of all reported mutations in HNPCC kindreds involve either the *MLH1* or *MSH2* gene, both implicated in the DNA mismatch repair machinery, essential to maintain fidelity during the DNA replication process. Microsatellite instability (MSI) is a genetic hallmark of tumors associated with HNPCC, as a result of DNA mismatch repair deficiency. The majority of ovarian cancer cases found in the context of HNPCC will show MSI[92], compared with approximately 10% in sporadic non-endometrioid-type cases[93-95]. In two studies, germ-line mutations in *MSH2* were significantly more frequently associated with extracolonic manifestations of the HNPCC syndrome compared with *MLH1* mutations[96,97]. The relative risk for women carrying *MSH2* mutations to develop ovarian cancer was estimated to 8.0[96]. Among 360 Finnish HNPCC mutation carriers, the cumulative ovarian cancer incidence was 12%[98]. Of note, in the latter study, only 3 out of the 50 HNPCC families were associated with *MSH2* germ-line mutations, all the others were families carrying *MLH1* alterations. In seven English and North

American HNPCC families carrying the single most common *MSH2* mutation (A→T at nt943+3), female carriers had a risk of 20% of developing a premenopausal ovarian cancer[55]. Thus it appears that both *MLH1* and *MSH2* germ-line mutations are associated with ovarian cancer, but that the relative risk for each gene is unpredictable and may be mutation or population specific. Wijnen *et al.* assessed the prevalence of *MLH1* and *MSH2* mutations in 184 families with familial clustering of colorectal cancer or other cancers associated with HNPCC and evaluated which clinical findings can predict the outcome of genetic testing[100]. The presence of a family history positive for ovarian cancer was not retained as a clinical factor associated with the identification of germ-line *MLH1* or *MSH2* mutations in this series. An earlier age of onset of ovarian cancer in HNPCC has been reported, with a mean age at diagnosis of 45 years, compared to 59 years in sporadic cases[47]. In another series of 13 ovarian cancers among Finnish HNPCC families the median age was 47 years[98].

Rubin *et al.* screened a series of 116 consecutive unselected ovarian cancer patients for germ-line *MLH1* and *MSH2* mutations[101]. Single strand conformation analysis was used to screen *MLH1* and *MSH2* among the 23% of tumors showing MSI in at least one marker. One germ-line mutation (a large genomic deletion) was detected in each of the two mismatch repair genes, but detailed family history was not available.

In summary, relative risk for ovarian cancer in HNPCC syndrome varies between 3.5 and 13[96,98,102]. The lifetime risk is approximately 12%[98]. In ovarian cancer unselected for family history, the prevalence of germ-line mutations in *MLH1* and *MSH2* is very low[101,103].

2.3.4. Other Syndromes

Very few cases of ovarian cancer have been reported in association with other inherited genetic syndromes (Table 2). Only two case reports have mentioned association of germ-line *TP53* mutations and ovarian cancer[104,105], and ovarian is not considered as a feature of the Li-Fraumeni syndrome[106-108]. Familial aggregation of ovarian germ cell cancer has been rarely reported[109].

2.4. Clinico-Pathological Characteristics

Clinico-pathological characteristics of ovarian tumor have been evaluated in familial aggregation of ovarian cancers or among patients with *BRCA1/2* germ-line mutation (hereditary ovarian cancer). Few data are available for ovarian cancer associated with other inherited genetic syndromes. Young age of onset is often considered as a hallmark of most of the hereditary cancers. As discussed above, in some studies, the average age of onset for familial or hereditary ovarian cancer was significantly lower (about 5 years) than that of ovarian cancer in the general population[23,47,110-114]. This significant difference in age of onset has not consistently been found[19,70,87,115-118]. The apparent excess of early onset disease in some families may in fact be due to ascertainment biases resulting from preferential referral of young women with ovarian cancer to familial tumor registries or cancer clinics. Interestingly, among *BRCA1/2*-related ovarian cancer, some evidence suggests an earlier age of onset restricted to women carrying the *BRCA1* mutations, but not for women with *BRCA2* mutations[26,80,114,119,120].

The existence of premalignant lesion for epithelial ovarian cancer is uncertain[121]. Careful histopathological analysis of prophylactic oophorectomy specimens among high-risk women, either because they have been identified as *BRCA1/2* mutation carriers or based on their family history, gave conflicting results regarding the presence of histological alterations susceptible to evolve in invasive carcinoma[122-125]. Papillary serous adenocarcinoma is the predominant histological type and a lower proportion of mucinous and borderline tumors were found among familial/hereditary ovarian cancer cases when compared with sporadic cases[19,44,70,110-112,115,120,126-133]. In a comprehensive study of the Gilda Radner Familial Ovarian Cancer Registry, the most important difference between familial and sporadic ovarian cancer was that mucinous adenocarcinomas were rarely seen in familial cases (1.4% versus 12.7% in unselected ovarian cancers from the SEER database)[111]. In a hospital-based series, 83% of patients with familial ovarian cancer and only 49% of matched controls had a serous cystadenocarcinoma ($P = 0.0025$)[115]. However, the difference in histological subtypes distribution between familial/hereditary ovarian cancers and the sporadic cases has not always been observed[114,116,134]. Boyd *et al.* conducted a large retrospective cohort study of Ashkenazi Jewish women with invasive epithelial ovarian cancer[114]. The mean age at diagnosis of eighty-eight carriers of one of the Ashkenazi Jewish *BRCA1/2* founder mutations, was significantly younger for *BRCA1*- (54 years) when compared with *BRCA2*-mutation carriers (62 years; $P = 0.04$), but no differences were noted regarding histological type, grade and stage between hereditary and sporadic cases. Of note, no well-differentiated tumors were observed in the *BRCA1/2* group and no mucinous subtypes were described. Despite these similarities, the authors showed a better survival for the hereditary cases, particularly for those receiving platinum-containing chemotherapy. Comparable results from a similarly designed study were reported[135]. Based on various epidemiological and mutation-based studies, it appears that the cancer risk to relatives of cases of mucinous or borderline ovarian tumors is less than for other forms[19,25,35,111,136].

Histological types of ovarian cancer associated with HNPCC have been rarely studied. In a Finnish series, ovarian cancers were all adenocarcinomas, but of 4 different sub-types, the most common being serous and mucinous[98].

Of note, in one study, rare granulosa cell tumors were associated with the highest familial risks of any histological subtype[16]. This finding must be treated with caution, as granulosa cell tumors have only been associated with the rare hereditary Peutz Jeghers syndrome. Familial occurrence of small-cell ovarian carcinoma has been anecdotally reported[137,138].

No difference in grade was found between site-specific familial ovarian cancer or *BRCA1/2*-associated ovarian cancer and sporadic ovarian tumors[26,112,114,132,139]. Four studies showed significantly more FIGO stages III and IV for familial/hereditary ovarian cases, when compared to a national cancer registry or population controls[113,118,132,133].

The occurrence of peritoneal papillary serous carcinoma indistinguishable histologically or macroscopically from ovarian cancer among carriers of ovarian cancer susceptibility genes, particularly *BRCA1/2*, represents a major threat to the efficacy of prophylactic oophorectomy[73,122,140-143]. The potential increased risk of malignant transformation of the entire peritoneal surface is thought to reflect the common origin of the ovarian epithelium and peritoneum from embryonic mesoderm. However, the peritoneum on the surface of the ovary may be particularly vulnerable to malignant transformation as a result of repeated injury following ovulation and/or high levels of local estrogen exposure[144,145]. Preliminary evidence suggests that some peritoneal carcinomas may arise multifocally, particularly in the context of *BRCA1* mutations[146]. Moreover, a recent publication showed some evidence in favor of a unique molecular pathogenesis of *BRCA1*-related papillary serous carcinoma of the peritoneum[147]. Males who carry *BRCA1* or *BRCA2* mutation are at low, but measurable risk of breast cancer[66,148-150]. Despite this, there has never been a reported case of peritoneal cancer in a male *BRCA1* or *BRCA2* mutation carrier. It is not clear why this is, but understanding the biology of the normal peritoneum in *BRCA1* and *BRCA2* mutation carriers is likely to shed light on this troublesome issue.

2.5. Risk-Prediction Models

Detailed pedigree drawing is an essential step in cancer risk evaluation. Relying on family history information to identify cases of ovarian cancer cases in relatives is permissible[37,151]. Nevertheless, it is important to get pathological reports or death certificates to confirm the family history whenever possible, particularly to adequately evaluate cancer risks and discuss the option of genetic testing.

Several empiric risk estimation models have been developed for breast cancer. These have been designed to estimate the cumulative risk (or the risk during a given period of follow-up time) of developing the disease, based on the family history (number of breast cancer cases, age of diagnosis)[152-154] or additional variables (current age, age of menarche, age at first childbirth, number of breast biopsies)[155]. Interestingly, these statistical models, based on large population-based epidemiological studies do not integrate ovarian cancer diagnosed in relatives. Moreover, these models are not appropriate for families that manifest an autosomal dominant pattern of breast cancer cases[156].

Tables for estimating the probability that an individual or a family carries a *BRCA1/2* mutation have been derived from analyses of genotype/phenotype correlation among individuals identified as *BRCA1/2* carriers[67,157]. Key clinical factors are age of onset for breast cancer and ovarian cancer occurrence. The recent BRCAPRO computer program uses a Bayesian calculation to estimate the probability that either a *BRCA1* or a *BRCA2* mutation is present in a family based on first- and second-degree family history of breast and ovarian cancer[158]. Key variables include the prevalence of mutations and age-specific penetrance estimate. The latter cannot be altered.

In summary, there is currently no risk assessment model specifically built to accurately estimate ovarian cancer risk. Thus, ovarian cancer risk evaluation rely on epidemiological studies and must consider the wide range of risk for ovarian cancer that has been attributed to *BRCA1* and *BRCA2* mutation carriers.

3. GENETIC TESTING

In 1996, the American Society of Clinical Oncology recommended that cancer predisposition testing be offered only in case of a strong family history of cancer or very early age of onset of disease, correlating with a greater than 10% probability of carrying a germ-line mutation in a cancer predisposing gene[159]. Statistical models discussed in the previous section estimate whether an individual is likely to satisfy this criteria and thus might be a candidate for genetic testing[67,157,158].

With the localization of *BRCA1* to chromosome 17q2[60], linkage analysis could be applied to establish risk in family members. This technique usually requires blood samples from both affected and asymptomatic family members over at least 3 generations. As sporadic disease cannot be unequivocally distinguished from hereditary breast cancer, absence of linkage cannot rule out the possibility of genetic basis for a particular family. The characterization of the major genes responsible for hereditary ovarian cancer facilitates genetic counseling and identification of mutation carriers. Results of *BRCA1/2* mutation screening among different groups of women affected with ovarian cancer are summarized in Table 4. Germ-line mutations in *BRCA1*, *BRCA2*, *MLH1* and *MSH2* contribute to only the minority of cases of unselected epithelial ovarian cancer[101] or early onset cases[103].

Table 4. Prevalence of BRCA1 and BRCA2 germ-line mutation in ovarian cancer.

A) Population- or hospital-based studies

Population studied	BRCA1/2 screening	Results (95% CI)	Reference
76 OC Japan	BRCA1: SSCA	4/76: 5% (1.5-13)	Matsushima et al., 1995[127]
115 OC USA	BRCA1: SSCA	7/115: 6% (2.5-12)	Takahashi et al., 1995[128]
50 OC Australia, UK, USA	BRCA2: HA, PTT	2/50: 4% (0.5-14)	Foster et al., 1996[160]
38 OC Iceland	BRCA2 999del5	3/38: 8% (1.7-21)	Johannesdottir et al., 1996[161]
55 OC UK, USA	BRCA2: SSCA, PTT	0/55	Lancaster et al., 1996[162]
130 OC USA	BRCA2: SSCA	4/130: 3% (0.8-7)	Takahashi et al., 1996[119]
374 OC < 70y UK	BRCA1: HA	13/374: 3.5% (2-6)	Stratton et al., 1997[70]
103 OC USA	BRCA1: sequencing	4/103: 4% (1-10)	Berchuck et al., 1998[131]
116 OC USA	BRCA1: SSCA BRCA2: SSCA	10/116: 9% (4-15) 1/116: 0.9% (0-5)	Rubin et al., 1998[101]
25 OC families The Netherlands	BRCA1: PTT + 185delAG BRCA2: PTT	9/25: 36% (18-57) 1/25: 4% (0.1-20)	Zweemer et al., 1998[113]
615 OC Sweden	BRCA1 1675delA BRCA1 1135insA	13/615: 2 (1-4) 5/615: 0.8 (0.3-2)	Dorum et al., 1999[163]
107 OC USA	BRCA1: CA	2/107: 2% (0.2-7)	Janezic et al., 1999[164]
101 OC < 30y UK	BRCA1: HA BRCA2: PTT	0/101 0/101	Stratton et al., 1999[103]
113 OC French Canadians	7 FC founder mutations*	8/113: 7% (3-13)	Tonin et al., 1999[120]
116 OC Japan	BRCA1: YSCA	7/116: 6% (2.5-12)	Yamashita et al., 1999[118]
90 OC Hungary	BRCA1:185delAG, 300T→G, 5382insC BRCA2: 6174delT, 9326insA	10/90: 11% (6-19) 0/90	van der Looij et al., 2000[165]

French Canadian founder mutations: BRCA1: C4446T, 2953del3+C, 3768insA; BRCA2: 2816insA, G6085T, 6503delTT, 8765delAG.

Abbreviation: CA, cleavage assay; HA, heteroduplex assay; SSCA, single strand conformation assay; OC, ovarian cancer; PTT, protein truncation test; YSCA, yeast stop codon assay.

B) Studies among Ashkenazi Jewish patients

Population studied	*BRCA1/2* screening	Results (%, 95% CI)	Reference
79 OC Israel	*BRCA1* 185delAG	15/79: 19% (11-29)	Modan et al., 1996[24]
31 OC USA	*BRCA1* 185delAG	6/31: 19% (7-37)	Muto et al., 1996[23]
21 OC Israel	AJ panel[#]	185delAG: 7/21 (33%, 15-57) 5382insC: 0/21 6174delT: 6/21 (29%, 11-52)	Abeliovich et al., 1997[78]
29 OC Israel	AJ panel[#]	185delAG: 8/29 (28%, 13-47) 5382insC: 4/29 (14%, 4-32) 6174delT: 5/29 (17%, 6-36)	Beller et al., 1997[166]
22 OC Israel	AJ panel[#]	185delAG: 5/22 (23%, 8-45) 5382insC: 2/22 (9%, 1-29) 6174delT: 3/22 (14%, 3-35)	Levy-Lahad et al., 1997[80]
59 OC Israel	*BRCA1* 185delAG *BRCA2* 6174delT	17/59: 29% (18-42) 2/59: 3% (0.4-12)	Gotlieb et al., 1998[25]
15 OC UK	AJ panel[#] + *BRCA1* 188del11	185delAG: 1/15 (7%, 0.2-32) 5382insC: 1/15 (7%, 0.2-32) 6174delT: 1/15 (7%, 0.2-32) *BRCA1* 188del11: 0/15	Hodgson et al., 1999[167]
32 OC USA	AJ panel[#]	185delAG: 8/32 (25%, 11-43) 5382insC: 0/32 6174delT: 6/32 (19%, 7-36)	Lu et al., 1999[136]
208 OC North America, Israel	AJ panel[#] + PTT	185delAG: 43/208 (21%, 15-27) 5382insC: 14/208 (7%, 4-11) 6174delT: 29/208 (14%, 9-19)	Moslehi et al., 2000[26]

[#]*AJ panel: BRCA1: 185delAG, 5382insC; BRCA2: 6174delT.*

When a reasonable probability of the presence of a cancer predisposing gene in a given family exists, genetic testing may be offered. Priority should be given to an affected family member, usually the person most likely to carry the mutation, e.g. youngest age of onset with characteristic pathobiological features. Notably, very early onset ovarian cancer is unlikely to be due to *BRCA1/2* germ-line mutation[103]. In the absence of a living affected individual, it is usually not possible to interpret a negative result in an asymptomatic family member. A negative test could be due to limitations of the nucleotide sequence analysis, mutation in other known or unknown genes, and familial aggregation of ovarian cancer cases due to chance or possibly due to shared environmental risk factors. Families in which mutations in cancer susceptibility genes are not found despite multiple cases of ovarian cancer remain problematic. In these cases, cancer geneticists must rely on the results of epidemiological studies performed on families with similar strong histories of ovarian cancer in order to estimate the risks. In families in which a disease-causing mutation has been identified, women who are determined not to be carriers can be reassured that their risk of ovarian cancer is similar to the general population. Another pitfall for the clinicians is the identification of genetic variant of undetermined clinical importance[168]. Segregation of the missense mutation with breast or ovarian cancer in affected family members suggests its significance as a disease-causing mutation rather than a rare polymorphism.

3.1. *BRCA1* and *BRCA2*

The breast-ovarian cancer susceptibility locus was localized to chromosome 17q21 in 1990[60] and the specific *BRCA1* gene was characterized in 1994[62]. *BRCA1*, composed of 5592 nucleotides within 24 exons, spreads over about 100 kb of genomic DNA, encodes a protein of 1863 amino acids whose cellular function remains unknown. Evidence suggests that BRCA1 may play a role in DNA repair and genetic recombination[169,170]. *BRCA1* may act as a caretaker gene, whose inactivation increases the frequency of DNA strand breaks, leading to alteration of other genes involved in carcinogenesis. A second major breast/ovarian cancer susceptibility gene was identified on chromosome 13q12 in 1995[64]. *BRCA2* is composed of 10,254 nucleotide pairs and 27 exons spanning over about 200 kb of genomic DNA. The BRCA2 protein (3418 amino acids) was found to have only slight homology with *BRCA1*. The frequency of mutations in the general population is estimated to be about 1 in 800 for *BRCA1* and somewhat less for *BRCA2*, but it can vary significantly among some ethnic groups or geographic regions. Thus, the prevalence of the 3 *BRCA1*/2 founder mutations among the Ashkenazim is approximately 1 to 50[171-173]. The Icelandic population carries the founder *BRCA2* 999del5 mutation at a frequency of 0.4%[161].

Several hundred different germ-line mutations in *BRCA1* and *BRCA2* have been reported (Breast Cancer Information Core (BIC) database: http:/www.nhgri.nih.gov/Intramural_research/Lab_transfer/Bic/). *De novo* germ-line mutations are thought to be rare in *BRCA1* and *BRCA2*[174]. Except for a few well characterized recurrent "founder mutations" in specific ethnic groups, the majority of *BRCA1*/2 mutations are unique and reported in only one family. Most *BRCA1* and *BRCA2* germ-line mutations are predicted to result in protein truncation caused by frameshift, nonsense, or splice-site alterations, and mutations are scattered throughout the genes. The large size and complexity of each gene, and the absence of clustering of mutations, have made the sequencing of the entire coding region, a costly and labor-intensive technique, the "gold standard" method of detecting mutations. Full-sequence analysis of the coding regions of *BRCA1* and *BRCA2* is commercially available (Myriad Genetics Laboratories, Salt Lake City, UT). As approximately 80 to 90% of *BRCA1/2* germ-line mutations result in the production of truncated proteins[175], the protein truncation test (PTT) is used as an option for mutation screening[176]. Single strand conformation assay has also been used for mutation screening (see Table 4). In the absence of reliable functional assays for *BRCA1* and *BRCA2*, the interpretation of sequence variations (missense mutation) is currently a major challenge for clinicians. Of 798 samples analyzed by automatic sequencing, 166 *BRCA1* mutations were detected, 38 (23%) were of unknown significance[175]. The DNA sequencing approaches have a high sensitivity, but do not detect all the *BRCA1/2* alterations. For example, large genomic alterations involving the *BRCA1* gene have been reported[177-180]. These alterations would not have been detected by the PCR-based techniques used to perform mutation screening.

Some *BRCA1* and *BRCA2* genotype/phenotype correlations have been reported. Mutations in the 3' portion of the *BRCA1* gene (exons 13 to 24) may be associated with a higher frequency of breast cancer relative to ovarian cancer in a series of 32 European families[181]. This observation has not been confirmed by larger studies[66,68,80,175,182,183]. In a series of 25 English breast/ovarian cancer families, ovarian cancer was more prevalent than breast cancer when *BRCA2* truncating mutations were located in a region of approximately 3.3 kb in exon 11 (the ovarian cancer cluster region [OCCR], nucleotides 3035 to 6629). Additional data from 45 *BRCA2* families ascertained outside the United Kingdom provided support for this clustering[72]. The analysis of 164 families with *BRCA2* mutations, 67 of whose had mutations in the OCCR has been recently reported[184]. The odds ratio for ovarian versus breast cancer in families with mutations in the OCCR, relative to non-OCRR mutations was 3.9 (P <0.0001), confirming the importance of the OOCR in term of ovarian cancer risk. The OCCR correspond to the coding region for a sequence of internal repeats in the BRCA2 protein which have been shown to interact with the DNA repair protein RAD51.

New technical approaches have been proposed to resolve the problems of *BRCA1/2* mutation screening, particularly to reduce the cost and increase sensitivity. A combination of extensive multiplex PCR amplification and two dimensional electrophoresis[185], denaturing high performance liquid chromatography[186], a yeast functional assay for mutations in the C terminal region of *BRCA1*[187], high density oligonucleotide arrays[188] and a mutagen sensitivity assay in peripheral lymphocytes[189] have been proposed. All these techniques need to be evaluated at a larger scale and compared with the currently used sequencing procedures. The widespread availability of commercial *BRCA1/2* testing is convenient, but the patent held by Myriad Genetics Laboratories could limit the development of newer, cheaper and more comprehensive non-gel based mutation screening methods.

3.2. *MLH1* and *MSH2*

MSI or replication error phenotype is a widely accepted hallmark of loss of DNA mismatch repair activity in the tumor cells. This is caused by mutations in one of the four mismatch repair genes involved in HNPCC: *MSH2*, *MLH1*, *PMS1*, and *PMS2*[89]. The identification of MSI in ovarian malignant tissue could be used as a screening tool to select cases for further DNA mismatch repair genes analysis[92,101]. Ovarian cancer has been rarely described in families with germ-line alterations in the fifth HNPCC causing gene *MSH6*[190,191]. Of note, mutations in *MSH6* may not be associated with MSI. It has yet to be determined whether all of these genes confer an increased risk of ovarian cancer.

The molecular diagnosis of HNPCC is usually based on nucleotide sequence screening in the 2 major DNA mismatch repair genes *MLH1* and *MSH2*, implicated in more than 90% of HNPCC families with characterized pathogenic germ-line mutations [International Collaborative group on HNPCC database: http://www.nfdht.nl/]. As for *BRCA1* and *BRCA2*, a major question for clinicians is the interpretation of missense mutations, which are particularly common in *MLH1* ($\geq 30\%$). Several assays have been developed to elucidate the functional significance of the missense mutations identified[192-194].

3.3. Founder Mutations

Founder effects have been described in populations which have grown rapidly from a small number of founders and without significant influx of people of different origins. The founder effect can occur when a relatively small group is genetically isolated from the rest of the population, because of geographic conditions or religious belief. If an individual in that isolated population carries a rare genetic alteration, the frequency of this allele in the next generations could increase in the absence of selection. Specific *BRCA1* and *BRCA2* mutations have been identified in diverse populations, such as in Ashkenazi Jewish, Icelandic, Swedish, Norwegian, Austrian, Dutch, British, Belgian, Russian, Hungarian, and French Canadian families[84,161,175,181,195-202]. The knowledge of well-characterized founder mutations in individuals of particular ethnic origins can simplify genetic counseling and testing, as the mutation screening can be limited to specific panels of mutations.

Three founder mutations (*BRCA1* 185delAG and 5382insC in *BRCA1*, *BRCA2* 6174delT) have been identified in the Ashkenazi Jewish families of Eastern European ancestry[68,203-205]. These mutations are carried by about 2.5% of the Ashkenazi Jewish population[171-173]. These founder mutations are particularly common in Ashkenazi Jewish women with ovarian cancer, even without a family history of breast/ovarian cancer (Table 4). Of note, the *BRCA1* 5382insC mutation is not restricted to the Ashkenazi Jewish ethnic group, as this mutation has been identified in other populations from Eastern Europe[201,206,207].
Founder mutations have also been described in mismatch repair genes[99,208,209].

3.4. Modifier Genes

The proportion of *BRCA1/2* carriers affected with ovarian cancer varies considerably among families and also among families with identical *BRCA1/2* mutations, one extreme being the site-specific ovarian cancer syndrome. For example, in two similarly designed study involving Ashkenazi Jewish women[26,82] the penetrance for ovarian cancer among the *BRCA1/2* founder mutation carriers was very different if the cases ascertained were breast cancer or ovarian cancer (12% *vs.* 41%). It has been proposed that several factors may contribute to the variable risk of ovarian cancer in carriers, such as other loci modifying the penetrance of *BRCA1/2* or gene-environment interaction. For example, it is possible that reproductive risk factors such as pregnancy or pill use, that affect ovarian cancer incidence in the general population, may also modify risk in *BRCA1/2* carriers[210,211]. Smoking could significantly decrease the risk of breast cancer among *BRCA1/2* mutation carriers, thus may allow ovarian cancer to become the main expression of the cancer predisposition[86,212].

In one study there was an association between rare *HRAS1* variable number of tandem repeat polymorphisms and an increased penetrance of *BRCA1*[182]. Although rare *HRAS1* alleles did not appear to modify risk of breast cancer in mutation carriers, the risk for ovarian cancer was 2.1-fold higher for *BRCA1* carriers with one or two rare *HRAS1* alleles than for carriers with only common alleles ($P = 0.015$). The precise mechanism of action of the *HRAS1* alleles in the pathogenesis of cancer is unclear. Interestingly, these rare *HRAS1* alleles may also increase the ovarian cancer risk in the general population[213].

The *APC* I1307K allele was identified as a founder mutation occurring in about 6% of the Ashkenazi population. This allele is present in a significantly higher proportion of Jewish colorectal cancer patients and in those with a family history of colorectal cancer[214-216]. The relative risk for colorectal cancer associated with the *APC* variant appears to be in the range of 1.5-2.0.

APC I1307K alone does not appear to confer a substantial risk of ovarian cancer in the Ashkenazi Jewish population generally[217,218]. Redston *et al.* reported that *APC* I1307K in the presence of germ-line *BRCA1* mutations moderately increased the prevalence of breast cancer[219], but subsequently a study did not reveal any clear clinicopathological features of breast tumor associated with *APC* I1307K[220]. Moreover, recent data suggest that *APC* I1307K allele does not confer an increased risk of ovarian cancer in association with germ-line *BRCA1/2* mutation among the Ashkenazi Jewish population[221].

Recently, Buller *et al.* reported that nonrandom X-chromosome inactivation was seen among a series of invasive epithelial ovarian cancer, but not among borderline tumors[222]. A significant relationship between nonrandom X-chromosome inactivation and *BRCA1*-associated ovarian cancer was noted in a small series of patients. It remains to be demonstrated how X-chromosome factors could modify the expression or function of the *BRCA1* gene product.

Genes implicated in carcinogens metabolism process have been evaluated in HNPCC with some evidence suggesting a role for *NAT2* variants as a modifier gene[223], but the role of polymorphisms in this gene in the variable spectrum of cancer seen in HNPCC syndrome is not established.

4. CONCLUSION

The ultimate aim of clinical predictive oncology is to have a beneficial impact on cancer morbidity and mortality by counseling individuals identified as possible cancer predisposing genes carriers, and providing specific recommendations for cancer surveillance and prevention[156]. Establishing an extensive verified family history is the essential step to identify individuals at risk of ovarian cancer and for whom genetic testing may be informative[224]. Cancer genetic susceptibility testing is now commercially available, but predictive oncology is still a relatively new field in medicine and consensus has not been reached regarding guidelines for testing in clinical practice. Based on an accurate personal and family history of cancer, including ethnicity and pathological confirmation of the cancer cases, empirical cancer risk estimates and mathematical models can usually adequately assess the ovarian cancer risk and the probability of a germ-line alteration in cancer susceptibility genes implicated in hereditary ovarian cancer. Because the benefits of genetic testing remain hypothetical, women should receive adequate counseling explaining the postulated risks and benefits of the genetic testing, including the ethical, legal and social implications of this type of analysis. It is highly desirable that such testing should take place in a setting that includes physicians trained in clinical cancer genetics and genetic counselors with specific experience in cancer risk assessment and counseling.

REFERENCES

1.   Hildreth NG, Kelsey JL, LiVolsi VA, et al. An epidemiologic study of epithelial carcinoma of the ovary. Am J Epidemiol 1981; 114:398-405.
2.   Parazzini F, Franceschi S, La Vecchia C, Fasoli M. The epidemiology of ovarian cancer. Gynecol Oncol 1991; 43:9-23.
3.   Whittemore AS, Harris R, Itnyre J. Characteristics relating to ovarian cancer risk: collaborative analysis of 12 US case-control studies. II. Invasive epithelial ovarian cancers in white women. Collaborative Ovarian Cancer Group. Am J Epidemiol 1992; 136:1184-1203.
4.   Amos CI, Struewing JP. Genetic epidemiology of epithelial ovarian cancer. Cancer 1993; 71:566-72.
5.   Godard B, Foulkes WD, Provencher D, et al. Risk factors for familial and sporadic ovarian cancer among French Canadians: a case-control study. Am J Obstet Gynecol 1998; 179:403-10.
6.   Cramer DW, Harlow BL, Willett WC, et al. Galactose consumption and metabolism in relation to the risk of ovarian cancer. Lancet 1989; 2:66-71.
7.   Whittemore AS, Wu ML, Paffenbarger RS, Jr., et al. Personal and environmental characteristics related to epithelial ovarian cancer. II. Exposures to talcum powder, tobacco, alcohol, and coffee. Am J Epidemiol 1988; 128:1228-40.
8.   Mori M, Harabuchi I, Miyake H, et al. Reproductive, genetic, and dietary risk factors for ovarian cancer. Am J Epidemiol 1988; 128:771-7.
9.   Parazzini F, Negri E, La Vecchia C, et al. Family history of reproductive cancers and ovarian cancer risk: an Italian case-control study. Am J Epidemiol 1992; 135:35-40.
10. Casagrande JT, Louie EW, Pike MC, Roy S, Ross RK, Henderson BE. "Incessant ovulation" and ovarian cancer. Lancet 1979; 2:170-3.
11. Cramer DW, Hutchison GB, Welch WR, et al. Determinants of ovarian cancer risk. I. Reproductive experiences and family history. J Natl Cancer Inst 1983; 71:711-6.
12. Franceschi S, Parazzini F, Negri E, et al. Pooled analysis of 3 European case-control studies of epithelial ovarian cancer: III. Oral contraceptive use. Int J Cancer 1991; 49:61-5.
13. Hankinson SE, Hunter DJ, Colditz GA, et al. Tubal ligation, hysterectomy, and risk of ovarian cancer. A prospective study. JAMA 1993; 270:2813-8.
14. Adami HO, Hsieh CC, Lambe M, et al. Parity, age at first childbirth, and risk of ovarian cancer. Lancet 1994; 344:1250-4.
15. Rosenberg L, Palmer JR, Zauber AG, et al. A case-control study of oral contraceptive use and invasive epithelial ovarian cancer. Am J Epidemiol 1994; 139:654-61.
16. Kerber RA, Slattery ML. The impact of family history on ovarian cancer risk. The Utah Population Database. Arch Int Med 1995; 155:905-12.
17. Purdie D, Green A, Bain C, et al. Reproductive and other factors and risk of epithelial ovarian cancer: an Australian case-control study. Survey of Women's Health Study Group. Int J Cancer 1995; 62:678-84.
18. Houlston RS, Collins A, Slack J, et al. Genetic epidemiology of ovarian cancer: segregation analysis. Ann Hum Genet 1991; 55:291-9.
19. Narod SA, Madlensky L, Bradley L, et al. Hereditary and familial ovarian cancer in southern Ontario. Cancer 1994; 74:2341-6.

50

20. Narod SA, Ford D, Devilee P, et al. An evaluation of genetic heterogeneity in 145 breast-ovarian cancer families. Breast Cancer Linkage Consortium. Am J Hum Genet 1995; 56:254-64.

21. Claus EB, Schildkraut JM, Thompson WD, Risch NJ. The genetic attributable risk of breast and ovarian cancer. Cancer 1996; 77:2318-24.

22. Whittemore AS, Gong G, Itnyre J. Prevalence and contribution of BRCA1 mutations in breast cancer and ovarian cancer: results from three U.S. population-based case-control studies of ovarian cancer. Am J Hum Genet 1997; 60:496-504.

23. Muto MG, Cramer DW, Tangir J, et al. Frequency of the BRCA1 185delAG mutation among Jewish women with ovarian cancer and matched population controls. Cancer Res 1996; 56:1250-2.

24. Modan B, Gak E, Sade-Bruchim RB, et al. High frequency of BRCA1 185delAG mutation in ovarian cancer in Israel. National Israel Study of Ovarian Cancer. JAMA 1996; 276:1823-5.

25. Gotlieb WH, Friedman E, Bar-Sade RB, et al. Rates of Jewish ancestral mutations in BRCA1 and BRCA2 in borderline ovarian tumors. J Natl Cancer Inst 1998; 90:995-1000.

26. Moslehi R, Chu W, Karlan B, et al. BRCA1 and BRCA2 mutation analysis of 208 Ashkenazi Jewish women with ovarian cancer. Am J Hum Genet 2000; 66:1259-72.

27. Claus EB, Schwartz PE. Familial ovarian cancer. Update and clinical applications. Cancer 1995; 76:1998-2003.

28. Parkin DM, Whelan SL, Ferlay J, Raymond L, Young J, editors. Cancer incidence in five continents vol. VII. Lyon: IARC Scientific Publications; 1997.

29. Greenlee RT, Murray T, Bolden S, Wingo PA. Cancer statistics, 2000. CA Cancer J Clin 2000; 50:7-33.

30. Hartge P, Whittemore AS, Itnyre J, and the collaborative ovarian cancer group. Rates and risks of ovarian cancer in subgroups of white women in the United States. Obstet Gynecol 1994; 84:760-4.

31. Lynch HT, Lynch JF. Hereditary ovarian carcinoma. Hematol Oncol Clin North Am 1992; 6:783-811.

32. Stratton JF, Pharoah P, Smith SK, et al. A systematic review and meta-analysis of family history and risk of ovarian cancer. Br J Obstet Gynaecol 1998; 105:493-9.

33. Wynder EL, Dodo H, Barber HR. Epidemiology of cancer of the ovary. Cancer 1969; 23:352-70.

34. Tzonou A, Day NE, Trichopoulos D, et al. The epidemiology of ovarian cancer in Greece: a case-control study. Eur J Cancer Clin Oncol 1984; 20:1045-52.

35. Schildkraut JM, Thompson WD. Familial ovarian cancer: a population-based case-control study. Am J Epidemiol 1988; 128:456-66.

36. Hartge P, Schiffman MH, Hoover R, et al. A case-control study of epithelial ovarian cancer. Am J Obstetr Gynecol 1989; 161:10-6.

37. Koch M, Gaedke H, Jenkins H. Family history of ovarian cancer patients: a case-control study. Int J Epidemiol 1989; 18:782-5.

38. Goldgar DE, Easton DF, Cannon-Albright LA, Skolnick MH. Systematic population-based assessment of cancer risk in first-degree relatives of cancer probands. J Natl Cancer Inst 1994; 86:1600-8.

39. Auranen A, Pukkala E, Makinen J, et al. Cancer incidence in the first-degree relatives of ovarian cancer patients. Br J Cancer 1996; 74:280-4.

40. Easton DF, Matthews FE, Ford D, et al. Cancer mortality in relatives of women with ovarian cancer - the OPCS study. Int J Cancer 1996; 65:284-94.

41. Hemminki K, Vaittinen P, Kyyronen P. Age-specific familial risks in common cancers of the offspring. Int J Cancer 1998; 78:172-5.

42. Sutcliffe S, Pharoah PDP, Easton DF, Ponder BAJ. Ovarian and breast cancer risks to women in families with two or more cases of ovarian cancer. Int J Cancer 2000; 87:110-7.

43. Schildkraut JM, Risch N, Thompson WD. Evaluating genetic association among ovarian, breast, and endometrial cancer: evidence for a breast/ovarian cancer relationship. Am J Hum Genet 1989; 45:521-9.

44. Greggi S, Genuardi M, Benedetti-Panici P, et al. Analysis of 138 consecutive ovarian cancer patients: incidence and characteristics of familial cases. Gynecol Oncol 1990; 39:300-4.

45. Amos CI, Shaw GL, Tucker MA, Hartge P. Age at onset for familial epithelial ovarian cancer. JAMA 1992; 268:1896-9.

46. Houlston RS, Bourne TH, Collins WP, et al. Risk of ovarian cancer and genetic relationship to other cancers in families. Hum Hered 1993; 43:111-5.

47. Lynch HT, Watson P, Lynch JF, et al. Hereditary ovarian cancer. Heterogeneity in age at onset. Cancer 1993; 71:573-81.

48. Vaittinen P, Hemminki K. Familial cancer risks in offspring from discordant parental cancers. Int J Cancer 1999; 81:12-9.

49. Jishi MF, Itnyre JH, Oakley-Girvan IA, et al. Risks of cancer among members of families in the Gilda Radner Familial Ovarian Cancer Registry. Cancer 1995; 76:1416-21.

50. Auranen A, Grenman S, Makinen J, et al. Borderline ovarian tumors in Finland: epidemiology and familial occurrence. Am J Epidemiol 1996; 144:548-53.

51. Rader JS, Neuman RJ, Brady J, et al. Cancer among first-degree relatives of probands with invasive and borderline ovarian cancer. Obstet Gynecol 1998; 92:589-95.

52. Prior P, Waterhouse JA. Multiple primary cancers of the breast and ovary. Br J Cancer 1981; 44:628-36.

53. Schildkraut JM, Thompson WD. Relationship of epithelial ovarian cancer to other malignancies within families. Genet Epidemiol 1988; 5:355-67.

54. Tulinius H, Olafsdottir GH, Sigvaldason H, et al. Neoplastic diseases in families of breast cancer patients. J Med Genet 1994; 31:618-21.

55. Olsen JH, Seersholm N, Boice JDJ, et al. Cancer risk in close relatives of women with early-onset breast cancer--a population-based incidence study. Br J Cancer 1999; 79:673-9.

56. Auranen A, Iselius L. Segregation analysis of epithelial ovarian cancer in Finland. Br J Cancer 1998; 77:1537-41.

57. Kasprzak L, Foulkes WD, Shelling AN. Forthnightly review: hereditary ovarian carcinoma. BMJ. 1999; 318:786-9.

58. Liber AF. Ovarian cancer in a mother and five daughters. Arch Pathol 1950; 49:280-90.

59. Go RC, King MC, Bailey-Wilson J, et al. Genetic epidemiology of breast cancer and associated cancers in high-risk families. I. Segregation analysis. J Natl Cancer Inst 1983; 71:455-61.

60. Hall JM, Lee MK, Newman B, et al. Linkage of early-onset familial breast cancer to chromosome 17q21. Science 1990; 250:1684-9.

61. Narod SA, Feunteun J, Lynch HT, et al. Familial breast-ovarian cancer locus on chromosome 17q12-q23. Lancet 1991; 338:82-3.

62. Miki Y, Swensen J, Shattuck-Eidens D, et al. A strong candidate for the breast and ovarian cancer susceptibility gene BRCA1. Science 1994; 266:66-71.

63. Wooster R, Neuhausen SL, Mangion J, et al. Localization of a breast cancer susceptibility gene, BRCA2, to chromosome 13q12-13. Science 1994; 265:2088-90.

64. Wooster R, Bignell G, Lancaster J, et al. Identification of the breast cancer susceptibility gene BRCA2. Nature 1995; 378:789-92.

52

65. Easton DF, Bishop DT, Ford D, Crockford GP. Genetic linkage analysis in familial breast and ovarian cancer: results from 214 families. The Breast Cancer Linkage Consortium. Am J Hum Genet 1993; 52:678-701.

66. Ford D, Easton DF, Stratton M, et al. Genetic heterogeneity and penetrance analysis of the BRCA1 and BRCA2 genes in breast cancer families. Am J Hum Genet 1998; 62:676-89.

67. Frank TS, Manley SA, Olopade OI, et al. Sequence analysis of BRCA1 and BRCA2: correlation of mutations with family history and ovarian cancer risk. J Clin Oncol 1998; 16:2417-25.

68. Tonin P, Weber B, Offit K, et al. Frequency of recurrent BRCA1 and BRCA2 mutations in Ashkenazi Jewish breast cancer families. Nat Med 1996; 2:1183-96.

69. Ligtenberg MJ, Hogervorst FB, Willems HW, et al. Characteristics of small breast and/or ovarian cancer families with germline mutations in BRCA1 and BRCA2. Br J Cancer 1999; 79:1475-8.

70. Stratton JF, Gayther SA, Russell P, et al. Contribution of BRCA1 mutations to ovarian cancer. N Engl J Med 1997; 336:1125-30.

71. Ford D, Easton DF, Peto J. Estimates of the gene frequency of BRCA1 and its contribution to breast and ovarian cancer incidence. Am J Hum Genet 1995; 57:1457-62.

72. Gayther SA, Mangion J, Russell P, et al. Variation of risks of breast and ovarian cancer associated with different germline mutations of the BRCA2 gene. Nat Genet 1997; 15:103-5.

73. Karlan BY, Baldwin RL, Lopez-Luevanos E, et al. Peritoneal serous papillary carcinoma, a phenotypic variant of familial ovarian cancer: implications for ovarian cancer screening. Am J Obstet Gynecol 1999; 180:917-28.

74. Ford D, Easton DF, Bishop DT, et al. Risks of cancer in BRCA1-mutation carriers. Breast Cancer Linkage Consortium. Lancet 1994; 343:692-5.

75. Antoniou AC, Gayther SA, Stratton JF, et al. Risk models for familial ovarian and breast cancer. Genet Epidemiol 2000; 18:173-90.

76. Richards WE, Gallion HH, Schmittschmitt JP, et al. BRCA1-related and sporadic ovarian cancer in the same family: implications for genetic testing. Gynecol Oncol 1999; 75:468-72.

77. Easton DF, Ford D, Bishop DT. Breast and ovarian cancer incidence in BRCA1-mutation carriers. Breast Cancer Linkage Consortium. Am J Hum Genet 1995; 56:265-71.

78. Abeliovich D, Kaduri L, Lerer I, et al. The founder mutations 185delAG and 5382insC in BRCA1 and 6174delT in BRCA2 appear in 60-percent of ovarian cancer and 30-percent of early-onset breast cancer patients among Ashkenazi women. Am J Hum Genet 1997; 60:505-14.

79. Easton DF, Steele L, Fields P, et al. Cancer risks in two large breast cancer families linked to BRCA2 on chromosome 13q12-13. Am J Hum Genet 1997; 61:120-8.

80. Levy-Lahad E, Catane R, Eisenberg S, et al. Founder BRCA1 and BRCA2 mutations in Ashkenazi Jews in Israel: frequency and differential penetrance in ovarian cancer and in breast-ovarian cancer families. Am J Hum Genet 1997; 60:1059-67.

81. Struewing JP, Hartge P, Wacholder S, et al. The risk of cancer associated with specific mutations of BRCA1 and BRCA2 among Ashkenazi Jews. N Engl J Med 1997; 336:1401-8.

82. Warner E, Foulkes W, Goodwin P, et al. Prevalence and penetrance of BRCA1 and BRCA2 gene mutations in unselected Ashkenazi Jewish women with breast cancer. J Natl Cancer Inst 1999; 91:1241-7.

83. Steichen-Gersdorf E, Gallion HH, Ford D, et al. Familial site-specific ovarian cancer is linked to BRCA1 on 17q12-21. Am J Hum Genet 1994; 55:870-5.

84.   Shattuck-Eidens D, McClure M, Simard J, et al. A collaborative survey of 80 mutations in the BRCA1 breast and ovarian cancer susceptibility gene. Implications for presymptomatic testing and screening. JAMA 1995; 273:535-41.

85.   Roth S, Kristo P, Auranen A, et al. A missense mutation in the BRCA2 gene in three siblings with ovarian cancer. Br J Cancer 1998; 77:1199-202.

86.   Liede A, Tonin PN, Sun CC, et al. Is hereditary site-specific ovarian cancer a distinct genetic condition? Am J Med Genet 1998; 75:55-8.

87.   Gayther SA, Russell P, Harrington P, et al. The contribution of germline BRCA1 and BRCA2 mutations to familial ovarian cancer: No evidence for other ovarian cancer-susceptibility genes. Am J Hum Genet 1999; 65:1021-9.

88.   Santarosa M, Dolcetti R, Magri MD, et al. BRCA1 and BRCA2 genes: role in hereditary breast and ovarian cancer in Italy. Int J Cancer 1999; 83:5-9.

89.   Lynch HT, de la Chapelle A. Genetic susceptibility to non-polyposis colorectal cancer. J Med Genet 1999; 36:801-18.

90.   Vasen HF, Mecklin JP, Khan PM, Lynch HT. The International Collaborative Group on Hereditary Non-Polyposis Colorectal Cancer (ICG-HNPCC). Dis Colon Rectum 1991; 34:424-5.

91.   Vasen HF, Watson P, Mecklin JP, Lynch HT. New clinical criteria for hereditary nonpolyposis colorectal cancer (HNPCC, Lynch syndrome) proposed by the International Collaborative group on HNPCC. Gastroenterology 1999; 116:1453-6.

92.   Ichikawa Y, Lemon SJ, Wang S, et al. Microsatellite instability and expression of MLH1 and MSH2 in normal and malignant endometrial and ovarian epithelium in hereditary nonpolyposis colorectal cancer family members. Cancer Genet Cytogenet 1999; 112:2-8.

93.   Fujita M, Enomoto T, Yoshino K, et al. Microsatellite instability and alterations in the hMSH2 gene in human ovarian cancer. Int J Cancer 1995; 64:361-6.

94.   Arzimanoglou II, Lallas T, Osborne M, et al. Microsatellite instability differences between familial and sporadic ovarian cancers. Carcinogenesis 1996; 17 :1799-804.

95.   Allen HJ, DiCioccio RA, Hohmann P, et al. Microsatellite instability in ovarian and other pelvic carcinomas. Cancer Genet Cytogenet 2000; 117:163-6.

96.   Vasen HF, Wijnen JT, Menko FH, et al. Cancer risk in families with hereditary nonpolyposis colorectal cancer diagnosed by mutation analysis. Gastroenterology 1996; 110:1020-7.

97.   Lin KM, Shashidharan M, Ternent CA, et al. Colorectal and extracolonic cancer variations in MLH1/MSH2 hereditary nonpolyposis colorectal cancer kindreds and the general population. Dis Colon Rectum 1998; 41:428-33.

98.   Aarnio M, Sankila R, Pukkala E, et al. Cancer risk in mutation carriers of DNA-mismatch-repair genes. Int J Cancer 1999; 81:214-8.

99.   Froggatt NJ, Green J, Brassett C, et al. A common MSH2 mutation in English and North American HNPCC families: origin, phenotypic expression, and sex specific differences in colorectal cancer. J Med Genet 1999; 36:97-102.

100. Wijnen JT, Vasen HF, Khan PM, et al. Clinical findings with implications for genetic testing in families with clustering of colorectal cancer. N Engl J Med 1998; 339:511-8.

101. Rubin SC, Blackwood MA, Bandera C, et al. BRCA1, BRCA2, and hereditary nonpolyposis colorectal cancer gene mutations in an unselected ovarian cancer population: relationship to family history and implications for genetic testing. Am J Obstet Gynecol 1998; 178:670-7.

102. Watson P, Lynch HT. Extracolonic cancer in hereditary nonpolyposis colorectal cancer. Cancer 1993; 71:677-85.

103. Stratton JF, Thompson D, Bobrow L, et al. The genetic epidemiology of early-onset epithelial ovarian cancer: a population-based study. Am J Hum Genet 1999; 65:1725-32.

54

104. Borresen AL. Oncogenesis in ovarian cancer. Acta Obstet Gynecol Scand 1992; 71 Suppl 155:25-30.
105. Jolly KW, Malkin D, Douglass EC, et al. Splice-site mutation of the p53 gene in a family with hereditary breast-ovarian cancer. Oncogene 1994; 9:97-102.
106. Buller RE, Skilling JS, Kaliszewski S, et al. Absence of significant germ line p53 mutations in ovarian cancer patients. Gynecol Oncol 1995; 58:368-74.
107. Kleihues P, Schauble B, zur Hausen, et al. Tumors associated with p53 germline mutations: a synopsis of 91 families. Am J Pathol 1997; 150:1-13.
108. Birch JM, Blair V, Kelsey AM, et al. Cancer phenotype correlates with constitutional TP53 genotype in families with the Li-Fraumeni syndrome. Oncogene 1998; 17:1061-8.
109. Stettner AR, Hartenbach EM, Schink JC, et al. Familial ovarian germ cell cancer: report and review. Am J Med Genet 1999; 84:43-6.
110. Bewtra C, Watson P, Conway T, et al. Hereditary ovarian cancer: a clinicopathological study. Int J Gynecol Pathol 1992; 11:180-7.
111. Piver MS, Baker TR, Jishi MF, et al. Familial ovarian cancer. A report of 658 families from the Gilda Radner Familial Ovarian Cancer Registry 1981-1991. Cancer 1993; 71:582-8.
112. Rubin SC, Benjamin I, Behbakht K, et al. Clinical and pathoological features of ovarian cancer in women with germ-line mutations of BRCA1. N Engl J Med 1996; 335:1413-6.
113. Zweemer RP, Verheijen RH, Gille JJ, et al. Clinical and genetic evaluation of thirty ovarian cancer families. Am J Obstet Gynecol 1998; 178:85-90.
114. Boyd J, Sonoda Y, Federici MG, et al. Clinicopathologic features of BRCA-linked and sporadic ovarian cancer. JAMA 2000; 283:2260-5.
115. Chang J, Fryatt I, Ponder B, et al. A matched control study of familial epithelial ovarian cancer: patient characteristics, response to chemotherapy and outcome. Ann Oncol 1995; 6:80-2.
116. Auranen A, Grenman S, Kleml PJ. Immunohistochemically detected p53 and HER-2/neu expression and nuclear DNA content in familial epithelial ovarian carcinomas. Cancer 1997; 79:2147-53.
117. Johannsson OT, Ranstam J, Borg A, Olsson H. Survival of BRCA1 Breast and Ovarian Cancer Patients: A Population-Based Study From Southern Sweden. J Clin Oncol 1998; 16:397-404.
118. Yamashita Y, Sagawa T, Fujimoto T, et al. BRCA1 mutation testing for Japanese patients with ovarian cancer in breast cancer screening. Breast Cancer Res Treat 1999; 58:11-7.
119. Takahashi H, Chiu HC, Bandera CA, et al. Mutations of the BRCA2 gene in ovarian carcinomas. Cancer Res 1996; 56:2738-41.
120. Tonin PM, Mes-Masson AM, Narod SA, et al. Founder BRCA1 and BRCA2 mutations in French Canadian ovarian cancer cases unselected for family history. Clin Genet 1999; 55:318-24.
121. Scully RE. Influence of origin of ovarian cancer on efficacy of screening. Lancet 2000; 355:1028-9.
122. Salazar H, Godwin AK, Daly MB, et al. Microscopic benign and invasive malignant neoplasms and a cancer-prone phenotype in prophylactic oophorectomies. J Natl Cancer Inst 1996; 88:1810-20.
123. Deligdisch L, Gil J, Kerner H, et al. Ovarian dysplasia in prophylactic oophorectomy specimens: cytogenetic and morphometric correlations. Cancer 1999; 86:1544-50.
124. Stratton JF, Buckley CH, Lowe D, Ponder BA. Comparison of prophylactic oophorectomy specimens from carriers and noncarriers of a BRCA1 or BRCA2 gene mutation. J Natl Cancer Inst 1999; 91:626-8.

125. Werness BA, Afify AM, Bielat KL, et al. Altered surface and cyst epithelium of ovaries removed prophylactically from women with a family history of ovarian cancer. Hum Pathol 1999; 30:151-7.

126. Narod SA, Tonin P, Lynch H, et al. Histology of BRCA1-associated ovarian tumours. Lancet 1994; 343:236.

127. Matsushima M, Kobayashi K, Emi M, et al. Mutation analysis of the BRCA1 gene in 76 Japanese ovarian cancer patients: four germline mutations, but no evidence of somatic mutation. Hum Mol Genet 1995; 4:1953-6.

128. Takahashi H, Behbakht K, McGovern PE, et al. Mutation analysis of the BRCA1 gene in ovarian cancers. Cancer Res 1995; 55:2998-3002.

129. Takano M, Aida H, Tsuneki I, et al. Mutational analysis of BRCA1 gene in ovarian and breast-ovarian cancer families in Japan. Jpn J Cancer Res 1997; 88:407-13.

130. Aida H, Takakuwa K, Nagata H, et al. Clinical features of ovarian cancer in Japanese women with germ-line mutations of BRCA1. Clin Cancer Res 1998; 4:235-40.

131. Berchuck A, Heron KA, Carney ME, et al. Frequency of germline and somatic BRCA1 mutations in ovarian cancer. Clin Cancer Res 1998; 4:2433-7.

132. Pharoah PD, Easton DF, Stockton DL, et al. Survival in familial, BRCA1-associated, and BRCA2-associated epithelial ovarian cancer. United Kingdom Coordinating Committee for Cancer Research (UKCCCR) Familial Ovarian Cancer Study Group. Cancer Res 1999; 59:868-71.

133. Sagawa T, Yamashita Y, Fujimoto T, et al. Clinicopathological comparisons of familial and sporadic cases in 219 consecutive Japanese epithelial ovarian cancer patients. Jpn J Clin Oncol 1999; 29:556-61.

134. Johannsson OT, Idvall I, Anderson C, et al. Tumour biological features of BRCA1-induced breast and ovarian cancer. Eur J Cancer 1997; 33:362-71.

135. Levy-Lahad E, Kaufman B, Eisenberg S, et al. Differential ovarian cancer survival in Ashkenazi BRCA1/BRCA2 carriers [abstract]. Am J Hum Genet 1999; 65 Suppl:135.

136. Lu KH, Cramer DW, Muto MG, et al. A population-based study of BRCA1 and BRCA2 mutations in Jewish women with epithelial ovarian cancer. Obstet Gynecol 1999; 93:34-7.

137. Lamovec J, Bracko M, Cerar O. Familial occurrence of small-cell carcinoma of the ovary. Arch Pathol Lab Med 1995; 119:523-7.

138. Longy M, Toulouse C, Mage P, et al. Familial cluster of ovarian small cell carcinoma: a new mendelian entity? J Med Genet 1996; 33:333-5.

139. Buller RE, Anderson B, Connor JP, Robinson R. Familial ovarian cancer. Gynecol Oncol 1993; 51:160-6.

140. Piver MS, Jishi MF, Tsukada Y, Nava G. Primary peritoneal carcinoma after prophylactic oophorectomy in women with a family history of ovarian cancer. A report of the Gilda Radner Familial Ovarian Cancer Registry. Cancer 1993; 71:2751-5.

141. Struewing JP, Watson P, Easton DF, et al. Prophylactic oophorectomy in inherited breast/ovarian cancer families. J Natl Cancer Inst Monograph 1995; 33-5.

142. Bandera CA, Muto MG, Schorge JO, et al. BRCA1 gene mutations in women with papillary serous carcinoma of the peritoneum. Obstet Gynecol 1998; 92:596-600.

143. Berchuck A, Schildkraut JM, Marks JR, Futreal PA. Managing hereditary ovarian cancer risk. Cancer 1999; 86:1697-704.

144. Fathalla MF. Incessant ovulation--a factor in ovarian neoplasia?. Lancet 1971; 2:163.

145. Eisen A, Weber BL. Primary peritoneal carcinoma can have multifocal origins: implications for prophylactic oophorectomy. J Natl Cancer Inst 1998; 90:797-9.

146. Schorge JO, Muto MG, Welch WR, et al. Molecular evidence for multifocal papillary serous carcinoma of the peritoneum in patients with germline BRCA1 mutations. J Natl Cancer Inst 1998; 90:841-5.

147. Schorge JO, Muto MG, Lee SJ, et al. BRCA1-related papillary serous carcinoma of the peritoneum has a unique molecular pathogenesis. Cancer Res 2000; 60:1361-4.

56

148. Struewing JP, Coriaty ZM, Ron E, et al. Founder BRCA1/2 mutations among male patients with breast cancer in Israel. Am J Hum Genet 1999; 65:1800-2.
149. Csokay B, Udvarhelyi N, Sulyok Z, et al. High frequency of germ-line BRCA2 mutations among Hungarian male breast cancer patients without family history. Cancer Res 1999; 59:995-8.
150. Haraldsson K, Loman N, Zhang QX, et al. BRCA2 germ-line mutations are frequent in male breast cancer patients without a family history of the disease. Cancer Res 1998; 58:1367-71.
151. Douglas FS, O'Dair LC, Robinson M, et al. The accuracy of diagnoses as reported in families with cancer: a retrospective study. J Med Genet 1999; 36:309-12.
152. Ottman R, Pike MC, King MC, Henderson BE. Practical guide for estimating risk for familial breast cancer. Lancet 1983; 2:556-8.
153. Anderson DE, Badzioch MD. Risk of familial breast cancer. Cancer 1985; 56:383-7.
154. Claus EB, Risch N, Thompson WD. Autosomal dominant inheritance of early-onset breast cancer. Implications for risk prediction. Cancer 1994; 73:643-51.
155. Gail MH, Brinton LA, Byar DP, et al. Projecting individualized probabilities of developing breast cancer for white females who are being examined annually. J Natl Cancer Inst 1989; 81:1879-86.
156. Weitzel JN. Genetic cancer risk assessment: putting it all together. Cancer 1999; 86:1663-72.
157. Couch FJ, DeShano ML, Blackwood MA, et al. BRCA1 mutations in women attending clinics that evaluate the risk of breast cancer. N Engl J Med 1997; 336:1409-15.
158. Parmigiani G, Berry D, Aguilar O. Determining carrier probabilities for breast cancer-susceptibility genes BRCA1 and BRCA2. Am J Hum Genet 1998; 62:145-58.
159. Statement of the American Society of Clinical Oncology: genetic testing for cancer susceptibility. J Clin Oncol 1996; 14:1730-6.
160. Foster KA, Harrington P, Kerr J, et al. Somatic and germline mutations of the BRCA2 gene in sporadic ovarian cancer. Cancer Res 1996; 56:3622-5.
161. Johannesdottir G, Gudmundsson J, Bergthorsson JT, et al. High prevalence of the 999del5 mutation in Icelandic breast and ovarian cancer patients. Cancer Res 1996; 56:3663-5.
162. Lancaster JM, Wooster R, Mangion J, et al. BRCA2 mutations in primary breast and ovarian cancers. Nat Genet 1996; 13:238-40.
163. Dorum A, Hovig E, Trope C, et al. Three per cent of Norwegian ovarian cancers are caused by BRCA1 1675delA or 1135insA. Eur J Cancer 1999; 35:779-81.
164. Janezic SA, Ziogas A, Krumroy LM, et al. Germline BRCA1 alterations in a population-based series of ovarian cancer cases. Hum Mol Genet 1999; 8:889-97.
165. Van der Looij M, Szabo C, Besznyak I, et al. Prevalence of founder BRCA1 and BRCA2 mutations among breast and ovarian cancer patients in Hungary. Int J Cancer 2000; 86:737-40.
166. Beller U, Halle D, Catane R, et al. High frequency of BRCA1 and BRCA2 germline mutations in Ashkenazi Jewish ovarian cancer patients, regardless of family history. Gynecol Oncol 1997; 67:123-6.
167. Hodgson SV, Heap E, Cameron J, et al. Risk factors for detecting germline BRCA1 and BRCA2 founder mutations in Ashkenazi Jewish women with breast or ovarian cancer. J Med Genet 1999; 36:369-73.
168. Frank TS. Laboratory identification of hereditary risk of breast and ovarian cancer. Curr Opin Biotechnol 1999; 10:289-94.
169. Welcsh PL, Owens KN, King MC. Insights into the functions of BRCA1 and BRCA2. Trends Genet 2000; 16:69-74.
170. Haber D. BRCA1: an emerging role in the cellular response to DNA damage. Lancet 2000; 355:2090-1.

171. Struewing JP, Abeliovich D, Peretz T, et al. The carrier frequency of the BRCA1 185delAG mutation is approximately 1 percent in Ashkenazi Jewish individuals. Nat Genet 1995; 11:198-200.

172. Oddoux C, Struewing JP, Clayton CM, et al. The carrier frequency of the BRCA2 6174delT mutation among Ashkenazi Jewish individuals is approximately 1 percent. Nat Genet 1996; 14:188-90.

173. Roa BB, Boyd AA, Volcik K, Richards CS. Ashkenazi Jewish population frequencies for common mutations in BRCA1 and BRCA2. Nat Genet 1996; 14:185-7.

174. Tesoriero A, Andersen C, Southey M, et al. De novo BRCA1 mutation in a patient with breast cancer and an inherited BRCA2 mutation. Am J Hum Genet 1999; 65:567-9.

175. Shattuck-Eidens D, Oliphant A, McClure M, et al. BRCA 1 sequence analysis in women at high risk for susceptibility mutations-risk factor analysis and implications for genetic testing. JAMA 1997; 278:1242-50.

176. Hogervorst FB, Cornelis RS, Bout M, et al. Rapid detection of BRCA1 mutations by the protein truncation test. Nat Genet 1995; 10:208-12.

177. Petrij-Bosch A, Peelen T, van Vliet M, et al. BRCA1 genomic deletions are major founder mutations in Dutch breast cancer patients. Nat Genet 1997; 17:341-5.

178. Swensen J, Hoffman M, Skolnick MH, Neuhausen SL. Identification of a 14 kb deletion involving the promoter region of BRCA1 in a breast cancer family. Hum Mol Genet 1997; 6:1513-7.

179. Montagna M, Santacatterina M, Torri A, et al. Identification of a 3 kb Alu-mediated BRCA1 gene rearrangement in two breast/ovarian cancer families. Oncogene 1999; 18:4160-5.

180. Puget N, Stoppa-Lyonnet D, Sinilnikova OM, et al. Screening for germ-line rearrangements and regulatory mutations in BRCA1 led to the identification of four new deletions. Cancer Res 1999; 59:455-61.

181. Gayther SA, Warren W, Mazoyer S, et al. Germline mutations of the BRCA1 gene in breast and ovarian cancer families provide evidence for a genotype-phenotype correlation. Nat Genet 1995; 11:428-33.

182. Phelan CM, Rebbeck TR, Weber BL, et al. Ovarian cancer risk in BRCA1 carriers is modified by the HRAS1 variable number of tandem repeat (VNTR) locus. Nat Genet 1996; 12:309-11.

183. Stoppa-Lyonnet D, Laurent-Puig P, Essioux L, et al. BRCA1 sequence variations in 160 individuals referred to a breast/ovarian family cancer clinic. Institut Curie Breast Cancer Group. Am J Hum Genet 1997; 60:1021-30.

184. Thompson DJ, Easton DF, Breast Cancer Linkage Consortium. Evidence for genotype-phenotype correlations in BRCA2 [abstract]. Am J Hum Genet 1999; 65 Suppl:327.

185. van Orsouw NJ, Dhanda RK, Elhaji Y, et al. A highly accurate, low cost test for BRCA1 mutations. J Med Genet 1999; 36:747-53.

186. Wagner T, Stoppa-Lyonnet D, Fleischmann E, et al. Denaturing high-performance liquid chromatography detects reliably BRCA1 and BRCA2 mutations. Genomics 1999; 62:369-76.

187. Humphrey JS, Salim A, Erdos MR, et al. Human BRCA1 inhibits growth in yeast: potential use in diagnostic testing. Proc Natl Acad Sci USA 1997; 94:5820-5.

188. Hacia JG, Brody LC, Chee MS, et al. Detection of heterozygous mutations in BRCA1 using high density oligonucleotide arrays and two-colour fluorescence analysis. Nat Genet 1996; 14:441-7.

189. Rothfuss A, Schutz P, Bochum S, et al. Induced micronucleus frequencies in peripheral lymphocytes as a screening test for carriers of a BRCA1 mutation in breast cancer families. Cancer Res 2000; 60:390-4.

190. Wijnen J, de Leeuw W, Vasen H, et al. Familial endometrial cancer in female carriers of MSH6 germline mutations. Nat Genet 1999; 23:142-4.

58

191. Wu Y, Berends MJ, Mensink RG, et al. Association of hereditary nonpolyposis colorectal cancer-related tumors displaying low microsatellite instability with MSH6 germline mutations. Am J Hum Genet 1999; 65:1291-8.
192. Andreutti-Zaugg C, Scott RJ, Iggo R. Inhibition of nonsense-mediated messenger RNA decay in clinical samples facilitates detection of human MSH2 mutations with an in vivo fusion protein assay and conventional techniques. Cancer Res 1997; 57:3288-93.
193. Shimodaira H, Filosi N, Shibata H, et al. Functional analysis of human MLH1 mutations in Saccharomyces cerevisiae. Nat Genet 1998; 19:384-9.
194. Polaczek P, Putzke AP, Leong K, Bitter GA. Functional genetic tests of DNA mismatch repair protein activity in Saccharomyces cerevisiae. Gene 1998; 213:159-67.
195. Johannsson O, Ostermeyer EA, Hakansson S, et al. Founding BRCA1 mutations in hereditary breast and ovarian cancer in southern Sweden. Am J Hum Genet 1996; 58:441-50.
196. Andersen TI, Borresen AL, Moller P. A common BRCA1 mutation in Norwegian breast and ovarian cancer families?. Am J Hum Genet 1996; 59:486-7.
197. Wagner TM, Moslinger R, Zielinski C, et al. New Austrian mutation in BRCA1 gene detected in three unrelated HBOC families. Lancet 1996; 347:1263.
198. Dorum A, Moller P, Kamsteeg EJ, et al. A BRCA1 founder mutation, identified with haplotype analysis, allowing genotype/phenotype determination and predictive testing. Eur J Cancer 1997; 33:2390-2.
199. Peelen T, van Vliet M, Petrij-Bosch A, et al. A high proportion of novel mutations in BRCA1 with strong founder effects among Dutch and Belgian hereditary breast and ovarian cancer families. Am J Hum Genet 1997; 60:1041-9.
200. Gayther SA, Harrington P, Russell P, et al. Frequently occurring germ-line mutations of the BRCA1 gene in ovarian cancer families from Russia. Am J Hum Genet 1997; 60:1239-42.
201. Ramus SJ, Kote-Jarai Z, Friedman LS, et al. Analysis of BRCA1 and BRCA2 mutations in Hungarian families with breast or breast-ovarian cancer. Am J Hum Genet 1997; 60:1242-6.
202. Tonin PN, Mes-Masson A-M, Futreal PA, et al. Founder *BRCA1* and *BRCA2* mutations in French Canadian breast and ovarian cancer families. Am J Hum Genet 1998; 63:1341-51.
203. Friedman LS, Szabo CI, Ostermeyer EA, et al. Novel inherited mutations and variable expressivity of BRCA1 alleles, including the founder mutation 185delAG in Ashkenazi Jewish families. Am J Hum Genet 1995; 57:1284-97.
204. Berman DB, Costalas J, Schultz DC, et al. A common mutation in BRCA2 that predisposes to a variety of cancers is found in both Jewish Ashkenazi and non-Jewish individuals. Cancer Res 1996; 56:3409-14.
205. Neuhausen SL, Mazoyer S, Friedman L, et al. Haplotype and phenotype analysis of six recurrent BRCA1 mutations in 61 families: results of an international study. Am J Hum Genet 1996; 58:271-80.
206. Csokay B, Tihomirova L, Stengrevics A, et al. Strong founder effects in BRCA1 mutation carrier breast cancer patients from Latvia. Mutation in brief no. 258. Hum Mutat 1999; 14:92.
207. Gorski B, Byrski T, Huzarski T, et al. Founder Mutations in the BRCA1 Gene in Polish Families with Breast-Ovarian Cancer. Am J Hum Genet 2000;66:1963-8.
208. Nystrom-Lahti M, Kristo P, Nicolaides NC, et al. Founding mutations and Alu-mediated recombination in hereditary colon cancer. Nat Med 1995; 1:1203-6.
209. Hutter P, Couturier A, Membrez V, et al. Excess of hMLH1 germline mutations in Swiss families with hereditary non-polyposis colorectal cancer. Int J Cancer 1998; 78:680-4.
210. Narod SA, Goldgar D, Cannon-Albright L, et al. Risk modifiers in carriers of BRCA1 mutations. Int J Cancer 1995; 64:394-8.

211. Narod SA, Risch H, Moslehi R, et al. Oral contraceptives and the risk of hereditary ovarian cancer. Hereditary Ovarian Cancer Clinical Study Group. N Engl J Med 1998; 339:424-8.
212. Brunet JS, Ghadirian P, Rebbeck TR, et al. Effect of smoking on breast cancer in carriers of mutant BRCA1 or BRCA2 genes. J Natl Cancer Inst 1998; 90:761-6.
213. Weitzel JN, Ding S, Larson GP, et al. The HRAS1 minisatellite locus and risk of ovarian cancer. Cancer Res 2000; 60:259-61.
214. Laken SJ, Petersen GM, Gruber SB, et al. Familial colorectal cancer in Ashkenazim due to a hypermutable tract in APC. Nat Genet 1997; 17:79-83.
215. Gryfe R, Di Nicola N, Lal G, et al. Inherited colorectal polyposis and cancer risk of the APC I1307K polymorphism. Am J Hum Genet 1999; 64:378-84.
216. Rozen P, Shomrat R, Strul H, et al. Prevalence of the I1307K APC gene variant in Israeli Jews of differing ethnic origin and risk for colorectal cancer. Gastroenterology 1999; 116:54-7.
217. Abrahamson J, Moslehi R, Vesprini D, et al. No association of the I1307K APC allele with ovarian cancer risk in Ashkenazi Jews. Cancer Res 1998; 58:2919-22.
218. Woodage T, King SM, Wacholder S, et al. The APCI1307K allele and cancer risk in a community-based study of Ashkenazi Jews. Nat Genet 1998; 20:62-5.
219. Redston M, Nathanson KL, Yuan ZQ, et al. The APC I1307K allele and breast cancer risk. Nat Genet 1998; 20:13-4.
220. Yuan ZQ, Begin LR, Wong N, et al. The effect of the I1307K APC polymorphism on the clinicopathological features and natural history of breast cancer. Br J Cancer 1999; 81:850-4.
221. Maresco DL, Arnold PH, Sonoda Y, et al. The APC I1307K allele and BRCA-associated ovarian cancer risk. Am J Hum Genet 1999; 64:1228-30.
222. Buller RE, Sood AK, Lallas T, et al. Association between nonrandom X-chromosome inactivation and BRCA1 mutation in germline DNA of patients with ovarian cancer. J Natl Cancer Inst 1999; 91:339-46.
223. Heinimann K, Scott RJ, Chappuis P, et al. N-acetyltransferase 2 influences cancer prevalence in hMLH1/hMSH2 mutation carriers. Cancer Res 1999; 59:3038-40.
224. Narod SA. Should a family history be taken from every woman with ovarian cancer. Arch Intern Med 1995; 155:893-4.

Acknowledgements

P.O. Chappuis is funded by grants from the Ligue Genevoise contre le Cancer et Cancer et Solidarité Fondation, Geneva, Switzerland.

Chapter 3

EARLY DETECTION OF OVARIAN CANCER: PROMISE AND REALITY

Robert C. Bast, Jr., Nicole Urban, Viji Shridhar, David Smith, Zhen Zhang, Steven Skates, Karen Lu, Jinsong Liu, David Fishman, and Gordon Mills
Departments of Experimental Therapeutics, Molecular Therapeutics, Gynecologic Oncology and Anatomic Pathology, University of Texas M.D. Anderson Cancer Center, Houston, TX 77030; The Fred Hutchinson Cancer Center, Seattle, WA 98101; Mayo Clinic, Rochester, MN 55905; Medical University of South Carolina, Charleston, SC 29425; Massachusetts General Hospital, Boston, MA 02114; and Northwestern University Medical School, Chicago, IL 60611

1. INTRODUCTION – THE RATIONALE FOR EARLY DETECTION

One of the most promising approaches to the control of many epithelial malignancies is to detect cancers before they have metastasized. Effective screening strategies have been developed and are widely utilized in clinical practice to detect cervical, breast, prostate and colorectal cancers. In the case of epithelial ovarian cancer, the ability to cure early stage disease provides an attractive rationale for the development of similarly effective screening strategies. Despite the improvement in median survival achieved with contemporary cytoreductive surgery and combination chemotherapy, ovarian cancer that has spread beyond the pelvis at the time of diagnosis can be cured in no more than 20% of cases. By contrast, when ovarian cancer is detected in Stage I, before it has spread from the ovaries, 90% of women can be cured with currently available therapy. At present, however, only 25% of ovarian cancers are diagnosed in Stage I (Ries et. al, 1999). Consequently, detection of preclinical disease at an earlier stage in a larger fraction of women might improve overall survival.

2. BIOLOGICAL REQUIREMENTS FOR EARLY DETECTION

The expectation that screening for ovarian cancer will impact favorably on survival depends critically upon several assumptions regarding the biology of this neoplasm. To screen effectively: 1) most epithelial ovarian cancers should arise as clonal tumors from the progeny of single cells in the ovary; 2) most advanced stage cancers should develop from clinically detectable stage I lesions; and 3) the duration that ovarian cancers remain localized to the ovary in Stage I should be sufficiently long to permit screening at practical intervals. Most ovarian cancers are thought to arise from a single layer of epithelial cells that cover the ovary or that line cysts immediately beneath the ovarian surface. The majority of ovarian cancers present with multiple nodules of cancer studding the peritoneal surface. In many cases, one or both ovaries are replaced by cancer, but in some cases involvement of the ovary is less striking. For many years pathologists debated whether all peritoneal tumor nodules had metastasized from the ovary or whether ovarian cancer was a polyclonal "field disease" with multiple primary tumors, some of which arose from the peritoneum. With the advent of molecular techniques, it was possible to determine whether ovarian cancer was indeed a clonal disease. When primary ovarian and peritoneal nodules were compared for loss of heterozygosity on multiple chromosomes, X chromosome inactivation and specific mutations in p53, more than 90% of sporadic ovarian cancers were found to be clonal (Jacobs et. al 1992; Mok et. al, 1992). Interestingly, primary peritoneal carcinoma (Muto et. al, 1995) and borderline tumors (Lu et. al, 1998) are more frequently polyclonal.

If 90% of sporadic ovarian cancers arise from the progeny of a single cell in the ovary, detection of malignancy prior to metastasis is at least a theoretical possibility. Whether most metastases occur from clinically apparent stage I lesions remains to be determined. Stage I cancers that grow large enough to be detected clinically without metastasizing may or may not be the precursors of cancers that metastasize. If ovarian cancer is a clonal disease, current theory suggests that multiple mutations, possibly 4-7, must occur in the progeny of a normal epithelial cell to produce an invasive malignancy during ovarian oncogenesis. Some of these mutations may predispose to proliferation and invasion, whereas others could contribute to metastasis. Stage I lesions should have mutations that predispose to proliferation, survival and invasion, but not to metastasis. If stage I lesions are the precursors of metastatic disease, both early and late stage cancers should share many of the same mutations that predispose to proliferation, survival and invasion. Advanced stage lesions should have additional genetic abnormalities related to metastatic potential. In this regard, mutations of p53 are found in a majority of advanced lesions, but in only 15% of clinically diagnosed stage I cancers (Kohler et. al, 1993). If p53 is associated with metastatic potential, discovery of p53 mutations in morphologically normal epithelial cells within inclusions cysts (Hutson et. al, 1995) and adjacent to certain developing ovarian cancers (Pathuri et. al, 2001) suggests that a fraction of cancers might acquire metastatic potential at an early stage in oncogenesis. Whether cancers with p53 mutations would metastasize prior to formation of clinically detectable stage I tumors is not known. Recent studies with expression array analysis and comparative genomic hybridization (CGH) suggest that poorly differentiated stage I lesions and stage III lesions have a very similar pattern of gene expression and of CGH abnormalities, consistent with the possibility that at least a fraction of stage III lesions could arise from clinically detected stage I precursors (Shridhar et. al, in press).

Whatever the mechanisms underlying progression of ovarian cancer, efficacy of screening will depend critically on the duration of the interval prior to conventional clinical detection and particularly on the interval during which cancer remains localized to the ovary. To place this interval of preclinical disease in perspective, Skates and Singer (1991) had developed a stochastic model for ovarian cancer screening with annual CA125 testing using a fixed threshold of 35 U/ml. According to this model, annual CA125 screening could produce sufficient stage shifts (largely III to I) to save 3.4 years of life per case, if the disease remained in Stage I for an average of 9 months with an average preclinical interval of 1.3 years. The benefit depended critically on the mean duration in stage I and on the coefficient of variation about the mean, with increasing benefit accruing with increasing duration. Neither the average preclinical interval nor the duration in stage I is known. In anecdotal cases (Bast et. al, 1985) and in trials from Stockholm (Zurawski et. al, 1988; Einhorn et. al, 1992) and the U.K. (Jacobs et. al, 1996; Jacobs et. al, 1999), CA 125 values appear to fluctuate around a stable mean in healthy women, but to rise exponentially prior to the clinical detection of ovarian cancer. Skates and coworkers (Skates et. al, 1999) analyzed CA 125 values obtained from 28 patients with ovarian cancer detected during the longitudinal screening trial conducted by Jacobs in 22,000 women in the United Kingdom between 1986 and 1995 (Jacobs et. al, 1999). Assuming an exponential increase in CA 125 in the presence of ovarian cancer, serial CA 125 values were fitted using a longitudinal change point model to estimate the preclinical interval from tumor inception to clinical detection. The mean estimated duration of preclinical cancer was 1.9 +/- 0.4 years, indicating that the stochastic model's assumptions and predictions of more than 3 years of life saved per case were conservative (Skates et. al, 1991).

3. EPIDEMIOLOGICAL REQUIREMENTS FOR EARLY DETECTION

Ovarian cancer is neither a common nor a rare disease. During the year 2001 in the United States, some 23,400 cases of ovarian cancer will be diagnosed (Greenlee 2001). The prevalence of ovarian cancer in the population of women over age 50 is 40 per 100,000. Given the prevalence of ovarian cancer, an extremely specific screening test is required to achieve an acceptable positive predictive value. A positive predictive value of 10% has often been cited as a reasonable standard in this setting. As the consequence of a positive screen is often a laparotomy or a laparoscopy, a positive predictive value of 10% would require 10 operations for each case of ovarian cancer detected. A positive predictive value of 10% requires a specificity of 99% assuming that sensitivity is at least 67% and the prevalance is 40 per 100,000.

4. SCREENING FOR OVARIAN CANCER WITH ULTRASOUND

For more than a decade, ultrasonography has been evaluated for early detection of ovarian cancer. Major studies are summarized in Table 1 (Campbell et. al, 1989; Bourne et. al, 1993; Van Nagell et. al 2000; Sato et. al, 2000). Early studies utilized transabdominal techniques (Table 1A), whereas more recent studies have employed transvaginal sonography (TVS) (Table 1B). As anticipated, ultrasonography has substantial sensitivity. In the 3 trials of TVS, 45 cancers were detected among 67,620 women screened, including 34 invasive and 11 borderline lesions. In addition, 6 ovarian or primary peritoneal cancers were diagnosed within 12 months of screening, consistent with an overall sensitivity of 88% for all stages of disease. Among the tumors detected by TVS, 73% were in stage I. As these studies included both prevalent and incident cases, the sensitivity of repeated annual screening for stage I disease might be even higher. On the other hand, not all of the stage I cancers detected were invasive cancers that were likely to metastasize over a short interval in the absence of signs or symptoms that would have prompted diagnosis by conventional methods. Of the 32 Stage I cancers detected in the 3 trials, only 18 (56%) were invasive epithelial cancers. TVS detected 9 borderline lesions, 4 granulosa cell tumors and one yolk sac tumor. Borderline and granulosa cell tumors metastasize less frequently before conventional diagnosis.

Specificity of TVS appears greater than that of transabdominal sonography. In two of the three major studies of TVS, positive predictive value has approached 10% (Bourne et. al, 1993; Van Nagell et. al, 2000). Overall, however, the positive predictive value has averaged 8.0%, suggesting that 12-13 operations might be required to detect each cancer. Consequently, TVS exhibits promising sensitivity, but provides specificity at the margin of an acceptable level. In widespread clinical use, specificity might be further compromised. In this regard, more precise definition of criteria for abnormal TVS may help to minimize unnecessary surgery. Size (<8.8 mL) and morphology are generally considered in differentiating benign from malignant lesions in postmenopausal women (Menon et. al, 2000). Simple cysts (single, thin walled, anechoic cysts with no septa or papillary projections) must be distinguished from other abnormalities ("complex morphology"). In one study, 741 women with abnormal CA 125 values underwent 1219 scans and 20 index cases of ovarian cancer occurred during a median followup of 6-8 years (Menon et. al, 2000). A sensitivity of 100% was achieved when both

Table 1. Ultrasound for Early Detection of Ovarian Cancer

TRIAL	MODE	#	OPERATIONS	OVARIAN CANCERS		PPV	STAGE I
				TOTAL	INVASIVE		
A. TRANSABDOMINAL SONOGRAPHY							
CAMPBELL 1990 (16)	TAS	5,479	326	5	5	1.5%	5 (100%)
B. TRANSVAGINAL SONOGRAPHY TVS							
BOURNE 1993 (17)	TVS	1,601	61	6	3	9.8%	5 (83%)
VAN NAGELL 2000 (18)	TVS	14,469	180	17	12	9.9%	11 (65%)
SATO 2000 (19)	TVS	51,550	324	22	19	7.4%	17 (77%)
TOTAL (TVS)		67,620	565	45	34	8.0%	33 (73%)

size and complex morphology were considered, compared to 89.5% for abnormal volume and 84% for complex morphology alone. The highest specificity (97%) and positive predictive value (37.2%) was achieved using complex morphology.

Attempts to utilize Doppler ultrasound to distinguish benign and malignant lesions have improved specificity in many, but not all studies (Karlan et. al, 1994; Valentin et. al, 1994; Tailor et. al, 1998). Color Doppler provides a spectral display that reflects flow toward and away from the ultrasound transducer. In early studies, data were processed to calculate impedance, resistive index (RI), and pulsatility index (PI). An initial report suggested that a color Doppler RI of < 0.4 predicted ovarian cancer with 100% sensitivity and 99% specificity (Kurjak et. al, 1991). Subsequent studies found the RI less accurate for distinguishing benign and malignant adnexal masses (Karlan et. al, 1994; Valentin et. al 1994; Tekay and Jouppila, 1995). Notably, 43% of benign premenopausal tumors contained vessels with an RI of < 0.4 during the follicular phase of the menstrual cycle (Tekay and Jouppila, 1995). In addition to pulsatility and resistance indices, recent analysis has focused on time-averaged maximum velocity (TAMXV) as a useful parameter. One recent study performed TVS and color Doppler in 67 women with adnexal masses (Tailor et. al, 1997). When 10 variables were subjected to regression analysis, only age, papillary projection score and TAMXV contributed significantly to the presence or absence of malignancy. The best sensitivity and specificity were 93.3 and 90.4% respectively at a 25% probability of malignancy. When the same data were analyzed with an artificial neural network (ANN), a sensitivity of 100% (95% confidence limits 78.2%-100%) and a specificity of 98.1% (95% confidence limits 89.5-100%) was achieved (Tailor et. al, 1999). In a similar study of 173 patients, ANN analysis was compared to a risk of malignancy index and to regression analysis using age, CA 125 and sonographic findings that included a semi-quantitative assessment of flow velocity to distinguish benign from malignant pelvic masses (Timmerman et. al, 1999). ANN proved slightly superior to the other methods of analysis, providing an area under the ROC curve of 0.979 with a sensitivity of 95.9% and a specificity of 93.5%. Each of these approaches requires confirmation in prospective studies.

Recent advances in ultrasound technology may improve the accuracy of pre-operative diagnosis and simplify the evaluation of patients with adnexal masses. Power Doppler measures the energy of a returning Doppler signal rather than displaying the changes in velocity detected by color Doppler. Use of power Doppler permits a more careful evaluation of vessels with low velocity blood flow. When PI and TAMX were calculated with color Doppler and power Doppler, similar specificities and sensitivities were found (Tailor et. al, 1998). When power Doppler was used to confirm results of conventional TVS, however, a power Doppler evaluation of the presence or absence of vascularity within solid portions or excrescences of a cyst improved accuracy when compared to an RI for the entire mass (Guerriero et. al, 1998). Most reported studies have been performed with two-dimensional (2-D) imaging. Three-dimensional (3-D) power Doppler ultrasound has recently been used to improve specificity after detection of pelvic masses with 2-D TVS (Cohen et. al, submitted). Three-dimensional imaging can facilitate measurement of blood flow within the solid areas and excrescences of complex cysts. In a trial of 71 women with pelvic masses, 14 masses were found to be malignant at laparotomy. All 14 had been detected by TVS, yielding 100% sensitivity, but only a 54% specificity. Examination of solid lesions and excrescences with 3-D power Doppler confirmed all 14 malignant masses and improved specificity from 54% to 75%.

5. SCREENING FOR OVARIAN CANCER WITH CA 125

In population based studies from Norway (Zurawski et. al, 1988) and Maryland (Helzlsouer et. al, 1993), elevations of CA 125 have been observed up to 5 years prior to diagnosis of ovarian cancer. Whether elevated CA 125 reflects the presence of early stage ovarian cancer or simply correlates with risk of disease is not known. In anecdotal cases it has been possible to document an exponential increase in CA 125 10-12 months prior to the clinical diagnosis of ovarian cancer (Figure 1) (Bast et. al, 1985). Screening studies from Stockholm (Zurawski et. al, 1988; Einhorn et. al, 1992) and the United Kingdom (Jacobs et. al; 1996, Jacobs et. al, 1999) have also documented exponentially rising CA 125 up to 21 months prior to diagnosis of ovarian cancer. Consequently, it appears that progressively rising CA 125 might provide substantial lead-time for detecting a fraction of ovarian cancers. Serum CA 125 values have, however, been elevated (>35 U/mL) in only 58% of 187 clinically detected stage I patients included in some 17 studies (Jacobs et. al, 1989; Woolas et. al, 1993; Van Haaften-Day et. al, 2001). Consequently, the sensitivity of CA 125 using a threshold of 35 U/ml for clinically detected early stage disease is more limited than that of TVS.

Figure 1. CA125 values prior to diagnosis of an epithelial ovarian cancer.

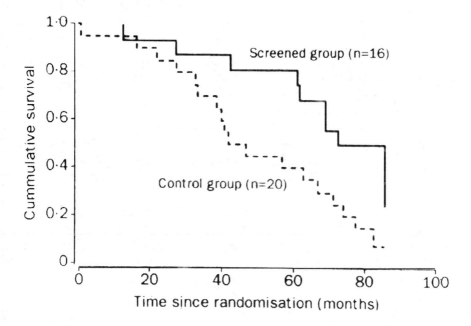

With a cutoff of 35 U/mL, the specificity of individual CA 125 values is 98-99% for a group of apparently healthy individuals without gynecologic symptoms. Although this is adequate for monitoring known ovarian cancer, it does not approach the 99.7% specificity required for screening to achieve a positive predictive value of 10%. A number of benign conditions can elevate CA 125 including endometriosis, adenomyosis, ovarian cysts, uterine fibroids, hepatic disease, renal failure, pancreatitis, and any other condition that can irritate serosal surfaces in the peritoneum, pericardium or pleura. In a small fraction of individuals, menstruation alone appears to elevate CA 125 in the absence of clinically apparent endometriosis. CA 125 values are higher and the specificity of CA 125 is lower in premenopausal women when compared to postmenopausal women (Westhoff et. al, 1990). As the majority of epithelial ovarian cancers occur in postmenopausal women, this is not necessarily a disadvantage for early detection of sporadic disease, but may further compromise attempts using a fixed CA125 threshold to screen premenopausal women who are at increased hereditary risk.

Given the limitations in specificity of CA 125 and of TVS, an NCI Consensus Development Panel (1995) recommended that neither test be used routinely to screen women at conventional risk for ovarian cancer outside of clinical trials. For women who are members of families with a strong history of ovarian and breast cancer, surveillance with both TVS and CA 125 is recommended, ideally in the context of a clinical screening trial.

6. STRATEGIES TO IMPROVE THE SPECIFICITY OF CA 125

The specificity of CA 125 can be improved by combination with ultrasound. In a study of 4000 apparently healthy women, Jacobs, et al, compared the specificities of CA 125, transabdominal ultrasound and pelvic exam, individually and in combination (Jacobs et. al, 1988). The specificity of CA 125 alone was 98.3%; pelvic examination alone was 97.7%; and a combination of pelvic examination plus ultrasound was 99.4%. A combination of CA 125 plus ultrasound achieved a specificity of 99.9%, exceeding the limit of 99.7% required to produce a positive predictive value of 10%.

Given the expense and inconvenience of performing ultrasound evaluations on all women over the age of 50, sequential use of CA 125 and ultrasound has been evaluated in a two stage screening strategy. A two stage screening strategy in ovarian cancer is analogous to strategies that have proven successful in screening for cancer at other sites. In screening for cervical cancer, Papanicolou smears have a relatively low specificity that is improved dramatically by serial monitoring and particularly by colposcopy. Similarly, mammography has a relatively low specificity that is enhanced by fine needle aspiration or core needle biopsy.

CA 125 and transabdominal ultrasound were combined in a trial conducted in Stockholm by Nina Einhorn and Kristen Sjovall (Zurawski et. al, 1988). Among 1082 women 40 years of age or older, CA 125 was greater than 35 U/mL in 3.3% and greater than 65 U/mL in 1%. On serial followup of elevated CA 125 values, only two women exhibited a doubling over time. In the one woman where an increase in antigen levels was sustained, stage III ovarian cancer was detected 21 months after the initial elevation of CA 125. In a subsequent trial that included 5550 apparently healthy women, only 1.5 % of women 50 years of age and over had CA 125 values greater than 35 U/mL, whereas 5.5% of women less than age 50 had a similar elevation (Einhorn et. al, 1992). Women whose CA 125 values were elevated (>30-35 U/mL) and an equal number of age matched controls with normal values were followed with serial CA 125, transabdominal ultrasound and pelvic examination. Among those with elevated CA 125 values, ovarian cancer was diagnosed in 6 women over the age of 50 with two each in stages IA, IIB and IIIC. During the next year, three premenopausal women with CA 125 in a normal range were subsequently found to have ovarian cancer through the Swedish tumor registry.

In a trial conducted in the United Kingdom between 1986 and 1995 Jacobs and coworkers randomized postmenopausal women 45 years of age to a control group (10,977) or to a screened group (10, 985) (Jacobs et. al, 1996; Jacobs et.al 1999). For the screened group, three annual CA125 values were obtained. If CA 125 was >30 U/mL, abdominal ultrasound was performed. If ultrasound was abnormal, laparotomy was undertaken. Among 10, 985 women screened, 29 operations were performed to detect 6 cancers, providing a positive predictive value of 21%. During 7 years of followup, 10 more ovarian cancers were diagnosed in the screened group. In the same interval 20 ovarian carcinomas were diagnosed in the control group. Median survival (Figure 2) in the screened group (72.9 months) was significantly greater (P = 0.0112) than in the control group (41.8 months). These data suggest that a two stage screening strategy might impact on survival.

7. DEVELOPMENT AND EVALUATION OF THE CA 125 ALGORITHM

Using data from the Stockholm study, Skates and colleauges (Skates et. al, 1995; Skates and Pauler, 2001) developed the risk of ovarian cancer calculation (ROCC), which uses a computer program to calculate the risk of having ovarian cancer given a screened subject's serial CA125 values. A screening test based on the ROCC distinguishes healthy individuals from most asymptomatic subjects with ovarian cancer in the Stockholm study. Serum samples cryopreserved from the trial were reanalyzed using the CA 125II assay. As there are multiple CA 125 determinants on a large glycoprotein, the original CA 125 assay had used the OC125 antibody to trap antigen on a bead and radiolabeled OC 125 antibody as a probe to detect bound antigen (Bast et. al, 1983). The CA 125II assay (Kenemans et. al, 1995) uses the M-11 antibody directed against an immunologically distinct epitope on the same molecule (Nap et. al, 1996) to trap antigen and radiolabeled OC 125 to detect bound antigen. The CA 125II has less variation over time within an individual than the original CA 125 assay, facilitating a more precise analysis of serial CA 125 values. To graphically present the additional information in CA125II values over time, a linear regression of log (CA125) versus time estimated the slope and the intercept which summarized the CA125 pattern over time for each subject in the Stockholm trial (Fig 3A).

Figure 2. *Survival of Patients Enrolled in a Randomized Trial for Early Detection Conducted in the United Kingdom between 1986 and 1995. (Jacobs et. al, 1999).*

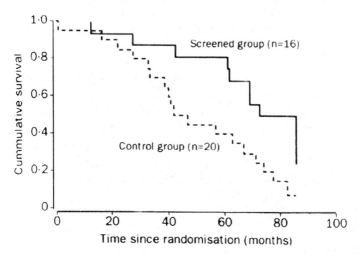

Healthy individuals, patients, with benign disease and women with non-gynecologic malignancy were found to have slopes close to horizontal, even when intercepts were above the normal cutoff of 30-35 U/mL (Fig 3B). Patients with ovarian cancer generally had linear increases of CA 125II on a logarithmic scale, consistent with an exponential increase in the source of antigen (Fig 3C). When the slopes and intercepts for each individual with or without ovarian cancer were plotted, the groups could be separated with a specificity of 99.9%, an apparent sensitivity of 83% and an estimated positive predictive value of 16% (Figure 4). As a single number summary of an individual's CA125 single or multiple values, the ROCC provided sensitivity and specificity values close to the test based on plots of the intercept and slope.

Following the encouraging analysis of the data from the Stockholm trial, an algorithm was developed where screening decisions were based on the single number summary of serial CA125 values provided by the ROCC. The risk of ovarian cancer algorithm (ROCA) obtains a CA125 value, calculates the ROCC, and triages the subject to normal, intermediate, or elevated risk decisions on the basis of the ROCC. For normal risk levels, the subject returns for a regular CA125II test, for intermediate risk levels the subject returns in 3 months for a further CA125II test, and for high-risk levels the subject is referred to TVS. Importantly, following each new CA125II test, the ROCC is recalculated, and the subject re-triaged. With such an approach where the risk is updated following each new CA125II test, subjects at high risk for having ovarian cancer based on serial CA125 patterns are rapidly triaged to TVS.

Figure 3A. CA125 Values in Patients with Ovarian Cancer, Benign Disease or without Illness. (Skates et. al, 1996).

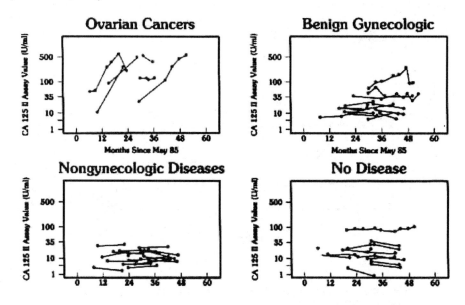

Figure 3B. Linear Progression of Log CA125II Assay Levels vs. Time for a Patient with Ovarian Cancer.

Linear Regression of Log CA 125 II Assay Levels vs Time

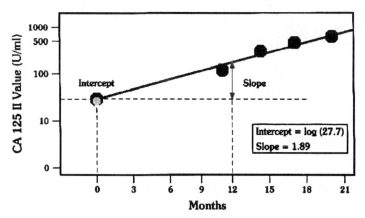

Figure 3C. Linear Regression of Log CA125II Assay Levels vs. Time for a Healthy Individual.

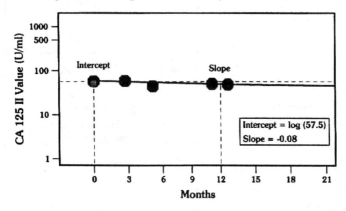

Figure 4. Slopes and Intercepts of CA125II for Healthy Individuals (o) and for Patients with Ovarian Cancer (•) from the Stockholm Trial. (Skates et. al, 1996).

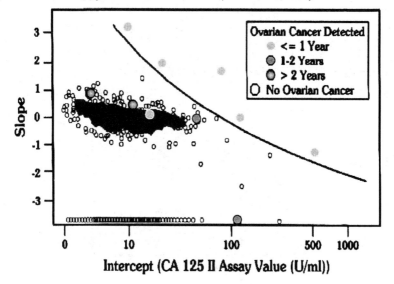

The algorithm has been applied prospectively in a pilot study of 10,000 postmenopausal women in the United Kingdom (Rosenthal et. al, 1998). Volunteers were randomized to a control group (5,046) and to a screened group (4, 954) using ROCA. In the screened group, 101 women were triaged to the elevated risk group and underwent TVS and 17 were referred to surgery where 4 ovarian cancers were found, including three invasive lesions in stage Ic (2), stage II (1) and one borderline tumor in stage Ia. Based on the early results and small number of cases of this study, the initial estimate of the positive predictive value was 23%. The prospective pilot trial of the ROC algorithm in the United Kingdom has made possible an analysis of serial CA125 values in healthy women (Pauler et. al, 2001). The only major determinent of CA125II level other than menopausal status was race. Black women had lower CA125II levels than white women.

8. RANDOMIZED CLINICAL STUDIES IN PROGRESS

The Medical Research Council in the United Kingdom has agreed to sponsor a trial in 200,000 women to evaluate different approaches to early detection of ovarian cancer with survival as an endpoint accrual has just begun. Fifty thousand women will be randomized to monitoring with the ROCA, where TVS follows CA125II testing if the risk of ovarian cancer calculation is sufficiently high. Fifty thousand will be randomized to screening every 12 months with TVS alone and 100,000 will be followed with conventional care. Management of any pelvic lesion is left to the discretion of the patient's local physician. The study will accrue patients over 3 years, screen for a mean of 6 years and require 10 years to complete. Sites throughout the United Kingdom will be utilized and blood will be couriered overnight at ambient temperature to London where sera will be separated and CA 125II analyzed.

The Prostate, Lung, Colon and Ovary (PLCO) Screening Trial was initiated in 1994 to study 37,000 men and an equal number of women who had been randomized for intervention. Design of the trial was originally optimized to evaluate the utility of PSA, digital rectal examination, chest film and sigmoidoscopy for early detection of prostate, lung and colorectal cancers. Ovarian cancer was added as an additional endpoint at a later date. Initially, only women over age 60 were included. Subsequently, the minimum age of participants was decreased to 55 years. CA125 is performed at entry and then annually for 5 years. TVS is performed at entry and annually for 3 years. Participants will be followed for 13 years. If CA 125 is elevated or a pelvic lesion encountered, patients are returned to their local physicians for management. A serum and plasma bank has been maintained at collaborating sites where samples are separated promptly.

If positive, the randomized trials will be of considerable value. A negative outcome would not, however, rule out the utility of screening. Patients in both trials will not necessarily be treated in a consistent, nor optimal manner. In the PLCO trial women between 50 and 55 years will be excluded, eliminating a group that might best tolerate the most intensive surgery and chemotherapy. Each of these factors might contribute to minimizing the impact of early detection.

9. COST-EFFECTIVENESS OF ONE AND TWO STAGE SCREENING STRATEGIES

A stochastic simulation model was developed by Urban and coworkers to identify an efficient ovarian cancer screening protocol (Urban et al., 1997). Estimates were made of effectiveness and cost-effectiveness of selected single modality and multimodal screening strategies applied to a hypothetical cohort of 1 million women aged 50 at the initiation of screening. A multimodal strategy involving CA 125 with a threshold for positivity of either elevation above 35U/mL or doubling since the previous screen, followed by TVS only if CA 125 is positive, was found to be efficient in the sense that no other strategies saved as many years of life at lower cost per year of life saved. Used annually, this strategy cost under $100,000 per year of life saved over a range of assumptions. The multimodal strategy used annually or every six months was efficient compared to either ultrasound or CA 125 used alone, over a wide range of assumptions.   In a more recent analysis, the cost and effectiveness of different screening strategies have also been modeled in a simulated trial of 800,333 women. In Table 2 annual (12 month) and semi-annual (6 month) screening strategies have been compared. For annual screening, TVS as a single modality has been compared to using CA125 as an initial step followed by TVS as indicated by rising CA 125 values. For semi-screening, CA 125 followed by TVS as indicated has been compared to alternating annual CA 125 and TVS so that one or the other procedure was performed every 6 months. Alternating CA 125 or TVS every 6 months produced the highest reduction in mortality and the greatest number of years of life saved among the four strategies. Some 15 operations would be performed, however, for each case of ovarian cancer detected, a figure that exceeds the frequently quoted limit of 10 operations per case detected. The cost per year of life saved depended critically on assumptions regarding the cost of TVS. As the cost of TVS was increased from $25 to $250, the cost per year of life saved with this strategy increased from $44,800 to $125,900. Use of CA 125 every 6 months followed by TVS for rising values produced fewer years of life saved and less reduction in mortality than alternating CA 125 and TVS, but was superior to annual TVS, particularly in years of life saved.

Table 2. *Cost efficacy of different screening strategies.*

Strategy	Surgeries/ Detected Cancer	Cost/Yr of Life Saved Discounted 3%	Mortality Reduction	Yrs of Life Saved
Annual				
CA125—TVS	3.8	$27,100-30,900	28.4%	2.0
TVS	17.7	$46,900-155,400	43.1%	2.1
Semi-Annual Alternating				
TVS&CA125	15.3	$44,800-125,900	58.8%	4.1
CA125—TVS	5.9	$42,885-49,000	44.7%	3.3

Moreover, semiannual CA 125 followed by TVS as needed prompted only 6 operations per case of ovarian cancer detected and cost at most $49,000 per year of life saved. This value does not exceed the benchmark of $50,000 per year of life saved for many widely used screening tests and interventions such as mammography. At present in the United States, the retail cost of TVS is greater than $250 in most communities. Arguably, the efforts of technicians might be used to a greater extent if TVS became a widely used primary screen for ovarian cancer, reducing the cost per examination. In the absence of such changes, however, two stage screening with serum or plasma assays triggering TVS may be more cost effective.

If semi-annual screening appears superior to annual screening, it remains to be seen whether women will participate consistently in more frequent screening. Women at increased risk in hereditary ovarian and breast cancer families may well be willing to undergo testing every 3 to 6 months. Whether women at average risk would be willing to undergo screening more often than once a year remains to be determined.

Cost-effectiveness analysis is of course, based on many assumptions, some of which are difficult to verify. In particular, the relationship between stage shift and mortality reduction has not been demonstrated in a randomized controlled trial and the length of the detectable preclinical phase of the disease is not known.

10. IMPROVING THE SENSITIVITY OF TWO STAGE SCREENING STRATEGIES

Use of CA 125 as an initial stage in screening limits the sensitivity of the entire two-stage strategy. At the time of conventional diagnosis, CA 125 levels are >35 U/mL in 50-60% of patients with Stage I disease. Using an algorithm that measures increases in CA 125 from the patient's own baseline, early stage disease might be detected when rising CA 125 is still less than 35 U/mL, increasing sensitivity above 60%. In 20% of ovarian cancers, however, CA 125 cannot be detected in tissue sections using immuno-histochemical techniques. Consequently the sensitivity of a screening strategy based on CA 125 alone cannot exceed 80%. In addition, certain histotypes might be detected preferentially by CA 125. While CA 125 can be expressed by all histotypes of ovarian cancer, mucinous cancers are less frequently positive.

Greater sensitivity and specificity might be achieved with multiple serum markers than with CA 125 alone. A large number of markers have been evaluated for their ability to detect cancers missed by CA 125 or to improve the specificity of the CA 125 assay for distinguishing malignant from benign lesions (Table 3). Serum, plasma and urine markers have included oncofetal antigens, mucin-like proteins, enzymes, co-enzymes, enzyme inhibitors, receptors, cytokines, peptide hormones, other proteins, phospholipids and sialylated lipids. With the possible exception of lysophosphatidic acid (LPA), markers evaluated to date have not proven consistently more sensitive than CA 125 for detecting different ovarian cancers when used as individual tests. At least 27 markers have been reported to enhance the sensitivity or specificity of CA 125 for the identification of patients with ovarian cancer. Serum, plasma or urine has often been obtained at the time of clinical presentation. Controls in many studies have included apparently healthy women or patients with benign pelvic masses.

Table 3. Association of CA 125 with Other Serum, Plasma and Urine Markers for Epithelial Ovarian Cancer

Oncofetal Antigens

• Carcinoembryonic Antigen	*Bast et al, 1983*; Erdekens et al, 1985; **Negishi et al 1987**; *Panza et al, 1988*; **Koebl et al, 1989**; **Lundqvist et al, 1989**; **Tholander et al, 1990a**; Tholander et al, 1990b; **Inoue et al, 1992**; *de Bruijin et al, 1993*; Kudoh et al, 1999; *Zakrzewska et al, 1999*; Tuxen et al, 1999; Engelen et al, 2000
• Placental Alkaline Phosphatase	Erdekins et al 1985; Heinonen et al, 1987*; **Ward et al, 1987***; De Broe and Pollet, 1988*; **Stigbrand et al, 1990**; *Hording et al, 1990*; *Tholander, 1990a*; *Tholander et al, 1990b*; Bast et al, 1991; ***Toftager-Larsen, et al, 1992****; Ind et al, 1997

Mucin-Associated Antigens

• CA15-3	**Einhorn et al, 1989**; **Benedetti et al, 1989**; **Gadducci et al, 1990**; Barrenetxea et al, 1990; **Lotzniker et al, 1991**; **Bast et al, 1991**; **Jacobs et al, 1992**; *Jacobs et al, 1993*; **Devine et al, 1994**; **Woolas et al, 1999**

- CA19-9 — **Negishi et al, 1987**; Koebl et al, 1989; *Barrenetxea et al, 1990*; **Gadducci et al 1990**; Bast et al, 1991; *Woolas et al, 1995*; Kudoh et al, 1999; **Woolas et al, 1999; Engelen et al, 2000**

- CA 50 — **Gadducci et al, 1990**

- CA 54-61 — Berek and Bast, 1995

- CA 72-4 (TAG72) — Gadducci et al 1989; **Einhorn et al, 1989**; *Scambia et al, 1990*; **Gadducci et al, 1990; Bast et al, 1991; Jacobs et al, 1992**; *Jacobs et al, 1993*; **Hasholzner et al, 1994**; Stenman et al 1995; **Nishida et al, 1995; Gaudagni et al, 1995; Hasholzner et al, 1996**; Gonzalez et al, 1997*; **Schutter et al, 1998; Fayed et al, 1998**; Zakrzewska et al, 1999; **Woolas et al, 1999**

- CA 195 — de Bruijin et al, 1993

- CASA — **McGuckin et al, 1990; Ward et al, 1993; Hasholzner et al, 1994; Devine et al, 1994; Meisel et al, 1995; Sliutz et al 1995; Kierkegaard et al, 1995; Hogdall et al, 1996**; Ind et 1997; **Oehler et al, 1999**; *Hogdall et al, 2000*

- HMFG-1 — Bast et al, 1991

- HMFG-2 — **Ward et al, 1987***; Bast et al, 1991; Berek and Bast, 1995

- Mucin-like Carcinoma Antigen (MCA) — Koebl et al, 1989; Bon et al, 1996

- Ovarian Serum Antigen (OSA) — **McGuckin et al, 1990**

- OVX1 — **Xu et al, 1993; Woolas et al, 1993; Woolas et al, 1995**; *Zhang et al, 1999; Hogdall et al, 2000*

- Sialyl TN (STN) — Kudoh et al, 1999

Enzymes, Co-Enzymes and Enzyme Inhibitors

- Galactosyltransferase — Goldhirsch et al, 1988; Nozawa et al, 1990*; *Sichel et al, 1994*

- Cathepsin L — **Nishida et al, 1995***

- Matrix Metalloproteinase 2 — **Garzetti et al, 1996**

- Prostasin — Mok et al, 2001*

- Kallekrein 6 and 10 — Diamandis et al, 2000; Luo et al, 2001*

- Tetranectin — Blaakaer et al, 1995*; **Hogdall et al, 1996, Hogdall et al, 1998**; *Hogdall et al, 2000*

- Alpha-1-antitrypsin — **Koebl et al, 1988**

- Tumor Associated Trypsin Inhibitor (TATI) — **Halila et al 1988; Mogensen et al, 1990a, 1990b; Gadducci et al, 1990**; de Bruijn et al, 1993; **Stenman et al, 1995; Peters-Engl, 1995; Medl et al, 1995**

Receptors

- p110 EGFR — Baron et al, 1999, **Boardman et al, 2000**

- ErbB-2 (HER-2-neu) McKenzie et al, 1993; Crump et al, 2000
- Tumor Necrosis Factor Receptor Grosen et al, 1993*; *Onsrud et al, 1996*
  (TNFR)
- Soluble Fas **Helfer et al, 2001**
- IL-2 Receptor **Ferdeghini et al, 1993**; Barton et al, 1993*;
  Hurteau et al, 1994; **Hurteau et al, 1995**; *de Bruijn et al, 1998*

Cytokines
- IL-6 **Berek et al, 1991**; Rustin et al, 1993; Plante et al, 1994*; Scambia et al, 1994; Scambia et al, 1995; Berek and Bast, 1995
- IL-8 Mayerhofer et al, 2001*
- IL-10 Rustin et al 1993; Berek and Bast, 1995;
- Macrophage Colony Stimulating **Xu et al, 1991**; **Woolas et al 1993**; **Woolas et al**
  Factor (M-CSF, CSF-1) **1995**; Zhang et al, 1999; **Zhang et al, 2001**

Hormones
- Beta chain – hCG Panza et al, 1988; Ind et al, 1997
- Inhibin Stenman et al 1995; Phocas et al, 1996; **Lambert-Messerlian et al, 1997**; **Robertson et al, 1999**; Ala-Fossi et al, 2000
- Urinary Gonadotropin Peptide **Wang et al, 1988**; Schwartz et al, 1991; **Walker et al, 1994**; **Schutter et al, 1999**; Crump et al, 2000*

Other Proteins and Peptides
- Ceruloplasmin *Koebl et al, 1988*
- C Reactive Protein (CRP) **Koebl et al, 1988**
- CYFRA21-1 Hasholzner et al, 1994; *Tempfer et al 1998*
- Immunosuppressive Acidic **Negishi et al, 1987**; **Castelli et al, 1987**; **Koebl et**
  Protein (IAP) **al, 1988**; *Mogensen et al, 1989*; **Castelli et al, 1991**
- NB/70K **Knauf and Bast, 1988**; *Petru et al, 1990*; Bast et al, 1991; Schwartz et al, 1991; Cane et al, 1995; Crump et al, 2000
- Tissue Peptide Antigen (TPA) Panza et al, 1988; **Lindqvist et al, 1989**; *Stigbrand et al, 1990*; *Hording et al, 1990*; **Gazizadeh et al, 1990**; Tholander, 1990a; **Tholander et al, 1990b**; *Toftager-Larsen et al, 1992*; Sliutz et al, 1995; Kudoh et al, 1999; Tuxen et al, 1999;

Lipids and Sialylated Lipids
- Lipid Associated Sialic Acid **Schwartz et al, 1987**; Szarka et al, 1988; *Patsner et*
  (LASA) *al, 1988*; **Vardi et al, 1999**; *Petru et al, 1990*; Schwartz et al, 1991; **Woolas et al, 1995**; Cane et al, 1995; Crump et al, 2000
- Lysophosphatidic Acid (LPA) Xu et al, 1998*

Bold references indicate additive sensitivity or specificity when a marker is used in combination with CA 125. *Italicized* references indicate a lack of additional sensitivity or specificity when a marker is used in combination with CA 125. ***Bold and italicized*** references indicate increased sensitivity but markedly decreased specificity when a marker is used in combination with CA 125. An asterisk (*) indicates a lack of correlation between a marker and CA 125 when individual patients are considered.

Simultaneous elevation of CA 125 with other markers in sera from patients with ovarian cancer can substantially increase specificity (Bast et. al, 1991). False positive values for several markers appear to be distributed independently in healthy women (Crump et. al, 2000). Consequently, simultaneous elevation of two or more markers occurs less frequently in healthy individuals than in women whose ovarian cancers co-express multiple markers. Coordinate expression of multiple markers can occur in benign neoplasms, but this must occur less frequently than in ovarian cancers, given the ability of multiple markers to distinguish malignant from benign pelvic masses (Woolas et. al, 1995; Zhang et. al 1999). This approach, however, has limitations in practice. As the sensitivity of most markers for ovarian cancer does not equal that of CA 125 (70-80%), the fraction of true positive tests for nearly all markers is smaller than that for CA 125 at a given level of specificity. Even when the sensitivity of other markers approaches that of CA 125, coordinate elevation may not be observed in all cases. Consequently, use of the coordinate elevation of two markers to improve specificity has generally been associated with a significant loss of sensitivity. However, as more markers are validated, elevation of multiple markers out of a larger set may increase both sensitivity and specificity.

Complementary expression of different markers, where resykts are considered positive when any marker is elevated, might increase sensitivity. More than 20 different markers have been found elevated in the serum, plasma or urine of individual ovarian cancer patients whose CA 125 values are within normal limits. Complementarity of novel markers with CA 125 has often related to the ability of these markers to detect different histotypes of epithelial ovarian cancer. CA 125 levels can be elevated in all histotypes, but are most frequently elevated in serous and least frequently elevated in mucinous cancers. Several markers are elevated more frequently than CA 125 in patients with mucinous neoplasms, including CA 19-9 (Gadducci et. al, 1992; Kudoh et. al, 1999; Engelen et. al, 2000), CA 72.4 (Gadducci et. al, 1989; Gadducci et. al, 1992; Gonzalez et. al, 1997), CA 195 (de Bruijn et. al, 1993), tumor associated trypsin inhibitor (TATI) and inhibin (Halila et. al, 1988; Medl et. al, 1995; Pettersson and McGuckin, 1999). CEA can also be elevated in mucinous tumors (Tholander et. al, 1990b), although levels are not sufficiently elevated to be of use in all studies (Zakrzewska et. al, 1999). Endometrioid cancers are associated with elevations of CA 125 (Kudoh et. al, 1999), CA 72.4 (Gonzalez et. al, 1997) and placental alkaline phosphatase (PLAP) (Stigbrand et. al, 1990). In clear cell cancers, levels of Sialyl TN

(Kudoh et. al, 1999) and galactosyltransferase (Nozawa et. al, 1990) have been elevated in the highest fraction of cases.

In general, however, increases in sensitivity with combinations of markers have been modest, improving the sensitivity of CA 125 by 5-10%, often at the expense of marked decreases in specificity. Most reports have studied a limited number of serum, plasma or urine specimens and have not evaluated early stage disease. Exceptions to this generalization include OVX1, macrophage colony stimulating factor (M-CSF, CSF-1) and lysophosphatidic acid (LPA).

OVX1 is a Lewis$_x$ determinant detected on a high molecular weight (>1000 kD) tumor associated mucin (Xu et. al, 1991). OVX1 is elevated in 48% of sera from ovarian cancer patients (Xu et. al, 1993) and is not an optimal stand-alone marker. It does, however, complement CA 125. OVX1 levels are elevated in 47% of patients with clinically evident ovarian cancer despite normal levels of CA 125 (Xu et. al, 1993). OVX1 is also elevated in 27% of patients with a positive second look and normal CA 125 levels. When serum is separated and frozen promptly OVX1 levels remain stable. If blood is permitted to stand at room temperature for more than a day, OVX1 levels are artificially increased (Hogdall et. al, 1999).

M-CSF is a cytokine dimer of 70 kD that binds to the CSF-1 receptor encoded by the *fms* proto-oncogene. Normal ovarian surface epithelial cells express low levels of M-CSF (Lidor et. al, 1993), but expression of the cytokine is upregulated during malignant transformation as is the expression of the *fms* proto-oncogene (Kacinski et. al, 1990). Elevated levels of M-CSF are found in 70% of patients with ovarian cancer (Xu et. al, 1991). Once again, complementarity has been observed with CA 125. M-CSF is elevated in 56% of patients with patients with clinically evident ovarian cancer despite normal levels of CA 125. M-CSF is also elevated in 31% of ovarian cancer patients with positive second look operations and normal levels of CA 125 (Xu et. al, 1991).

A combination of OVX1, M-CSF and CA 125 can detect a greater fraction of patients with stage I ovarian cancer than can CA 125 alone. Data were evaluated from two separate studies that measured the three markers in sera drawn preoperatively from a total of 89 women with stage I ovarian cancer (Woolas et. al, 1993; Van Haaften-Day et. al, 2001). When both retrospective trials are taken together, CA 125 was elevated in 69% of patients with stage I disease, whereas one of the three markers (OVX1, M-CSF and CA 125) was elevated in 84%. While the potential increase in sensitivity is encouraging, there was an additive effect on false positives, providing a specificity of 89% compared to a specificity of 99% for CA 125 alone.

A distinctive form of SN2 LPA has been found in ascites and plasma of patients with ovarian cancer (Xu et. al, 1995; Xu et. al, 1998). SN2 LPA is a potent stimulant of ovarian cancer cell growth and prevents apoptosis of cancer cells in the presence of certain cytotoxic drugs such as cisplatin (Fang et. al, 2000). SN2 LPA differs chemically and functionally from the SN1 LPA found in platelets, but the SN1 form can interfere with assays for the SN2 form necessitating the study of plasma from which platelets have been removed, rather than serum that contains platelet derived lipids. LPA is present in ascites fluid from >95% of patients with advanced ovarian cancer. The LPA concentration is less than 1 uM in plasma from 95% of healthy women. Using this threshold, elevated levels of LPA have been detected in 80% of women with stage I ovarian cancer. Complementarity has been observed with CA 125. In contrast to CA 125, however, the range of LPA elevation is generally narrow. When the threshold of normal values is raised to exclude 99% of healthy women, sensitivity is markedly reduced. Two clinical trials are in progress testing the ability of LPA to distinguish between benign and malignant pelvic masses.

11. POTENTIAL SERUM OR PLASMA MARKERS THAT ARE NOT YET FULLY CHARACTERIZED

Several markers and new strategies have recently been reported that might increase the sensitivity for early detection of ovarian cancer observed with CA 125 alone. To date too few stage I cases have been examined to determine their utility for early detection. Individual markers include the 110 kD component of the extracellular domain of the epidermal growth factor receptor (p110EGFR), kallikrein 6 and kallikrein 10 (NES-1). New technologies have also been applied to the identification of novel markers. RNA expression array analysis has already identified NES-1, prostasin, HE4 and creatine kinase B as potential markers for ovarian cancer. Surface enhanced laser desorption and ionization (SELDI) provides a method for studying patterns of protein expression. in contrast to most serum markers that are elevated in the presence of cancer, levels of p110EGFR are decreased in the presence of ovarian cancer (Baron et. al, 1999). Women with Stage III-IV ovarian cancer have significantly lower levels of p110EGFR than do healthy women. Complementarity with CA 125 has been observed (Boardman et. al, 2000). Whether p110EGFR detects a sufficient number of patients with early stage disease to be useful remains to be determined. Through a systematic study of kallikreins associated with ovarian cancer, two members of this family have shown promise as markers. Kallikrein 6 levels were elevated in 66% of 53 patients with ovarian cancer (Daimandis et. al, 2000). Similarly, kallikrein 10 levels were elevated in 56% of patients with ovarian cancer (Luo, et. al, 2001). Sensitivity for early stage disease has not yet been determined.

New technologies promise to increase the number of potential markers dramatically. In some cases these technologies have detected the same markers discovered by other approaches. Using expression array analysis the

NES-1 gene was found upregulated in mRNA from ovarian cancers when compared to normal ovarian epithelial cells. Kallikrein 10 encoded by this message was expressed by 91% of serous ovarian cancers, 73% of non-serous ovarian cancers and 73% of primary peritoneal cancers in tissue section (Schvartsman et. al, 2001). Another serine protease gene, prostasin, has been found upregulated in ovarian cancer cell lines by array analysis (Mok et. al, 2001). Serum prostasin levels from ovarian cancer patients were approximately double those of healthy controls. No correlation was found with CA 125 levels, consistent with the possibility that use of both assays might provide additional information. Creatine kinase B (CKB) message was also upregulated on expression array analysis. Serum CKB enzyme activity could distinguish ovarian cancer patients from women with benign pelvic masses (p=0.046) and from healthy donors (p=0.0004). Each of 3 patients with stage I ovarian cancer had elevated enzyme levels (Gibson et. al, 2001).

Whereas kallikrein 10, prostasin and CKB had been identified as serum markers in other contexts, novel genes have been identified by array analysis. The HE4 gene was found to be upregulated in ovarian cancers using an array analysis of 28,000 cDNAs (Schummer et. al, 1999). The HE4 gene is expressed by 86% of 29 serous cancers, each of 10 endometrial cancers and only 1 of 10 clear cell ovarian cancers in tissue section (Schmandt et. al, 2001). A serum assay for this marker is currently being developed. Similarly, mesothelin/megakaryocyte potentiating factor mRNA was forum upregulated on expression arrays (Wane et. al, 1999) and the mesothelin protein has been detected in sera from ovarian cancer patients (Scholter et. al, 1999).

SELDI analysis separates polypeptides with different molecular weights and charges on matrices. Using laser desorption, peptides are ionized and selectively resolved by atomic mass spectroscopy. Complex patterns of peptide expression can be identified in sera of ovarian cancer patients that differ from those in normal sera, even when the identity of the peptides is not known. Using a heuristic computer algorithm of peptide expression, sera from normal individuals could be correctly distinguished from those of ovarian cancer patients in each of 200 samples. Whether this will apply to early stage disease is currently being evaluated (Ardekani et. al, 2001).

12. MATHEMATICAL ANALYSIS OF MULTIPLE MARKERS

Use of multiple markers may increase sensitivity for early detection of ovarian cancer. As in the case of individual markers, increased sensitivity is generally associated with decreased specificity. Given the requirement for 99.7% specificity to attain a positive predictive value of 10%, any decrease in specificity for an initial screening step might generate an unacceptable number of false positives. With a two stage screening strategy, the initial stage can exhibit a more modest specificity, but must not trigger an impractical number of second stage tests. In the second Stockholm trial, for example, a CA 125 cutoff of <30-35 U/mL prompted ultrasound examinations in 2% of participants (Einhorn et. al, 1992). Ultrasound and clinical examination, in turn, provided an acceptable positive predictive value. Use of markers in combination for an initial stage in screening will depend upon the specificity of each assay, the variation of each assay over time and the possible overlap of false positive values for different markers in the same patient. Different mathematical approaches have been used to increase the sensitivity of combined markers without sacrificing or even improving specificity.

Studies to date have generally considered combinations of multiple markers at a single point in time. An early study considered different statistical techniques for combining 8 different preoperative serum markers to distinguish benign from malignant pelvic masses in 429 patients, 192 of whom had malignant histology (Woolas et. al, 1995). The sensitivity and specificity of CA 125 alone (>35 U/mL) were 78.1% and 76.8%, respectively. A panel consisting of CA 125, OVX1, lipid associated sialic acid (LASA), CA 15-3 and CA 72-4 had a sensitivity of 83.3% and a specificity of 84%, when two or more markers were elevated. Using logistic regression analysis, concentrations of these five markers produced a sensitivity of 85.4% and a specificity of 83.1%. Considering the values of markers in different sequences, classification and regression tree analysis substantially improved the sensitivity to 90.6% and the specificity to 93.2%.

Using the same data set, a panel of the four markers selected based on their discriminatory power, CA 125II, CA 72-4, CA 15-3 and LASA was analyzed collectively with an artificial neural network (ANN) to differentiate malignant from benign pelvic masses (Zhang et. al, 2001). A prototype ANN classifier was developed using a subset of the data which included 73 patients with malignant conditions and 101 patients with benign conditions. The ANN classifier demonstrated a much improved sensitivity over that of the CA 125II assay alone (87.5% vs. 68.4%) while maintaining a statistically comparable specificity (79.0% vs. 82.4%) in discriminating malignant from benign pelvic masses in an independent validation test using data from the remaining 255 patients which had been set aside and kept blinded to the developers of the ANN system. The ANN system was further tested using additional serum specimens collected from 196 apparently healthy women. The ANN system had a specificity of 100% compared to that of 94.8% with the CA 125II assay alone. In a more recent study, serum specimens from patients with stage I ovarian cancer were analyzed for CA125II, CA72-4, CA15-3, and macrophage colony stimulating factor (M-CSF) (Zhang et. al, in press). The four tumor marker values were then used as inputs to an Artificial Neural Network (ANN) to detect stage I epithelial ovarian cancer. The ANN was derived using a training set from 100 apparently healthy women, 45 women with benign conditions arising from the ovary, and 62 epithelial ovarian cancer patients (24 stage I, 3 stage II, and 35 late stage cases). A separate in-training cross-validation set from 27 apparently healthy women, 56 women with benign conditions, and 38 women with various types of malignant pelvic masses was used to monitor the ANN's generalization performance during training. The selection of individual patients for both datasets was randomized. An independent test dataset from 98 apparently healthy women and 60 early stage epithelial ovarian cancer patients (51 stage I, 6 stage II, and 3 stage IIIa cases) was used to evaluate the ANN. ROC analysis using the whole test set confirmed the overall superiority of the ANN over CA125II alone (p=0.05). At a fixed specificity of 98%, the ANN has a sensitivity of 67% (40/60) for detecting early stage epithelial ovarian cancer, and 63% (32/51) for stage I cases only. In comparison, CA125II alone at a cutoff chosen to match the 98% specificity, has a sensitivity of 45% (27/60) for all early stage epithelial ovarian cancer cases and 43% (22/51) for stage I cases only. The results suggest that the combined use of tumor markers through ANN may be a better choice than the use of CA125II alone in a two-step approach for population screening in which a secondary test such as ultrasound is used to keep the overall specificity at an acceptable level. As in the case of CA 125 alone, greater specificity for multiple markers might be attained if the trend of their values were studied over time. Serial measurements of CA 125, HER-2/neu, urinary gonadotropin peptide, LASA and Dianon NB 70/K were measured during six years of follow-up of 1257 healthy women at risk of ovarian cancer (Crump et. al, 2000). These five markers behaved approximately independently in asymptomatic healthy women, suggesting that the combined false positive rate from screening with multiple markers may be estimated by the sum of the individual false positive rates. Studies are underway to develop algorithms that would include multiple markers over time, increasing sensitivity while maintaining adequate specificity.

13. OPTIMIZATION OF A SECOND STAGE IN SCREENING

If we can identify an optimal initial stage of screening with greater than 90 sensitivity and at least 98 specificity, it will be necessary to define an optimal second stage in screening that improves specificity to 99.7% without sacrificing sensitivity. TVS has improved specificity in trials to date in Stockholm and in the United Kingdom. Imaging might be improved by better defining criteria for malignancy. Regression analysis and neural network analysis have been applied to differentiating malignant from benign pelvic lesions. More sophisticated power 3D Doppler ultrasound may aid in distinguishing malignant from benign masses, although additional prospective trials are needed to establish its utility. For effective screening in the community, Doppler instruments and the expertise for their use must be widely available. Other technologies might prove useful in this setting. The role of positron emission tomography (PET) remains to be defined. Optical imaging that utilizes fluorescence, scatter and Raman spectra might help to define pre-malignant as well as malignant lesions. An "ovarian pap smear" obtained at laparoscopy might attain the same goal, depending, in part, on how often lesions are found on the ovarian surface. Each of these modalities might detect primary peritoneal disease as well as lesions localized to the ovary.

14. FUTURE EXPECTATIONS FOR OVARIAN CANCER SCREENING

The randomized trials that are currently being conducted will require 7-10 years or more to complete. Both the trial in the United Kingdom and the PLCO trial in the United States may yield false negative results. In both trials, therapy of ovarian cancer once diagnosed is at the discretion of local physicians and may or may not be optimal. In the PLCO trial, only women over age 55 are included, eliminating younger women with ovarian cancer who may tolerate best and most benefit from aggressive surgery and intensive chemotherapy. In addition, the control groups may do better than expected, if they have access to CA125 and TVS outside of the clinical trial setting, as may be the case in the United States. Against this possibility, however, is a survey from the State of Washington that indicates screening for ovarian cancer occurred in 2% of respondents (Drescher et. al, 2000).

Both of the major trials include women at conventional risk of developing ovarian cancer. Hereditary ovarian cancer may or may not be amenable to early detection using CA 125 algorithms or TVS. Such lesions can be polyclonal and can arise from the peritoneum. Primary peritoneal carcinoma can develop even after oophorectomy. The incidence of primary peritoneal disease is not completely defined, although recent reports suggest that primary peritoneal cancer may be only 5 to 10 % as prevalent as primary ovarian neoplasms. Studies from Cedars-Sinai Hospital in Los Angeles suggest that there may be only a short clinical interval between development of a primary peritoneal cancer and the clinical presentation of metastatic disease. Several patients have presented with advanced stage ovarian cancer within 6 months of a normal CA 125. Aside from the issues of sensitivity and lead-time, hereditary ovarian cancers occur at a slightly earlier age, necessitating screening of premenopausal women. Screening in a premenopausal population produces a high incidence of false positive CA 125 values (Westhoff et al, 1990). Conversely, levels of several markers are increased in healthy postmenopausal women, including lipid associated sialic acid

(LASA), NB/70K, urinary gonadotropin peptide (UGP), HER-2 and tissue peptide antigen (TPA) (Cane et. al, 1995; Tuxen et. al, 1999). Consequently, clinical trials in both heredity and sporadic cancer will be required. It will not be possible to assume that methods used in screening for sporadic ovarian cancer will apply to hereditary disease and vice versa. In this regard, it is appropriate that the Cancer Genetics Network is piloting the use of the CA125 algorithm in a high-risk population of women who will be tested every 3 months.

15. REQUIREMENTS FOR TRANSFORMING PROMISE INTO REALITY

Optimal progress in developing effective strategies for early detection of ovarian cancer will require a number of factors and reagents. Larger banks of serum, plasma, urine and tumor samples should be established from patients with stage I cancer at the time of initial surgery. Serum and plasma samples, promptly frozen, are needed from women screened over time to evaluate the specificity, variation and ultimately the sensitivity of different strategies. In the United Kingdom, where samples are sent via overnight courier at ambient temperature, levels of labile markers may be artifactually lost or even increased as observed with LPA and OVX1 (Hogdall et. al, 1999). Promptly frozen specimens of serum and plasma have been established around the PLCO trial and should prove useful. In addition, institutions funded by NCI Specialized Programs of Research Excellence (SPORE) grants are developing serum and plasma banks from women at conventional risks. The Early Detection Research Network and the Cancer Genetics Network are also collecting valuable reagents and data. New technologies including expression arrays, SAGE and SELDI are likely to identify hundred of candidates for new markers. An effective strategy must be developed to select and prioritize these markers. Regulatory change would also be desirable. In the past, the United States Food and Drug Administration (FDA) has required that new tumor markers be capable of "standing alone" for monitoring or detection. From currently available data, it appears that complementary rather than "stand alone" markers will be required to improve the sensitivity of an initial step in screening for ovarian cancer. Regulatory approval of tests based on surrogate endpoints could also facilitate more rapid progress. In this regard, regulatory and funding agencies might plan for success. At present, we should develop plans and pilots for the next generation of randomized studies. Such studies might be funded and initiated when the current generation of screening trails exhibits a shift toward detecting ovarian cancer at an earlier stage of disease. Despite a substantial gap between the promise and reality of screening for ovarian cancer, with the progress that has been made to date and with the impact of new technologies, the next decade may well see the emergence and validation of an effective strategy for early detection of this disease.

ACKNOWLEDGEMENT
This review has been supported in part by a grant from the National Cancer Institute, Department of Health and Human Services 1P50 CA83638-02.

REFERENCES:
Ala-Fossi SL, Maenpaa J, Blauer M, Tuohimaa P, Punnonen R. (2000). Inhibin A, B and pro-alpha C in serum and peritoneal fluid in postmenopausal patients with ovarian tumors, Eur J Endocrinol 142, 334-9.

Ardekani AM, Hitt B, Brown MR, Fishman DA, Mills G, Liotta L, Petricoin EF, Kohn EC. (2001). A high throughput proteomic approach to serum marker development for discriminition between ovarian cancer patients and unaffected individuals, Proc Soc Gynecol Oncol 32:102.

Avall Lundqvist E, Nordstrom L, Sjovall K, Eneroth P. (1989). Evaluation of seven different tumour markers for the establishment of tumour marker panels in gynecologic malignancies, Eur J Gynaecol Oncol 10, 395-405.

Baron AT, Lafky JM, Boardman CH, Balasubramaniam S, Suman VJ, Podratz KC, Maihle NJ. (1999). Serum sErb B1 and epidermal growth factor levels as tumor biomarkers in women with stage III or IV epithelial ovarian cancer, Can Epid Bio Prev 8, 129-37.

Baron AT, Lafky JM, Boardman CH, Balasubramaniam S, Suman VJ, Podratz KC, Maihle NJ. (1999). Serum sErbB1 and epidermal growth factor levels as tumor biomarkers in women with stage III or IV epithelial ovarian cancer, Cancer Epidemiol Biomarkers 8, 129-37.

Barton DP, Blanchard DK, Michelini-Norris B, Nicosia SV, Cavanagh D, Djeu JY. (1993). High serum and ascitic soluble interleukin-2 receptor alpha levels in advanced epithelial ovarian cancer, Blood 81, 424-9.

Barrenetxea G, Martin-Mateos M, Barzazan Mj, Montoya F, Matia JC, Rodriquez-Escudero FJ. (1990). Serum CA 125, CA 15.3 and CA 19.9 levels and surgical findings in patients undergoing second look operations for ovarian carcinomas, Eur J Gynaecol Oncol,11, 369-74.

Bast RC Jr, Klug TL, St. John E, Jenison E, Niloff JM, Lazarus H, Berkowitz RS, Leavitt T, Griffiths CT, Parker L, Zurawski VR Jr, Knapp RC. (1983). A radioimmunoassay using a monoclonal antibody to monitor the course of epithelial ovarian cancer, New Engl J Med 309, 883-887.

Bast RC jr, Knauf S, Epenetos A, Khokia B, Daly L, Tanner M, Soper J, Creasman W, Gall S, Knapp RC. (1991). Coordinate elevation of serum markers in ovarian cancer but not in benign disease, Cancer 68, 1758-63.

Bast RC Jr, Siegal FP, Runowicz C, Klug TL, Zurawski VR Jr, Schonholz D, Cohen CJ, Knapp RC. (1985). Elevation of serum CA 125 prior to diagnosis of an epithelial ovarian carcinoma, Gynecol Oncol 22, 115-120.

Bell R, Petticrew M, Sheldon T. (1998). The performance of screening tests for ovarian cancer: results of a systematic review, Br J Obstet Gynaec 105, 1136-47.

Ben-Arie A, Hagay Z, Ben-Hur H, Open M, Dgani R. (1999). Elevated serum alkaline phosphatase may enable early diagnosis of ovarian cancer, Eur J Obstet Gynecol Reprod Biol 86, 69-71.

Beneditti Panici P, Scambia G, Baiocchi G, Iacobelli S, Mancuso S. (1989). Predictive value of multiple tumor marker assays in second-look procedures for ovarian cancer, Gynecol Oncol 35, 386-9.

Berek JS, Bast RC Jr. (1995). Ovarian cancer screening. The use of serial complementary tumor markers to improve sensitivity and specificity for early detection, Cancer 76, 2092-6.

88

Berek JS, Chung C, Kaldi K, Watson JM, Knox RM, Martinez-Maza O. (1991). Serum interleukin-6 levels correlate with disease status in patients with epithelial ovarian cancer, Am J Obstet Gynecol 164, 1038-42.

Blaakaer J, Hogdall CK, Micic S, Toftager-Larsen K, Hording U, Bennett P, Bock J. (1995). Ovarian carcinoma serum markers and ovarian steroid activity—is there a link in ovarian cancer? A correlation of inhibin, tetranectin and CA125 to ovarian activity and the gonadotropin levles, Eur J Obstet Gynecol Reprod Biol 59, 53-6.

Boardman CH, Baron AT, Lafky JM, Metzinger D, Sunman VJ, Fishman DA, Podratz KC, Maihle NJ. (2000). Soluble ERBB/EGFR as a tumor biomarker in women with epithelial ovarian cancer, Proceedings American Association for Cancer Research, 41, Abstract #4635, 730.

Bon GG, Verheijen RH, Zuetenhorst JM, van Kamp GJ, Verstraeten AA, Kenemans P. (1996). Mucin-like carcinoma-associated antigen serum levels in patients with adenocarcinomas originating from ovary, breast and colon, Gynecol Obstet Invest 42, 58-62.

Bourne TH, Campbell S, Reynolds KM, Whitehead MI, Hampson J, Royston P, Crayford TJB, Collins WP. (1993). Screening for early familial ovarian cancer with transvaginal ultrasonography and colour blood flow imaging, Br Med J 306, 1025-9.

Bourne TH, Campbell S, Reynolds KM, Whitehead MI, Hampson J, Royston P, Crayford T, Collins WP. (1993). Screening for early familial ovarian cancer with transvaginal ultrasonography and colour blood flow imaging, Br Med J 306, 1025-9.

Campbell S, Ghan V, Royston P, Whitehead M, Collins W. (1989). Transabdominal ultrasound screening for early ovarian cancer, Br Med J 299, 1363-7.

Cane P, Azen C, Lopez E, Platt LD, Karlan BY. (1995). Tumor marker trends in asymptomatic women at risk for ovarian cancer: relevance for ovarian cancer screening, Gynecol Oncol 57, 240-5.

Castelli M, Battaglia F, Scambia G, Panici PB, Ferrandina G, Mileo AM, Mancuso S,

Ferrini U. (1991). Immunosuppressive acidic protein and CA 125 levels in patients with ovarian cancer, Oncology 48, 13-7.

Castelli M, Romano P, Atlante G, Pozzi M, Ferrini U. (1987). Immunosuppressive acidic protein and CA 125 levels in patients with ovarian cancer, Oncology 48, 13-7.

Cohen LS, Escobar PF, Scharm C, Glimco B, Fishman DA. Three-dimensional power doppler ultrasound improves the diagnostic accuracy for ovarian cancer prediction, submitted for publication.

Collins WP, Bourne TH, Campbell S. (1998). Screening strategies for ovarian cancer, Curr Opin Obstet Gynecol, 10, 33-9.

Consensus Development Panel on ovarian cancer. (1995). JAMA 273, 491-7.

Crump C, McIntosh MW, Urban N, Anderson G, Karlan BY. (2000). Ovarian cancer tumor marker behavior in asymptomatic healthy women: implications for screening, Cancer Epidemiol Biomarkers Prevent, 9, 1107-11.

De Brujin HW, ten Hoor KA, Boonstra H, Marink J, Krans M, Aalders JG. (1993). Cancer-associated antigen CA 195 in patients with mucinous ovarian tumours: a comparative analysis with CEA, TATI, and CA 125 in serum specimens and cyst fluids, Tumour Biol 14, 105-15.

De Brujn HW, ten Hoor KA, van der Zee AG. (1998). Serum and cystic fluid levels of soluble interleukin-2 receptor-alpha in patients with epithelial ovarian tumors are correlated, Tumour Biol 19, 160-6.

De Broe ME, Pollet DE. (1988). Multicenter evaluation of human placental alkaline phosphatase as a possible tumor-associated antigen in serum, Clin Chem 34, 1995-9.

Devine PL, McGuckin MA, Quin RJ, Ward BG. (1994). Serum markers CASA and CA 15-3 in ovarian cancer: all MUC1 assays are not the same, Tumour Biol 15, 337-44.

Diamandis EP. (2001). Two new ovarian cancer biomarkers, Tumor Markers: A New Era, Santa Barbara, CA.

Diamandis EP, Yousef GM, Soosaipillai AR, Bunting P. (2000). Human kallikrein 6 (zyme/portease M/neurosin): a new serum biomarker of ovarian carcinoma 33, 579-83.

Drescher C, Holt SK, Andersen MR, Anderson G, Urban N. (2000). Reported ovarian cancer screening among a population-based sample in Washington State, Obstet Gynecol 96, 70-4.

Eerdekens MW, Nouwen EJ, Pollet DE, Briers TW, De Broe ME. (1985). Placental alkaline phosphatase and cancer antigen 125 in sera of patients with benign and malignant diseases, Clin Chem 31, 687-90.

Einhorn N, Knapp RC, Bast RC, Zurawski VR Jr. (1989). CA 125 assay used in conjunction with CA 15.3 and TAG-72 assays for discrimination between malignant and non-malignant diseases of the ovary, Acta Oncol 28, 655-7.

Einhorn N, Sjovall K, Knapp RC, Hall P, Scull RE, Bast RC, Zurawski VR. (1992). Prospective evaluation of serum CA 125 levels for early detection of ovarian cancer, Obstet Gynecol 80, 14-8.

Engelen MJ, de Bruijn HW, Hollema H, ten Hoor KA, Willemse PH, Aalders JG, van der Zee AG. (2000). Serum CA 125, carcinoembryonic antigen, and CA 19-9 as tumor markers in borderline ovarian cancer, Gynecol Oncol 78, 16-20.

Fang X, Gaudette D, Furui T, Mao M, Estrella V, Eder A, Pustilnik T, Sasagwa T, Lapushin R, Yu S, Jaffe RB, Wiener JR, Erickson JR, Mills GB. (2000). Lysophospholipid growth factors in the initiation, progression, metastases, and management of ovarian cancer, Ann NY Acad Sci 905, 188-208.

Fayed ST, Ahmad SM, Kassim SK, Khalifa A. (1998). The value of CA 125 and CA 72-4 in management of patients with epithelial ovarian cancer, Dis Markers 14, 155-60.

Ferdeghini M, Gadducci A, Prontera C, Malagnino G, Fanucchi A, Annicchiarico C, Facchini V, Bianchi R. (1993). Serum soluble interleukin-2 receptor assay in epithelial ovarian cancer, Tumour Biol 14, 303-9.

Fishman DA, Cohen LS. (2000). Is transvaginal ultrasound effective for screening asymptomatic women for the detection of early-stage epithelial ovarian carcinoma, Gynecol Oncol 77, 347-49.

Gadducci A, Ferdeghini M, Ceccarini T, Prontera C, Faccini V, Bianchi R, Fioretti P. (1989). The serum concentrations of TAG-72 antigen measured with CA 72-4 IRMA in patients with ovarian carcinoma, J Nucl Med Allied Sci 33, 32-6.

Gadducci A, Ferdeghini M, Ceccarini T, Prontera C, Facchini V, Bianchi R, Fioretti P. (1990). A comparative evaluation of the ability of serum CA 125, CA 19-9, CA 15-3, CA 50, CA 72-4 and TATI assays in reflecting the course of disease in patients with ovarian carcinoma, Eur J Gynaecol Oncol 11, 127-33.

Gadducci A, Ferdeghini M, Prontera C, Moretti L, Mariani G, Bianchi R, Fioretti P. (1992). The concomitant determination of different tumor markers in patients with epithelial ovarian cancer and benign ovarian masses: relevance for differential diagnosis, Gynecol Oncol 44, 147-54.

Garzetti GG, Ciavattini A, Lucarini G, Goteri G, RomaniniC, Biagini G. (1996). Increased serum 72 Kda metalloproteinase in serous ovarian tumors: comparison with CA 125, Anticancer Res 16, 2123-7.

Ghazizadeh M, Sasaki Y, Oguro T, Aihara K, Tenjin H, Araki T. (1990). Combined immunohistochemical study of tissue polypeptide antigen and cancer antigen 125 in human ovarian tumours, Histopathology 17, 123-8.

Gibson HE, Wong KK, Yiu GK, Muto MM, Berkowitz RS, Cramer DW, Mok SC. Clinical applications of microarray technology: Creatine kinase B is an upregulated gene in epithelial ovarian cancer and shows promise as a serum marker, Society of Gynecologic 32nd Annual Meeting, Abstract 8, 43.

Goldhirsch A, Berger E, Muller O, Maibach R, Misteli S, Buser K, Roesler H, Brunner K. (1988). Ovarian cancer and tumor markers: sialic acid, galactosyltransferase and CA-125, Oncology 45, 281-6.

Gonzalez A, Vizoso F, Vazquez J, Ruibal A, Balibrea JL. (1997). Clinical significance of preoperative serum levels of CA 125 and TAG-72 in ovarian cancer, Int J Biol Markers 12, 112-7.

Grosen EA, Granger GA, Gatanaga M, Ininns EK, Hwang C, DiSaia P, Berman M, Manetta A, Emma D, Gatanaga T. (1993). Meausrement of the soluble membrane receptors for tumor mecrosis factor and lymphotoxin in the sera of patients with gynecologic malignancy, Gynecol Oncol 50, 68-77.

Greenlee RT, Hill-Harmon MB, Murray T, Thun M. (2001). Cancer statistics, 2001, CA Journ Clin 51, 15-37.

Guadagni F, Roselli M, Cosimelli M, Ferroni P, Spila A, Cavaliere F, Casaldi V, Wappner G, Abbolito MR, Greiner JW. (1995). CA 72-4 serum marker – a new tool in the management of carcinoma patients, Cancer Invest 13, 227-38.

Guerriero S, Ajossa S, Risalvato A, Lai MP, Mais V, Angiolucci, Melis GB. (1998) Diagnosis of adnexal malignancies by using color Doppler energy imaging as a secondary test in persistent masses. Ultrasound Obstet Gynecol 11, 277-82.

Halila H, Lehtovirta P, Stenman UH. (1988). Tumour-associated trypsin inhibitor (TATI) in ovarian cancer, Br J Cancer 57, 304-7.

Hasholzner U, Baumgartner L, Steiber P, Meier W, Hofmann K, Fateh-Moghadam A. (1994). Significance of the tumour markers CA 125 II, CA 72-4, CASA and CYFRA 21-1 in ovarian carcinoma, Anticancer Res 14, 2743-6.

Hasholzner U, Baumgartner L, Steiber P, Meier W, Reiter W, Pahl H, Fateh-Moghadam A. (1996). Clinical significance of the tumour markers CA 125 II and CA 72-4 in ovarian carcinoma, Int J Cancer 69, 329-34.

Healy DL, Mamers P, Bangah M, Burger HG. (1993). Clinical and pathophysiologocical aspects of inhibin, Human Reprod, Suppl 2, 138-40.

Hefler L, Mayerhofer K, Nardi A, Reinthaller A, Kainz C, Tempfer C. (2000). Serum soluble Fas levels in ovarian cancer, Obstet Gynecol 96, 65-9.

Heinonen PK, Kallioniemi OP, Koivula T. (1987). Comparison of CA 125 and placental alkaline phophatase as ovarian tumor markers, Tumori 73, 301-2.

Helzlsouer KJ, Bush TL, Albert AJ, Bass KM, Zacur H, Comstock GW. (1993). Prospective study of serum CA 125 levels as markers of ovarian cancer, JAMA 269, 123-6.

Hogdall CK. (1998). Human tetranectin: methodological and clinical studies, APMIS Suppl 86, 1-31.

Hogdall CK, Hogdall EV, Hordin U, Toftager-Larsen K, Arends J, Norgaard-Pedersen B, Clemmensen I. (1996). Use of tetranectin, CA-125 and CASA to predict residual tumor and survival at second-and third-look operations for ovarian cancer, Acta Oncol 35, 63-9.

Hogdall EVS, Hogdall CK, Kjaer SK, Iles R, Xu FJ, Yu, Y, Bast RC Jr, Blaakaer J, Jacobs I. (1999). OVX1 radioimmunoassay results are dependent on the method of sample collection and storage, Clin Chem 45, 692-694.

Hogdall EV, Hogdall CK, Tingulstad S, Hagen B, Nustad K, Xu FJ, Bast RC, Jacobs IJ. (2000). Predictive values of serum tumours markers tetranectin, OVX1, CASA and CA125 in patients with a pelvic mass, Int J Cancer 89, 519-23.

Hording U, Toftager-Larsen K, Dreisler A, Lund B, Daugaard S, Lundvall F, Arends J, Winkel P, Rorth M. (1990). CA 125, placental alkaline phophatase, and tissue polypeptide antigen in the monitoring of ovarian carcinoma. A comparative study of three different tumor markers, Gynecol Obstet Invest 30, 178-83.

Hurteau JA, Woolas RP, Jacobs IJ, Oram DC, Kurman CC, Rubin LA, Nelson DL, Berchuck A, Bast RC Jr, Mills GB. (1995). Soluble interleukin-2 receptor alpha is elevated in sera of patients with benign ovarian neoplasms and epithelial ovarian cancer, Cancer 76, 1615-20.

Hurteau JA, Simon HU, Kurman C, Rubin L, Mills GB. (1994). Levels of soluble interleukin-2 receptor-alpha are elevated in serum and ascitic flluid from epithelial ovarian cancer patients, Am J Obstet Geynecol 170, 918-28.

Hutson R, Ramsdale J, Wells M. (1995). p53 protein expression in putative precursor lesions of epithelial ovarian cancer, Histopathology 27, 367-71.

Ind T, Iles R, Shepard J, Chard T. (1997), Serum concentrations of cancer antigen 125, placental alkaline phosphatase, cancer-associated serum antigen and free beta human chorionic gonadotrophin as prognostic markers for epithelial ovarian cancer, Br J Obstet Gynaecol 104, 1024-9.

Inoue M, Fujita M, Nakazawa A, Ogawa H, Tanizawa O. (1992). Sialyl-Tn, sialyl-Lewis Xi, CA 19-9, CA 125, carcinoembryonic antigen, and tissue polypeptide antigen in differentiating ovarian cancer from benign tumours, Obstet Gynecol 79, 434-40.

Jacobs I, Bast RC Jr. (1989). CA125 tumour-associated antigen: A review of the literature, Hum Reprod 4, 1-12.

Jacobs IJ, Rivera H, Oram DH, Bast RC Jr. (1993). Differential diagnosis of ovarian cancer with tumour markers CA 125, CA 15-3 and TAG 72.3, Br J Obstet Gynaecol 100, 1120-4.

Jacobs IJ, Oram DH, Bast RC Jr. (1992). Strategies for improving the specificity of screening for ovarian cancer with tumour-associated antigens CA 125, CA 15-3 and TAG 72.3, Obstet Gynecol 80, 396.9.

Jacobs I, Stabile I, Bridges J, Kemsley P, Reynolds C, Grudzinskas J, Oram D. (1999). Multimodal approach to screening for ovarian cancer, The Lancet, 268-71.

Jacobs I. (1988). Screening for ovarian cancer by CA 125 measurements. The Lancet, 889

Jacobs IJ, Kohler MF, Wiseman RW, Marks JR, Whitaker R, Kerns BA, Humphrey P, Berchuck A, Ponder BA, Bast RC Jr.. (1992). Clonal origen of epithelial ovarian cancer: Analysis by loss of heterozigosity, p53 ,mutation and chromosome inactivation, J Natl Cancer Inst 84, 1793-8.

Jacobs IJ, Rivera H, Oram DH, Bast RC Jr. Differential diagnosis of ovarian cancer with tumour markers CA 125, CA 15-3 and TAG 72.3, Br J Obstet Gynaecol 100, 1120-4.

Jacobs IJ, Skates S, Davies AP, Woolas RP, Jeyerajah, A, Weidemann P, Sibley K, Oram DH. (1996). Risk of diagnosis of ovarian cancer after raised serum CA 125 concentration: a prospective cohort study, Br Med J 313, 1355-8.

Kacinski BM, Carter D, Mittal K. (1990). Ovarian adenocarcinomas express fms-complementary transcripts and fms antigen, often with coexpression of CSF-1, Am J Path 137, 135-47.

Karlan BY, Plkatt LD. (1994). The current status of ultrasound and color doppler imaging in screening for ovarian cancer, Gynecol Oncol 55, S28-S33.

Kenemans P, Verstraeten AA, van Kamp Gj, von Mendsdorff-Pouilly S. (1995). The second generation CA 125 assays, Ann Med 27, 107-13.

Kierkegaard O, Mogensen O, Mogensen B, Jakobsen A. (1995). Predictive and prognostic valiules of cancer-associated serum antigen (CASA) and cancer antigen 125 (CA 125) levels prior to second-look laparotomy for ovarian cancer, Gynecol Oncol 59, 251-4.

Knauf S, Bast RC Jr. (1988). Tumor antigen NB/70K and CA 125 levels in the blood of preoperative ovarian cancer patients and controls: a preliminary report of the use of the NB12123 and CA125 radioimmunoassays alone and in combination, Int J Biol Markers 3, 75-81.

Koebl H, Schieder K, Neunteufel W, Bieglmayer C. (1989). A comparative study of mucin-like carcinoma-associated antigen (MCA), CA 125, A 19-9 and CEA in patients with ovarian cancer, Neoplasma 36, 473-8.

Koebl H, Tatra G, Bieglmayer C. (1988). A comparative study of immunosuppressive acidic protein (IAP), CA 125 and acute-phase proteins as parameters for ovarian cancer monitoring, Neoplasma 35, 215-20.

Kohler MF, Kerns BJM, Soper JT, Humphrey PA, Marks JR, Bast RC Jr, Berchuck A. (1993). Mutation and overexpression of p53 in early-stage epithelial ovarian cancer, Obstet Gynecol 81, 643-650.

Kudoh K, Kikuchi Y, Kita T, Tode T, Takano M, Hirata J, Mano Y, Yamamota K, Nagata I. (1999). Preoperative determination of several serum tumor markers in patients with primary epithelial ovarian carcinoma, Gynecol Obstet Invest 47, 52-7.

Kurachi H, Adachi H, Morishige K, Adachi K, Takeda T, Homma H, Yamamota T, Miyake A. (1996). Transforming growth factor-alpha promotes tumor markers secretion from human ovarian cancers in vitro, Cancer 78, 1049-54.

Kurjak A, Kupesic S, Breyer B. (1998).The assessment of ovarian tumor angiogensis: What does three-dimensional power Doppler add? Ultrasound Obstet Gynecol 12, 136-146.

Kurjak A, Zalud I, Alfirevic Z. (1991). Evaluation of adnexal masses with transvaginal color ultrasound. J Ultrasound Med 10, 295-7.

Lambert-Messerlian GM, Steinhoff M, Zheng W, Canick JA, Gajewski WH, Seifer DB, Schneyer AL. (1997). Multiple immunoreactive inhibin proteins in serum from postmenopausal women with epithelial ovarian cancer, Gynecol Oncol 65, 512-6.

Lidor YJ, Xu FJ, Martinez-Maza O, Olt GJ, Marks JR, Berchuck A, Ramakrishnan S, Berek JS, Bast RC Jr. (1993). Constitutive production of macrophage colony stimulating factor and interleukin-6 by human ovarian surface epithelial cells, Exp Cell Res 207, 332-339.

Lotzniker M, Pavesi F, Scarabvelli M, Vadacca G, Franchi M, Moratti R. (1991). Tumour associated antigens CA 15.3 and CA 125 in ovarian cancer, Int J Biol Markers 6, 115-21.

Lu KH, Bell DA, Welch WR, Berkowitz RS, Mok SC. (1998). Evidence for the multifocal origin of bilateral and advanced human serous borderline ovarian tumors, Cancer Res 58, 2328-30.

Luo L, Bunting P, Scorilas A, Diamandis EP. (2001). Human kallidrein 10: a novel tumor marker for ovarian carcinoma? Clin Chem Acta 306, 111-8.

Luo LY, Grass L, Howarth DJC, Pierre T, Ong H, Diamandis EP. (2001). Immunofluorometric assay of human kallikrein 10 and its identification in biological fluids and tissues, Clinical Chem 47, 237-46.

Mayerhofer K, Bodner K, Bodner-Adler B, Schindl M, Kaider A, Hefler L, Zeillinger R, Leodolter S, Armin E, Kainz C. (2001). Interleukin-8 serum level shift in patients with ovarian carcinoma undergoing paclitaxel-containing chemotherapy, Cancer 91, 388-93.

McGuckin MA, Layton GT, Bailey MJ, Hurst T, Kho9o SK, Ward BG. (1990). Evaluation of two new assays for tumor-associated antigens, CASA and OSA, found in the serum of patients with epithelial ovarian carcinoma—comparison with CA125, Gynecol Oncol 37, 165-71.

McKenzie SJ, DeSombre KA, Bast BS, Hollis DR, Whitaker RS, Berchuck A, Boyer CM, Bast RC Jr. (1993). Serum levels of HER-2 neu (C-erbB-2) correlate with overexpression of p185neu in human ovarian cancer, Cancer 71, 3942-6.

Medl M, Ogris E, Peters-Engl C, Leodolter S. (1995). TATI (tumour-associated trypsin inhibitor) as a marker of ovarian cancer, Br J Cancer 71, 1051-4.

Meisel M, Straube W, Weise J, Burkhardt B. (1995). A study of serum CASA and CA 125 levles in patients with ovarian cancer, Arch Gynecol Obstet 256, 9-15.

Menon U, Talaat A, Rosenthal AN, Macdonald ND, Jeyerajah AR, Skates SJ, Sibley K, Oram DH, Jacobs IJ. (2000). Performance of ultrasound as a second line test to serum CA125 in ovarian cancer screening, Br J Obstet Gynecol 107, 165-69.

Mogensen O, Mogensen B, Jakobsen A. (1990). Tumor-associated trypsin inhibitor and cancer antigen 125 in pelvic masses, Gynecol Oncol 38, 170-4.

Mogensen O, Mogensen B, Jakobsen A. (1990). Tumour-associated tyrpsin inhibitor (TATI) and cancer antigen 125 (CA 125) in mucinous ovarian tumours, Br J Cancer 61, 327-9.

Mogenson O, Mogensen B, Jakobsen A. (1989). Alpha 1-acid glucoprotein in ovarian cancer with a reference to immunosuppressive acidic protein and cancer antigen 125, Cancer 64, 1867-71.

Mok CH, Tsao SW, Knapp RC, Fishbaugh PM, Lau CC. (1992). Unifocal origin of advanced human epithelial ovarian cancer, Cancer Res 52, 5119-22.

Mok SC, Chao J, Skates S, Wong K, Yiu GK, Muto MG, Berkowitz RS, Cramer DW. (2001). Prostasin, an upregulated gene in ovarian cancer, identified through microaaray technology. Tumor Markers: A New Era, Santa Barbara, CA.

Muto MG, Welch WR, Mok SC, Bandera CA, Fishbauth PM, Tsao SW, Lau CC, Goodman HM, Knapp RC, Berkowitz. (1995). Evidence for a multifocal origin of papillary serous carcinoma of the peritoneum., Cancer Res 55, 490-2.

Nap M, Vitali A, Nustad K, Bast RC Jr, O'Brien TJ, Nilsson O, Seguin P, Suresh MR, Bormer OP, Saga T, de Bruijin HW, Nozawa S, Kreutz FT, Jette D, Sakahara H, Gadnell M, Endo K, Barlow EH, Warren D, Paus E, Hammarstrom S, Kenemans P, Hilgers J. (1996). Immunohistochemical characterization of 22 monoclonal antibodies against the CA125 antigen: 2nd report from the ISOBM TD-1 Workshop, Tumour Biol 17, 325-31.

Negishi Y, Furukawa T, Oka T, Sakamoto M, Hirata T, Okabe K, Matayoshi K, Akiya K, Soma H. (1987). Clinical use of CA 125 and its combination assay with other tumor marker in patients with ovarian carcinoma, Gynecol Obstet Invest 23, 200-7.

Nishida Y, Kohno K, Kawamata T, Morimitsu K, Kuwano M, Miyakawa I. Increased cathepsin L levels in serum in some patients with ovarian cancer: comparison with CA125 and CA72-4, Gynecol Oncol 56, 357-61.

Nozawa S, Yajima M, Sakuma T, Udagawa Y, Kiguchi K, Sakayori M, Narisawa S, Iizuka R, Uemura M. (1990). Cancer-associated galactosyltransferase as a new tumor marker for ovarian clear cell carcinoma, Cancer Res 50, 754-9.

Oehler MK, Sutterlin M, Caffier H. (1999). CASA and CA 125 in diagnosis and follow-up of advanced ovarian cancer, Anticancer Res 19, 2513-8.

Onsrud M, Shabana A, Austgulen R. (1996). Soluble tumor necrosis factor receptor and CA 125 in serum as markers for epithelial ovarian cancer, Tumour Biol 17, 90-6.

Panza N, Pacilio G, Campanella L, Peluso G, Battista C, Amoriello A, Utech W, Vacca G, Lombardi G. (1988). Cancer antigen 125, tissue polypeptide antigen, carcinoembryonic antigen, and beta-chain human chorionic gonadotropin as serum markers of epithelial ovarian carcinoma, Cancer 61, 76-83.

Pathuri B, Leitao M, Barakat RR, Akram M, Bogomolniy F, Olvera N, Lin O, Soslow R, Robson ME, Offit K, Boyd J. (2001). Genetic analysis of ovarian carcinoma histogenesis, Proc Soc Gyn Oncol 32:43.

Patsner B, Mann WJ, Visicchio M, Loesch M. (1988). Comparison of serum CA125 and lipid-associated sialic acid (LASA-P) in monitoring patients with invasive ovarian adenocarcinoma, Gynecol Oncol 30, 98-103.

Pauler DK, Menon U, MCIntosh MW, Symecko HL, Skates SJ. (2001). Factors influencing serum CA125II levels in healthy postmenopausal women, Cancer Epidemiol Biomarkers Prevention, in press.

Peters-Engl C, Medl M, Ogris E, Leodolter S. (1995). Tumor-associated trypsin inhibitor (TATI) and cancer antigen 125 (CA125) in patients with epithelial ovarian cancer, Anticancer Res 15, 2727-30.

Petru E, Sevin BU, Averette HE, Koechli OR, Perras JP, Hilsenbeck S. (1990). Comparison of three tumor markers –CA-125, lipid-associated sialic acid (LSA), and NB/70K—in monitoring ovarian cancer, Gynecol Oncol 38, 181-6.

Phocas I, Sarandakou A, Sikiotis K, Rizos D, Kalambokis D, Zourlas PA. (1996). A comparative study of serum alpha-beta a immunoreactive inhibin and tumor-associated antigens CA 125 and CEA in ovarian cancer, Anticancer Res 16, 3827-31.

Plante M, Rubin SC, Wong GY, Federici MG, Finstad CL, Gastl GA. (1994). Interleukin-6 level in serum and ascites as a prognostic factor in patients with epithelial ovarian cancer, Cancer 73, 1882-8.

Ries LAG, Kosary CL, Hankey BF, Miller BA, Clegg L, Edwards BK, (eds). (1999). SEER cancer statistics review 1973-1996, National Cancer Institute, Bethesda, MD.

Robertson DM, Cahir N, Burger HG, Mamers P, McCloud PI, Pettersson K, McGuckin M. (1999). Combined inhibin and CA125 assays in the detection of ovarian cancer, Clin Chem 45, 651-8.

Rosenthal AN, Jacobs IJ. (1998), The role of CA 125 in screening for ovarian cancer, Int J Biol Makers 13, 216-20.

Rosenthal A, Jacobs I, (1998). Ovarian Cancer Screening, Seminars Onc 25, 315-25.

Rustin GJ, van der Burg ME, Berek JS. (1993). Advanced ovarian cancer. Tumour markers, Ann Oncol 4, 71-7.

Santala M, Burger H, Ruokonen A, Stenback F, Kauppila A. (1998). Elevated serum inhibin and tumor-assocated trypsin inhibitor concentrations in a young woman with dysgerminoma of the ovary, Gynecol Oncol 71, 465-8.

Sato S, Yokoyama Y, Sakamota T, Futagami M, Saito Y. (2000). Usefulness of mass screening for ovarian carcinoma using transvaginal ultrasonography, Cancer 89, 582-8.

Scambia G, Benedetti Panici P, Perrone L, Sonsini C, Giannelli S, Gallo A, Natali PG, Mancuso S. (1990). Serum levels of tumour assocated glycoprotein (TAG 72) in patients with gynaecological malignancies, Br J Cancer 62, 147-51.

Scambia G, Testa U, Panici PB, Martucci R, Foti E, Petrini M, Amoroso M, Masciullo V, Peschle C, Mancuso S. (1994). Interleukin-6 serum levels in patients with gynecological tumors, Int J Cancer 57, 318-23.

Scambia G, Testa U, Benedetti Panici P, Foti E, Martucci R, Gadducci A, Perillo A, Facchini V, Peschle C, Mancuso S. (1995). Prognostic significance of interleukin 6 serum levels in patients with ovarian cancer, Br J Cancer 71, 354-6.

Schelling M, Braun M, Kuhn W. (2000). Combined transvaginal B-mode and color Doppler sonography for differential diagnosis of ovarian tumors: results of a multivariate logistic regression analysis, Gynecol Oncol 77, 78-86.

Schmandt RE, Clifford SL, Lee J, Lillie J, Deavers MT, Shaw P, Jung M, Levenback C, Bast RC, Mills GB, Gershenson DM, Lu KH. (2001). Differential expression of the secreted protease inhibitor, HE4, in epithelial ovarian cancer, Proc Soc Gynecol Oncol 32:103.

Scholler N, Fu N, Yang Y, Ye Z, Goodman GE, Hellström KE, Hellström I. (1999). Soluble member(s) of the mesothelin/mega potentiating family are detectable in same from patients with ovarian carcinoma. Proc Natl Acad Sci USA 96, 11531-36.

Schummer M, Ng WL, Bumgarner RE, Nelson PS, Schummer B, Hassel L, Rae Baldwin L, Karlan BY, Hood L. (1999). Comparative hybridization of an array of 21,500 ovarian cDNAs for the discovery of genes overexpressed in ovarian carcinomas, Gene 238, 375-385.

Schutter EM, Mijatovic V, Kok A, Van Kamp GJ, Verstraeten R, Verheijen RH. (1999). Urinary gonadotropin peptide (UGP) and serum CA 125 in gynaecologic practice, a clinical prospective study, Anticancer Res 19, 5551-7.

Schutter EM, Sohn C, Kristen P, Mobus V, Crombach G, Kaufmann M, Caffier H, Kreienberg R, Verstraeten AA, Kenemans P. (1998). Estimation of probability of malignancy using a logistic model combining physical examination, ultrasound, serum CA 125, and serum CA 72-4 in postmenopusal women with a pelvic mass: an international multicenter study, Gynecol Oncol 69, 56-63.

Schwarz PE, Chambers JT, Taylor KJ, Pellerito J, Hamers L, Cole LA, Yang-Feng TL, Smith P, Mayne ST, Makuch R. (1991). Early detection of ovarian cancer: preliminary results of the Yale Early Detection Program, Yale J Biol Med 64, 573-82.

Schwartz PE, Chambers SK, Chambers JT, Gutmann J, Katopodis N, Foemmel R. (1987). Circulating tumor markers in the monitoring of gynecologic malignancies, Cancer 60, 353-61.

Schvartsman HS, Lu KH, Le J, Lillie J, Deavers MT, Clifford SL, Wolf J, Mills GB, Bast RC, Gershenson DM, Schmandt RE. (2001). Over-expression of NES-1 in epithelial ovarian carcinoma, Society of Gynecologic 32nd Annual Meeting, Abstract, 103.

Shridhar V, Lee J, Pandita A, Iturria S, Avula R, Staub J, Morrissey M, Calhoun E, Sen A, James D, Kalli K, Keeney G, Roche P, Cliby W, Mills GB, Bast RC Jr, Couch FJ, Hartmann LC, Lillie J, Smith DI. (2001). Genetic analysis of early versus late stage ovarian tumors, Cancer Res in press.

Sichel F, Salaun V, Bar E, Gauduchon P, Malas JP, Goussard J, Le Talaer JY. (1994). Biological markers and ovarian carcinomas: galactosyltransferase, CA 125, isoenzymes of amylase and alkaline phosphatase, Clin Chim Acta, 227, 87-96.

Skates SJ, Jacobs IJ, MacDonald N, Rosenthal A, Menon U, Sibley K, Knapp RC. (1999). Estimated duration of pre-clinical ovarian cancer from longitudinal CA125 levels, Proc Amer Assoc Cancer Res 40:43 (A#288).

Skates SJ, Pauler DK. (2001). Screening based on the risk of cancer calculation from Bayesian Hierarchical change-point models of longitudinal markers, J Am Statist Assoc, in press.

Skates SJ, Singer DE. (1991). Quantifying the potential benefit of CA 125 screening for ovarian cancer, J Clin Epidemiol 44, 365-80.

Skates SJ, Xu F-J, Yu Y-H, Sjövall K, Einhorn N, Chang YC, Bast RC Jr, and Knapp RC. (1995). Toward an optimal algorithm for ovarian cancer screening with longitudinal tumor markers, Cancer 76, 2004-2010.

Sliutz G, Tempfer C, Kainz C, Mustafa G, Gitsch G, Koelbl H, Biegelmayer C. (1995). Tissue polypeptide specific antigen and cancer associated serum antigen in the follow-up of ovarian cancer, Anticancer Res 15, 1127-9.

Stenman UH, Alfthan H, Vartiainen J, Lehtovirta P. (1995). Markers supplementing CA 125 in ovarian cancer, Ann Med 27, 115-20.

Stigbrand T, Riklund K, Tholander B, Hirano K, Lalos O, Stendahl U. (1990). Placental alkaline phosphatase (PLAP)/ PLAP-like alkaline phosphatase as tumour marker in relation to CA 125 and TPA for ovarian epithelial tumours, Eur J Gynaecol Oncol 11, 351-60.

Szarka G, Pulay T, Csomor S, Tran-Phoung-Mai, Schumann B. (1988). The significance of neopterin determination as a tumour marker in ovarian cancer, Acta Chir Hung 29, 359-64.

Tailor A, Jurkovic D, Bourne TH, Collins WP, Campbell S. (1997). Sonographic predication of malignancy in adnexal masses using multivariate logistic regression analysis, Ultrasound Obstet Gynecol 10, 41-7.

Tailor A, Jurkovic D, Bourne TH, Collins WP, Campbell S. (1999). Sonographic prediction of malignancy in adnexal masses using an artificial neural network, Br J Obstet Gynaecol 106, 21-30.

Tailor A, Jurkovic D, Bourne T, Natucci M, Collins WP, Campbell S. (1998). Comparison of transvaginal color Doppler imaging and color Doppler energy for assessment of intraovarian blood flow. Obstet Gynecol 91, 561-7.

Tekay A, Jouppila P. (1995). Blood flow in benign ovarian tumors and normal ovaries during the follicular phase. Obstet Gynecol 86, 55-9.

Tempfer C, Hefler L, Heinzl H, Loesch A, Gitsch G, Rumpold H, Kainz C. CYFRA 21-1 serum levels in women with adnexal masses and inflammatory diseases, Br J Cancer 78, 1108-12.

Tholander B, Taube A, Lindgren A, Sjoberg O, Stendahl U, Tamsen L. (1990). Pretreatment serum levels of CA-125, carcinoembryonic antigen, tissue polypeptide antigen, and placental alkaline phophatase in patients with ovarian carcinoma: influence of histological type, grade of differentiation, and clinical stage of disease, Gynecol Oncol 39, 36-33.

96

Tholander B, Taube A, Lindgren A, Sjoberg O, Stendahl U, Kiviranta A, Hallman K, Holm L, Weiner E, Tamsen L. (1990). Pretreatment serum levels of CA-125, carcinoembryonic antigen, tissue polypeptide antigen, and placental alkaline phophatase, in patients with ovarian carcinoma, borderline tumors, or benign adnexal masses: relevance for differential diagnosis, Gynecol Oncol 39, 16-25.

Timmerman D, Verrelst H, Bourne TH, De Moor B, Collins WP, Vergote I, Vandewalle J. (1999). Artificial neural network models for the preoperative discrimination between malignant and benign adnexal masses, Ultrasound Obstet Gynecol, 13, 17-25.

Toftager-Larsen K, Hording U, Dreisler A, Daugaard S, Lund B, Bock J, Lundvall F, Frederiksen K, Norgaard-Pedersen B. (1992). CA-125, placental alkaline phosphatas and tissue polypeptide antigen as preoperative serum markers in ovarian carcinoma, Gynecol Obstet Invest 33, 177-82.

Tuxen MK, Soletormos G, Petersen PH, Schioler V, Dombernowski P. (1999). Assessment of biological variation and analytical imprecision of CA 125, CEA, and TPA in relation to monitoring of ovarian cancer, Gynecol Oncol 74, 12-22.

Urban N, Drescher C, Etzioni R, Colby C. (1997). Use of a stochastic simulation model to identify and efficient protocol for ovarian cancer screening, Controlled Clin Trials 18, 251-70.

Urban N. Screening for ovarian cancer. Br Med J 1999; 319:1317-8

Valentin L, Sladkevicius P, Marsal K. (1994). Limited contribution of Doppler velocimetry to the differential diagnosis of extrauterine pelvic tumors. Obstet Gynecol 83, 425-33.

Van Haaften-Day C, Xu F, Yu Y, Bast, RC Jr, Hacker N. (2001). OVX1, CA 125 and M-CSF as tumor markers for surface epithelial-stromal tumors of the ovary - a critical appraisal, Cancer In Revision.

Van Nagell JR, Depriest PD, Reedy MB, Gallion HH, Ueland FR, Pavlik EJ, Kryscio RJ. (2000). The efficacy of transvaginal sonographic screening in asymptomatic women at risk for ovarian cancer, Gynecol Oncol 77, 350-56.

Vardi JR, Tadros GH, Foemmel R, Shebes M. (1989). Plasma Lipid-associated sialic acid and serum CA 125 as indicators of disease status with advanced ovarian cancer, Obstet Gynecol 74, 379-83.

Walker R, Crebbin V, Stern J, Scudder S, Schwartz P. (1994). Urinary gonadotropin peptide (UGP) as a marker of gynecologic malignancies, Anticancer Res 14, 1703-9.

Wang K, Gan L, Jeffery E, Gayle M, Gown AM, Skelly M, Nelson PS, Ng WP, Schummer M, Hood L, Mulligan J. (1999). Monitoring gene expression profile changes in ovarian carcinomas using cDNA microarray, Gene 229:101-8.

Wang YX, Schwartz PE, Chambers JT, Cole LA. (1988). Urinary gonadotropin fragments (UGF) in cancers of the female reproductive system. II. Initial serial studies, Gyncol Oncol 31, 91-102.

Ward BG, Cruickshank DJ, Tucker DF, Love S. (1987). Independent expression in serum of three tumour-associated antigens: CA 125, placental alkaline phosphatase and HMFG2 in ovarian carcinoma, Br J Obstet Gynaecol 94, 696-8.

Ward BG, McGuckin MA, Ramm LE, Goglan M, Sanderson B, Tripcony L, Free KE. (1993). The management of ovarian carcinoma is improved by the use of cancer-associated serum antigen and CA 125 assays, Cancer 71, 430-8.

Westhoff C, Gollub E, Patel J, Rivera H, Bast R Jr. (1990). CA 125 levels in menopausal women, Obstet Gynecol 76, 428-431.

Woolas RP, Conaway MR, Fengji X, Jacobs IJ, Yu Y, Daly L, Davies AP, O'Briant K, Berchuck A, Soper JT, Clarke-Pearson DL, Rodriquez G, Oram DH, Bast RC. (1995). Combinations of multiple serum markers are superior to individual assays for discriminating malignant from benign pelvic masses, Gynecol Oncol 59, 111-16.

Woolas RP, Oram DH, Jeyarajah AR, Bast RC, Jacobs IJ. (1999). Ovarian cancer identified through screening with serum markers but not by pelvic imaging, Int J Gynecol Cancer 9, 497-501.

Woolas RP, Xu FJ, Jacobs IJ, Yu Y, Daly L, Berchuck A, Soper JT, Clark-Pearson DL, Oram DH, Bast RC. (1993) Elevation of multiple serum markers in patients with stage I ovarian cancer. J Natl Cancer Inst 85, 1748-51.

Xu FJ, Ramakrishnan S, Daly L, Soper JT, Berchuck A, Clarke-Pearson D, Bast RC Jr. (1991). Increased serum levels of macrophage colony-stimulating factor in ovarian cancer, Am J Obstet Gynecol 165, 1356-1362.

Xu F-J, Yu Y-A, Daly L, DeSombre K, Anselmino L, Hass GM, Berchuck A, Soper J, Clarke-Pearson D, Boyer C, Layfield LJ, Bast RC Jr. (1993). OVX1 radioimmunoassay complements CA-125 for predicting the presence of residual ovarian carcinoma at second-look surgical surveillance procedures, J Clin Oncol 11, 1506-1510.

Xu FJ, Yu YH, Li BY, Moradi M, Elg S, Lane C, Carson L, Ramakrishnan S. (1991). Development of two new monoclonal antibodies reactive to a surface antigen present on human ovarian epithelial cancer cells, Cancer Res 51; 4012-9.

Xu Y, Gaudette DC, Boynton JD, Frankel A, Fang XL, Sharma A, Hurteau J, Casey G, Goodbody A, Mellors A. (1995). Characterization of an ovarian cancer activating factor in ascites from ovarian cancer patients, Clin Cancer Res 1, 1223-32.

Xu Y, Shen Z, Wiper DW, Wu M, Morton RE, Elson P, Kennedy AW, Belinson J, Markman M, Casey G. (1998). Lysophosphatidic acid as a potential biomarker for ovarian and other gynecologic cancers, JAMA 280; 719-23.

Zakrzewska I, Borawska R, Poznanski J, Mackowiak B. (1999). Significance of some tumor markers in differential diagnosis of ovarian cancer, Rocz Akad Med Bialymst 44, 235-43.

Zhang Z, Barnhill SD, Zhang H, Xu F, Yu Y, Jacobs I, Woolas RP, Berchuck A, Madyastha KR, Bast RC. (1999). Combination of multiple serum markers using an artificial neural network to improve specificity on discriminating malignant from benign pelvic masses, Gynecol Oncol 73, 56-61.

Zhang Z, Xu F, Yu Y, Berchuck A, Havrilesky LJ, de Bruijn HWA, vader Zee AGJ, Woolas RP, Jacobs I, Bast RC. (2001). Use of multiple markers to detect stage I epithelial ovarian cancers: neural network analysis improves performance. Proc Amer Soc Clin Oncol, in press.

Zurawski VR Jr, Orjaseter H, Anderson A, Jellum E. (1988). Elevated serum CA 125 levels prior to diagnosis of ovarian neoplasia; relevance for early detection of ovarian cancer, Int J Cancer 42, 677-80.

Zurawski VR, Knapp RC, Einhorn N, Kenemans P, Mortel R, Ohmi K, Bast RC, Ritts RE, Malkasian G. (1988). An initial analysis of pre operative serum CA 125 levels in patients with early stage ovarian carcinoma, Gynecol Oncol 30, 7-14.

Chapter 4

CURRENT DIAGNOSIS AND TREATMENT MODALITIES FOR OVARIAN CANCER

Peter E. Schwartz
Yale University School of Medicine, Department of Obstetrics and Gynecology
333 Cedar Street, New Haven, Connecticut 06520

1. INTRODUCTION

Ovarian cancer is the major pelvic cancer health hazard for women. In 2000, the American Cancer Society estimates that 23,100 new ovarian cancer cases will be diagnosed and 14,000 women will have died of ovarian cancer (1). It is the fifth most common cancer in American women but the fourth most common cause of cancer death (1). The high mortality rate is due in part to a lack of obvious early warning symptoms, unavailability of sensitive early detection techniques and therapy of limited effectiveness. Despite improvements in management of women with epithelial ovarian cancer, the overall survival for this disease has been unchanged for at least the last 20 years (2). This chapter will concentrate on advances in the diagnosis and management of epithelial ovarian cancers, the form of ovarian cancer that represents at least 90% of all ovarian malignancies.

2. DIAGNOSIS OF OVARIAN CANCER

The lack of obvious early warning symptoms has been a major hurdle in trying to identify ovarian cancer in an early stage when it is highly curable. Approximately 70% of women are not diagnosed with ovarian cancer until it is in an advanced stage of disease. In an international survey performed on women who have experienced ovarian cancer, 95% of 1725 women with the disease experienced symptoms (3). These symptoms included abdominal (77%), gastrointestinal (70%), pain (58%), constitutional (50%), urinary (34%) and vaginal (26%). Only 11% of Stage I and II patients and 3% of Stage III and IV patients reported no symptoms prior to their diagnosis. Women who ignored their symptoms were much more likely to have had advanced disease than those who did not. Fifty-five percent of the women had their diagnosis made within 3 months of seeing a health care provider, but 26% did not have the diagnosis made until 6 months after seeing the health provider and 11% went more than a year before the diagnosis was established. Delay in diagnosis was associated with omission of a pelvic examination at the first visit, having a multitude of symptoms, being initially diagnosed with no problems, depression, stress, irritable bowel or gastritis and not initially undergoing diagnostic imaging studies or CA-125 testing (3). Being of a younger age also delayed the diagnosis. However, the type of doctor seen initially, their insurance and specific symptoms did not correlate with the delay in diagnosis. Early detection may be possible if both women and their physicians carefully evaluate abdominal and pelvic symptoms. Nevertheless, the symptoms that most women experience are subtle. The persistence of symptoms for more than 2 weeks should lead to evaluation.

Major research efforts in the past seeking to identify a circulating tumor marker had led to the recognition that serum CA-125 is elevated in over 80% of women with advanced ovarian cancer (4). It is now well established that serial serum CA-125 determinations in women who have advanced ovarian cancer accurately reflect the impact of therapy on the patient. Rising CA-125 levels indicates ineffective treatment. Declining CA-125 levels are associated with objective responses (4). These observations subsequently led to the use of serum CA-125 determinations for screening women at high risk for ovarian cancer (5-7).

CA-125 is a glycoprotein with a molecular weight of over 200,000 Daltons. It has never been fully characterized in terms of its molecular structure. It is frequently elevated in benign gynecologic processes that occur in reproductive age women. These processes include, endometriosis, uterine leiomyoma, benign ovarian cysts and pelvic inflammatory disease (4). It is also elevated in the first trimester of pregnancy. It may be elevated from any cause of peritoneal, pleural or pericardial inflammation. Any cause for ascites such as hepatopathies, congestive heart failure or severe myxedema may be associated with elevations of CA-125. In addition, while 80% of ovarian cancers in the original clinical publication were found to be associated with elevated CA-125 levels, almost 60% of pancreatic cancers and 20-25% of all other solid tumors were also associated with elevated CA-125 (4). Nevertheless, CA-125 remains the best of all clinically available circulating markers for determining the presence of ovarian cancer.

Ovarian cancer early detection programs in the United States have routinely employed CA-125 as the circulating tumor marker of choice to try and identify early ovarian cancer (5-7). A prospective study in the United Kingdom has followed 22,000 women and has demonstrated that CA-125 determinations can be used to identify the presence of early ovarian cancer (8). However, most patients with early stage ovarian cancer did not have elevated CA-125 levels (8). Current data suggests that CA-125 is elevated in approximately one third of women with Stage I ovarian cancer, but is routinely elevated in the majority of patients with advanced stage disease.

Lysophosphatidic acid (LPA) has been identified in ascites fluid and now has been studied in the plasma of healthy women, women with benign gynecologic conditions and women with ovarian cancer (9). Xu, et al demonstrated elevated LPA levels in the plasma of 9 of 10 patients with Stage I ovarian cancer and all 24 women with Stage II, III and IV ovarian cancer as well as all 14 women with recurrent ovarian cancer (9). In turn serum CA-125 was only elevated in 2 of the 9 patients with Stage I ovarian cancer and in 26 of the 38 women who had advanced stage or recurrent disease. Unfortunately, LPA levels were also elevated in 4 of 17 (23.5%) women with benign gynecologic disease and in 5 of 48 (10.4%) control women. LPA may be more effective in identifying early stage ovarian cancer than CA-125. There remains a dramatic need to identify a more specific circulating marker for ovarian cancer.

Diagnostic imaging has been employed for the early detection of ovarian cancer. While a spectrum of new technologies is available, the single most cost-effective technique to screen women is endovaginal ultrasound with color Doppler flow (10). Advances in ultrasound technology now enable us to look directly at the ovary in a more sensitive fashion. Ultrasound determined morphology remains the most important finding with composite tumors, i.e. tumors containing both solid and cystic elements, being characteristic for ovarian cancer. The additional finding of ascites substantially increases the likelihood of an ovarian malignancy being present. Simple ovarian cysts are usually benign, although on occasion an ovarian tumor of borderline malignant potential may appear to be a simple cyst. Completely solid masses in teenagers may be associated with benign fibromas or fibrothecomas or with dysgerminomas. Solid tumors in postmenopausal women are usually fibromas or fibrothecomas. Unfortunately, virtually all studies using ultrasound technology have a high false positive rate often leading to surgery for benign conditions (11-13). DePriest and colleagues have been able to demonstrate early ovarian cancers in a series of postmenopausal women followed at the University of Kentucky Medical Center (14). The cost effectiveness of this approach has not been confirmed. Three-dimensional ultrasound is now becoming available. It is hoped that 3-dimensional ultrasound incorporating color Doppler flow technology may allow for early detection of clinically occult ovarian cancer.

Identification of precursors for epithelial ovarian cancers has yet to be accomplished. Much more research needs to be performed to identify such a lesion. Until technology enhances our ability to detect ovarian cancer, we must rely on clinical histories, physical examinations, CA-125 determinations and ultrasound evaluations to aid us in the early detection of ovarian cancer.

At present surgery remains the mainstay in the diagnosis, staging and initial treatment of ovarian cancer.

3. SURGERY FOR THE DIAGNOSIS OF OVARIAN CANCER

Women found to have pelvic masses suspicious for ovarian cancer based on physical examination, diagnostic imaging studies or CA-125 determination, should be placed on a preoperative bowel preparation so that aggressive surgery including intestinal resections may be safely performed. Surgery should be performed through a vertical midline or paramedian incision that can be extended into the upper abdomen in order to have access to the entire peritoneal cavity. Upon entering the abdominal cavity, any fluid present should be aspirated and sent for cytologic evaluation. If no fluid is present, peritoneal cytology should be obtained by irrigating the pelvis and the right and left paracolic spaces with approximately 100 cc of normal saline, aspirating the irrigant and submitting it for cytology and cell block analysis. The abdominal cavity should then be explored looking for any intraperitoneal abnormalities suggestive of metastatic disease. The pelvic and para-aortic retroperitoneum should be carefully palpated looking for enlarged lymph nodes. The patient should then undergo staging and surgical treatment as indicated below.

4. STAGING AND SURGICAL TREATMENT OF OVARIAN CANCER

The International Federation of Obstetricians and Gynecologists (FIGO) staging system for ovarian cancer is presented in Table 1. Patients with clinically early stage ovarian cancer, i.e. limited to one ovary (Stage I), may undergo limited surgery in selected cases. The minimum initial surgery for women who appear to have early ovarian cancer should include a unilateral salpingo-oophorectomy, and surgical staging that includes a wedge biopsy of the contralateral ovary, omentectomy, appendectomy, pelvic and periaortic lymph node sampling, biopsies of the peritoneum including the cul-de-sac, paracolic spaces and diaphragm and washings of the pelvis and paracolic spaces. It is the author's routine to obtain a frozen section evaluation of the involved ovary. If an epithelial cancer is confirmed, the patient wishes to preserve reproductive function and there is no obvious cancer elsewhere, it is appropriate to stage the patient surgically and await the final pathology report before deciding on additional therapy. For women in whom preservation of reproductive function is not an issue, it is wisest to remove both ovaries and the uterus, thereby eliminating a second site of occult disease, the

Table 1: International Federation of Gynecology and Obstetrics Staging for Carcinoma of the Ovary

Stage I	Growth limited to ovaries
Stage IA	Growth limited to one ovary; no ascites present containing malignant cells. No tumor on the external surface; capsule intact
Stage IB	Growth limited to both ovaries; no ascites present containing malignant cells. No tumor on the external; capsules intact.
Stage IC	Tumor classified as either Stage IA or IB but with tumor the surface of one or both ovaries; or with ruptured (s); or with ascites containing malignant cells present or with positive peritoneal washings.
Stage II	Growth involving one or both ovaries, with pelvic extension.
Stage IIA	Extension and/or metastases to the uterus and/or tubes.
Stage IIB	Extension to the other pelvic tissues.
Stage IIC	Tumor either Stage IIA or IIB but with tumor on the surface one or both ovaries; or with capsule(s) ruptured; or with ascites containing malignant cells present or with positive peritoneal washings.
Stage III	Tumor involving one or both ovaries with peritoneal implants outside the pelvis and/or positive retroperitoneal or inguinal nodes. Superficial liver metastasis equals Stage III. Tumor is limited to the true pelvis but with histologically proven malignant extension to small bowel or omentum.
Stage IIIA	Tumor grossly limited to the true pelvis negative nodes but with histologically confirmed microscopic seeding of abdominal peritoneal surfaces
Stage IIIB	Tumor of one or both ovaries with histologically confirmed implants of abdominal peritoneal surfaces none exceeding 2 cm in diameter; nodes are negative.
Stage IIIC	Abdominal implants greater than 2 cm in diameter and/or positive retroperitoneal or inguinal nodes.
Stage IV -	Growth involving one or both ovaries with distant metastases. If pleural effusion is present, there must be positive cytology findings to allot a case to Stage IV. Parenchymal liver metastasis equals Stage IV.

Int J Gynecol Oncol 1989;28:189-190

contralateral ovary, and a large peritoneal surface, the uterus. Laparoscopic surgery is now being employed for surgical staging of women with early ovarian cancer (15). The surgical skills necessary to perform laparoscopic omentectomies and para-aortic lymphaden-ectomies of necessity will limit this approach to a few centers at least for the immediate future.

Surgery for bilateral ovarian cancer, or disease that has spread beyond the ovaries, should be aggressive cytoreductive surgery that includes removing both ovaries, the fallopian tubes and the uterus, a complete omentectomy, periaortic and pelvic lymph node sampling and an aggressive effort to remove all visible or palpable lesions in the abdominal cavity or in the retroperitoneal spaces. The rationale for cytoreductive surgery is based on empiric results originally described by Griffiths, *et al* (16). Their observations and many others support the concept that the less the volume of residual tumor left at the initial surgery, the greater the chances of the patients having prolonged survival and possibly being cured (17). Optimal cytoreductive surgery is leaving no gross residual tumor behind at the initial operation. Whether one leaves 1 cm or 3 cm maximum diameter of residual tumor has little impact in overall survival compared to that of no residual tumor (18-20). Ovarian cancer spreads locally, intraperitoneally and through lymphatic spaces. It has not routinely spread hematogenously at the time of diagnosis. Cytoreductive surgery may be accomplishable because the tumor will usually be confined to the abdominal cavity and/or the retroperitoneal spaces. No prospective randomized trials exist comparing cytoreductive surgery to non-cytoreductive surgery as part of the management of ovarian cancer. It is possible that women who can be successfully cytoreduced surgically represent a subgroup of women with less virulent tumor. Cytoreductive surgery can be aided using the ultrasonic aspirator, the argon beam coagulator or loop electrical excision to eliminate diffuse seedings or multiple small implants at the time of the initial surgery (21-23). A recent report failed to prove the hypothesis that cytoreductive surgery in patients with Stage III disease followed by platinum-based combination chemotherapy would allow patients presenting with large-volume ovarian cancer who were optimally cytoreduced to have the same chance for survival as patients initially found to have only small-volume ($\leq$ 1 cm) disease in the upper abdomen (24). Patients found to have extra-pelvic disease of 1 cm or less had a better recurrence-free interval and survival than those patients with large volume disease who were cytoreduced to disease of 1 cm or less (24). The value of systematic pelvic and para-aortic lymphadenectomy compared to lymph node sampling is now being evaluated (25,26).

5. MANAGEMENT OF BORDERLINE MALIGNANT POTENTIAL TUMORS OF THE OVARY

Borderline malignant potential tumors of the ovary are unusual in that they have the ability to metastasize yet are very effectively managed by surgery alone. Numerous series have confirmed that surgical management of this disease is overwhelmingly successful (27,28). A Yale University experience demonstrated that out of 95 consecutive patients treated, only 5 women died from borderline malignant potential tumors of the ovary (27). Two patients died from the complications of chemotherapeutic treatments rather than from the disease itself. Patients with borderline tumors who are routinely treated with additional therapy, usually in the form of chemotherapy, either have gross residual tumor left at the initial operation or have evidence of invasive metastases (29). The latter are rarely diagnosed and remain ill-defined by pathologic standards. Regrettably, there is no evidence demonstrating that chemotherapy treatment is effective in the management of borderline malignant potential tumors with invasive metastases. A clinical management problem that does arise is that borderline malignant potential tumors may be initially treated by ovarian cystectomy as the surgeon was not considering that an excised cyst had malignant potential. In this circumstance, Lim-Tan, et al have demonstrated that ovarian malignancies containing multiple cysts with borderline malignant potential tumors and that have a positive margin, i.e., the raw area where the ovarian cyst was separated from the underlying ovarian stroma, are at the greatest risk for recurrence (30). Microscopic foci of minimally invasive cancer have been identified in borderline malignant potential tumors of the ovary (31). These findings have the same clinical implications as finding pure borderline malignant potential tumors alone.

6. POSTOPERATIVE MANAGEMENT LIMITED INVASIVE CANCERS (STAGES I AND II)

Ahmed, et al have followed 194 women with invasive stage I ovarian cancer for a median time of 54 months (range 15-83) without administering adjuvant therapy (32). The relapse rate at 5 years for stage IA, IB, and IC disease was 12.8%, 34.7%, and 38.1% respectively. The survival rate at 5 years for patients with stage IA disease was 93.7%, for those with IB disease 92%, and for those with IC disease, 84% (32). A univariate analysis revealed the histologic grade, the presence of ascites, and the presence of surface ovarian tumor were significant independent prognostic factors. No factors reached statistical significance on multivariate analysis. Intra-operative rupture of tumor did not have a negative impact on survival. The data suggested a role for adjuvant therapy in women with grade 3 tumors or stage IC disease due to ascites or positive peritoneal washings. Young, *et. al* presented a series where Stage IA and IB, grade 1 and 2 patients were managed with surgery only or were randomized to receive melphalan (33). There was no difference in survival between the observation only and the melphalan treated group. Similar studies have been reported by other investigators (34). It would appear that adjuvant therapy in patients with these early lesions (without ascites) may be unnecessary except for women with clear cell carcinomas (33,34).

The Gynecologic Oncology Group randomized 204 patients to receive either intraperitoneal ^{32}P or three cycles of cis-platinum and cyclophosphamide chemotherapy (35). No statistical difference was recognized between the two groups (5-year survival 76% vs. 83% respectively). Bollis, *et al* randomized 85 patients with stage IA and IB, grade 2 or 3 to cisplatin or no further treatment, in one trial, and randomized 161 patients with Stage IC disease in another trial to cisplatin or intraperitoneal ^{32}P therapy (36). Cisplatin reduced the relapse rate by 65% in the first trial, and by 61% in the second. Survival was not significantly different, as those women who develop recurrences after adjuvant cisplatin almost always died of disease. Colombo, *et al* have reported on 56 stage I ovarian cancers treated with conservative surgery, i.e. unilateral salpingo-oophorectomy (37). Twelve women received cisplatin therapy. Two of 38 (5.3%) stage IA disease women recurred and died. Seventeen women desiring to procreate have had 26 pregnancies, resulting in 16 healthy babies, two ectopic pregnancies, four spontaneous abortions and four elective terminations.

7. POSTOPERATIVE MANAGEMENT OF ADVANCED INVASIVE CANCERS (STAGE III AND IV)

Survival for patients with advanced stage disease has significantly improved with the introduction of modern combination chemotherapy. Prior to that experience, women with advanced stage disease treated with surgery with or without additional radiation therapy had a 20 to 25 percent one year survival and virtually all patients succumbed by 5 years following diagnosis (38). In the current era, patient receiving cisplatin-based chemotherapy for advanced stage ovarian cancer have a 50 percent two year survival in most series (18-20). Unfortunately, the five-year survival for advanced disease is only about 20 percent at best. Patients with advanced disease most likely to be alive and disease-free at five years are those who had undergone complete surgical debulking (18-20). Other factors that significantly influence survival in multivariant analysis are the patient's age and performance status (18). Extremely poor results with stage IV disease has been well documented from studies from the Yale-New Haven Medical Center, M.D. Anderson Cancer

Center and the Brigham and Women's Hospital, but have been disputed by others (19, 39-43).

The modern chemotherapy era began in 1979 when cisplatin became available for routine use in ovarian cancer management. It very quickly became obvious that there were four drugs extremely important in the management of advanced ovarian cancer, cisplatin, adriamycin, cyclophosphamide and hexamethylmelamine. Adding one drug to cisplatin combination regimens was as effective as adding multiple drugs to these regimens. Cisplatin is highly emetogenic and is association with nephropathies and neuropathies at high doses. During the 1980's, the combination of cisplatin and cyclophosphamide became the routine combination of choice for managing women with advanced ovarian cancer (44). Carboplatin replaced cisplatin in the standard chemotherapy for ovarian cancer because of equivalency in efficacy but less toxicity (45,46). In general, patients received six cycles of combination therapy given every three to four weeks and were then reassessed to determine whether ovarian cancer was present. Reassessment included CT scans, CA 125 determinations and physical examinations. Attempts to demonstrate that longer treatment produces better overall results remain controversial (47,48). McGuire, et al has reported that modest increases in dose intensity, i.e. doubling cisplatin and cyclophosphamide doses from 50 and 500 mg to 100 and 1000 mg respectively, had no impact on patient outcome except for increasing toxicity (49).

A Gynecologic Oncology Group (GOG) study indicated that paclitaxel (Taxol) in combination with cisplatin gives superior results to that of cyclophosphamide in combination with cisplatin in women previously untreated with advanced stage III or IV disease (50). Advanced stage disease was defined as having residual tumor greater than 1 cm in maximum diameter. In that series of 386 eligible patients, women treated with paclitaxel and cisplatin had an 18.0 month median duration of progression-free interval whereas those women treated with cyclophosphamide and cisplatin had a 13 month median duration of progression-free interval ($p<0.001$). The overall survival for the women receiving paclitaxel and cisplatin was significantly longer (median 38 vs. 24 months, $p<0.001$,) but treatment appears to be palliative for the majority of women who receive it. A follow-up GOG study comparing higher dose cisplatin alone to higher dose paclitaxel alone and to the combination of cisplatin and paclitaxel revealed median survivals of 30.2, 26.0 and 26.6 months respectively with the highest toxicity in the cisplatin alone group (51). Unanswered questions remain about the optimum dose of paclitaxel per cycle and the optimum time of infusion (52). Carboplatin and paclitaxel has now become the standard therapy for the treatment of advanced ovarian cancer, in the United States.

8. CA-125 MONITORING

The tumor marker CA 125 has been very important in helping clinicians to assess ovarian cancer treatment success or failure. Regrettably failure is often easier to diagnose quickly than success. Women who fail to normalize their CA 125 level to below 35 U/mL in three months or have a CA 125 half-life of greater than 12 days, almost invariably will fail initial combination chemotherapy for ovarian cancer (53).

9. SECOND LOOK SURGERY

Second-look surgery was introduced in ovarian cancer management as a research technique to identify women with occult disease so that treatment could be changed (54). Unfortunately, in the original reports, only a 6.8% objective (complete and partial) response rate occurred with second-line chemotherapy treatment (55). The introduction of cisplatin yielded a 25% objective response rate but cisplatin was promptly moved up to become a first-line agent. Thus, women who undergo second-look surgery should be aware that the surgery itself may tell us that cancer is present but the surgery may have little or no impact on survival (56). If disease is found to be present and can be completely removed, patients appear to experience a better overall survival than those in whom tumor is present but is not able to be resected (54). A false-negative result ranging from 10 to 50 percent has been reported with negative second-look operations (57). CA 125 levels when elevated, have been routinely (>90%) associated with positive second-look operations. Unfortunately, when CA 125 levels have normalized, approximately 40 to 60 percent of women have persistent ovarian cancer at second-look surgery.

Casey, et al reported on 76 patients undergoing second-look laparoscopy and compared their results to 86 undergoing second-look laparotomies (58). Eleven percent of patients had their laparoscopies converted to laparotomies. The detection rate of persistent disease for patients undergoing second-look procedures was similar, 52.6% vs. 53.6%, as was the recurrence rate of 7 patients in each group. Laparoscopy was significantly less expensive due to shorter operating times and hospitalizations (58).

The approach to second-look surgery at the Yale-New Haven Medical Center is as follows. Women who have completed first-line chemotherapy have serum tumor markers drawn and undergo a CT scan and complete physical examination. If the CT scan is negative, the serum tumor markers are normal, the physical examination is normal and the patient is asymptomatic, the patient is followed without second-look surgery. Patients with stage I and II disease have a low incidence of positive second-look operations such that there is little purpose to performing the surgery. Patients who had stage IV disease almost invariably die of the cancer regardless of the second-look findings. Patients with stage III, grade 1 tumors that were completely cytoreduced, also have a very low incidence of positive findings at second-look surgery. Second-look surgery plays its greatest role in patients with stage III, grade 2 and grade 3 tumors with or without residual disease left at the initial operation. This group frequently will recur despite the patients being clinically free of disease. This is the group for whom second-look surgery is recommended and experimental second-line treatment is given if disease is present at surgery.

10. NEW APPROACHES TO TREATING ADVANCED AND REFRACTORY OVARIAN CANCER

Dose intensification regimens have recently become popularized as a result of work in part by Levin and Hryniuk, who demonstrated a relationship between the cisplatin dose and the response in terms of median survival for women with epithelial ovarian cancers (59). Two studies have looked at 50 versus 100 mg/m^2 of cisplatin in combination with cyclophosphamide. In a European study, the 100 mg/m^2 treated patients did significantly better, but they experienced greater toxicity, leading the investigators to recommend 75 mg/^{2} as the standard dose of cisplatin (60). However, a GOG study demonstrated no difference in survival between those treated with 50 and 100 mg/m^2 (61). In a prospective randomized trial 117 patients received carboplatin at an area under the concentration time curve (AUC) of 6 for 6 courses and 110 patients received carboplatin at an AUC of 12 (62). No difference in progression-free survival was noted. The overall survival at 5 years was 31% and 34% respectively. Significantly more toxicity was encountered in patients receiving carboplatin at an AUC of 12.

Hematologic toxicity may be ameliorated using granulocyte colony-stimulating factor (63). However, as doses of medications become higher, non-hematologic toxicities become manifest and are dose-limiting. These toxicities include nephropathies and neuropathies. Cisplatin and carboplatin combination therapy has also been assessed with or without either cyclophosphamide or with or without ifosfamide (64,65). It would appear that the response rates are similar to that seen with cisplatin-based chemotherapy using conventional doses in combination with cyclophosphamide. However, as one increases the number of agent, toxicities become dose limiting.

High dose chemotherapy with hematologic rescue in patients with previously untreated Stage III and IV ovarian cancer has been reported by Legros, et al (66). The investigators used autologous bone marrow transplantation (ABMT) or peripheral-blood stem cells (PBSC) to overcome myelosuppression. High dose melphalan (140 mg/m^2) was used in 23 patients and high dose carboplatin (140 mg/m²/d on days 1 to 4) and cyclophosphamide (1.6 G/m² on days 1-4) was used in 30 patients. The best results were achieved in 19 patients with pathologic complete responses at second-look surgery. They had a 74.2% 5-year overall survival and a 32.8% 5-year disease-free survival.

Aghajanian, *et al* have reported on high dose Taxol in combination with high dose carboplatin for 3 cycles and then one cycle of high dose melphalan for women with previously untreated Stage IIC-IV epithelial ovarian cancers (67). These investigators concluded that high dose chemotherapy regimens should be limited to research protocols in women who underwent optimum cytoreductive surgery at their initial surgery. Twelve of 22 (55%) patients had a pathologic complete response at second-look surgery and 6 of 22 (27%) had a surgical partial response in this series (67). However, only 3 of 15 (20%) suboptimally debulked patients had a pathologic complete response and none of the Stage IV patients achieved a pathologic complete response.

It is now recognized that management of cisplatin failures should be assessed in terms of when they occur in relation to the initial cisplatin chemotherapy regimen. Women who fail cisplatin-based chemotherapy while on the cisplatin chemotherapy are considered platinum refractory. Those who fail within a six months period of time following completion of the chemotherapy are platinum resistant (68). Those who failed cisplatin-based combination chemotherapy more than six months following completion of the cisplatin or carboplatin regimens can often be successfully retreated with these same agents and are considered platinum-sensitive (69). Stiff, *et al* reported on 100 consecutive women treated with high dose chemotherapy and with ABMT for persistent/relapsed ovarian cancer (70). The median progression-free and overall survivals were only 7 and 13 months respectively. The most important prognostic factors were patient age, bulk of tumor at transplant and platinum sensitivity.

Topotecan, a topoisomerase-1 inhibitor, has shown modest activity in patients who have failed cisplatin and paclitaxel therapy (71,72). These studies reported 13% and 14% objective rates respectively. Topotecan was more effective than paclitaxel in a second randomized study that used these agents as single agents following failure of one platinum-based regimen for ovarian cancer (72). The objective response rate for topotecan in patients previously treated with platinum-based chemotherapy was enhanced to 38% when the topotecan was given in a 21 day infusion (73). Topotecan was active in platinum resistant, refractory and sensitive tumors.

Vinorelbine has been reported to have a 21% objective response rate in a population of heavily pretreated and platinum-resistant ovarian cancer patients (74). Lonidamine potentiated cisplatin responses in 27 women previously treated with cisplatin resulting in objective responses in 5 of 18 (28%) platinum refractory or resistant patients and 5 of 9 (55%) late-relapse patients (75). Muggia, *et al* reported 9 clinical responses to liposomal doxorubicin (Doxil) in 35 patients (25.7%) who had failed platinum and paclitaxel regimens for ovarian cancer (76). The median progression-free survival was 5.6 months. Gemcitabine, a fluorinated derivative of cytarabine has been shown to have an objective response rate of 16-20% in recurrent ovarian cancer (77).

11. SECONDARY DEBULKING SURGERY

Secondary debulking surgery has recently been reassessed. Secondary debulking surgery is infrequently curative (78,79). However, prolonged survival can be achieved in some patients who have large persistent ovarian cancer that can be surgically cytoreduced. This is particularly true if the time from completion of the initial treatment to recurrence is greater than one year (78). Secondary cytoreductive surgery does not improve the results of ineffective initial cytoreductive surgery. Rather, it improves the results of that seen when no secondary cytoreductive surgery is performed. This surgery is palliative for the overwhelming majority of women.

Van der Burg, *et al* published the results of a prospective randomized trial for women with advanced ovarian cancer who had a maximum residual tumor >1 cm diameter at completion of initial surgery (80). All patients received three cycles of cyclophosphamide and cisplatin therapy. All patients (319) with objective responses or stable disease were then randomized to secondary debulking surgery or no surgery followed by three more cycles of chemotherapy. Sixty-five percent of the surgical patients had disease >1 cm at secondary surgery and 45 percent were cytoreduced to <1 cm. The progression-free and overall survival were statistically longer (p=0.01) in the group undergoing surgery. The difference in median survival was six months. In an update, the 5-year survival was 23% for the surgery group and 12% for the non-surgery group (80). The 5-year progression-free survival was 12% and 4.5% respectively.

12. INTRAPERITONEAL CHEMOTHERAPY

Intraperitoneal chemotherapy was popularized a decade ago as a method to deliver high dose chemotherapy directly to the tumor while minimizing systemic side effects (81). The ideal drug for this approach has a high peritoneal to plasma drug exposure ratio, a steep dose responsive relationship, does not irritate the peritoneum and is not cross-resistant with other drugs (81). Cisplatin was the first drug to be shown to be appropriate in the management of ovarian cancer by the intraperitoneal route. However, intraperitoneal chemotherapy should be limited to women who are optimally surgically debulked. Markman has evaluated reasons for intraperitoneal chemotherapy failure in women who are optimally cytoreduced to less than 1 to 2 cm of residual tumor (82). These reasons include diffuse intra-abdominal carcinomatosis, progressive disease while receiving initial cisplatin-based chemotherapy, the presence of extensive intra-abdominal adhesions that preclude adequate intra-abdominal distribution and disease in a non-accessible site such as the liver or lymph nodes (79).

A phase III prospective randomized trial comparing intraperitoneal cisplatin and Etoposide to intravenous cisplatin and cyclophosphamide failed to demonstrate any difference in survival between the two treatment arms with a median follow-up of 46 months (range 21-70 months) (83). A prospective randomized trial for patients with optimally cytoreduced advanced ovarian cancer compared 276 women who received intravenous cyclophosphamide and cisplatin to 263 women who received intraperitoneal cisplatin and intravenous cyclophosphamide (84). A statistical survival advantage (P=0.03) was achieved by the intraperitoneal chemotherapy treated patients as their median survival was 49 months (95% CI 43-55) compared to 41 months (95% CI 34-47) for those receiving intravenous chemotherapy.

13. IMMUNOTHERAPY

Other techniques that have shown promise in managing refractory ovarian cancer include intraperitoneal administration of autologous lymphokine-activated killer cells and intraperitoneal administration of tumor directed antibodies conjugated to toxins or radioisotopes (85-87). Only very preliminary results are available for these techniques. They may represent effective treatment in the future. Intraperitoneal recombinant interferon gamma demonstrated a 23% complete response rate among 98 assessable patients who received this treatment following documentation of residual disease at second-look surgery (88). In a study of intraperitoneal interferon α, 7 of 25 (28%) patients with platinum-sensitive tumors and minimum residual disease (<0.5 cm) at second-look laparotomy demonstrated objective responses (4 complete, 3 partial) while none of 21 platinum-resistant tumors responded to this treatment (89). In a second study intraperitoneal α interferon was given in an alternate sequential fashion with intraperitoneal cisplatin in women with residual disease (<0.5 cm) at second-look laparotomy (90). Five of 18 (28%) patients had a pathologic response.

14. NEOADJUVANT THERAPY

An approach currently being evaluated at the Yale-New Haven Medical Center is neoadjuvant chemotherapy for patients who (a) by diagnostic imaging techniques, have intra-abdominal carcinomatosis compatible with ovarian cancer that routinely would not be resectable to less than 2 cm residual tumor or are medically debilitated and unable to tolerate cytoreductive surgery and (b) have, by fine needle aspiration or cytologic techniques, disease compatible with an epithelial ovarian cancer (91). No difference in overall survival or progression-free survival was observed in 59 consecutive women with advanced malignancies compatible with ovarian cancer treated with neoadjuvant chemotherapy when compared to 206 consecutive women with Stage IIIC and IV epithelial ovarian cancers who underwent cytoreductive surgery followed by platinum-based combination chemotherapy (92). Similar results have recently been reported by Surwit, *et. al* (93). It is the author's opinion that women with findings compatible with non-cytoreducible, advanced stage III disease or stage IV ovarian cancer do better subjectively with neoadjuvant chemotherapy than with inadequate cytoreductive surgery followed by the same chemotherapy. The European Organization for Research and Treatment of Cancer has activated a protocol that will randomize 740 women to receive either conventional or neoadjuvant chemotherapy.

15. GENE THERAPY

Advances in molecular biology have led to the development of gene therapy approaches for treatment of women with epithelial ovarian cancers (94). The trials are currently in Phase 1 and employed in patients with recurrent disease. Trial strategies include the use of herpes simplex virus thymidine kinase (HSV-TK) gene followed by exposure to the antiviral drug ganciclovir which subsequently is converted into a triphosphate form leading to cell death. Other approaches include the injection of *in vitro* interluken-2(IL-2) gene modified ovarian cancer cells, tumor infiltrating lymphocytes using a chimeric antibody/T-cell receptor gene and an anti-erbB-2 fragment gene in patients with erbB-2 expressing ovarian cancers (94).

REFERENCES

1. Landis SH, Murray T, Bolden S, et al. Cancer statistics, 2000. CA Cancer J Clin 2000; 50: 8-13.
2. Yanik R. Ovarian cancer: Age contrasts in incidence, histology, disease stage at diagnosis and mortality. Cancer 1993; 71:517-523.
3. Goff BA, Mandel LS, Muntz HG, Melancon CH. Ovarian cancer diagnosis: Results of a National Ovarian Cancer Survey. Gynecol Oncol 2000; 76:231.
4. Bast RC Jr, Klug TJ, St John E, et al. A radioimmunoassay using a monoclonal antibody to monitor the course of epithelial ovarian cancer. N Engl J Med 1983; 309:883-7
5. Schwartz PE, Chambers JT, Taylor KJW, et al. Early detection of ovarian cancer: background, rationale and structure of the Yale Early Detection Program. Yale J Biol Med 1991; 64:557-71.

114

6. Karlan BY, Raffel LJ, Crvenkovic G, et al. A multidisciplinary approach to the early detection of ovarian carcinoma: rationale, protocol design and early results. Am J Obstet Gynecol 1993; 169:494-501.

7. Muto M, Cramer DW, Brown DL, et al. Screening for ovarian cancer: the preliminary experience of a familial ovarian cancer center. Gynecol Oncol 1993; 51:12-20.

8. Jacobs I, Davies AP, Bridges J, et al. Prevalence screening for ovarian cancer in postmenopausal women by CA-125 measurement and ultrasonography. BMJ 1993; 306:1030-4.

9. Xu Y, Shen Z, Wiper D, et al. Lysophosphatidic acid as a potential biomarker for ovarian and other gynecologic cancers. JAMA 1998; 280:719-723.

10. Taylor KJW, Schwartz PE. Screening for early ovarian cancer. Radiology 1994; 192:1-10.

11. Campbell S, Bhan V, Royston P, et al. Transabdominal ultrasound screening for ovarian cancer. BMJ 1989; 299:1363-7.

12. Campbell S, Bourne T, Bradley E. Screening for ovarian cancer by transvaginal sonography and colour Doppler. Eur J Obstet Gynecol Reprod Biol 1992; 49:33-34.

13. Van Nagell JR, Higgins RV, Donaldson ES, et al. Transvaginal sonography as a screening method for ovarian cancer: a report of the first 1000 cases screened. Cancer 1990; 65:573-7.

14. DePriest PD, Gallion HM, Paulik EJ, Kryscio RJ, Van Nagell JR Jr. Transvaginal sonography as a screening method for the detection of early ovarian cancer. Gynecol Oncol 1997; 65:408-417.

15. Childers JM, Lang J, Surwit EA, Hatch KO. Laparoscopic surgical staging of ovarian cancer. Gynecol Oncol 1995; 59:25-33.

16. Griffiths CT. Surgical resection of tumor bulk in the primary treatment of ovarian cancer. Mongr Natl Cancer Inst. 1975; 45:101-104.

17. Hoskins WJ. Surgical staging and cytoreduction surgery of epithelial ovarian cancer. Cancer 1993; 71:1534-40.

18. Shelley WE, Carmichael JC, Brown LB, et al. Adriamycin and cis-platinum in the treatment of stage III and IV epithelial ovarian cancer. Gynecol Oncol 1988; 29:208-221.

19. Schwartz PE, Chambers JT, Kohorn EI, Chambers SK, Weitzman H, Voynick M, MacLusky N, Naftolin F. Tamoxifen in combination chemotherapy with cytotoxic chemotherapy in advanced epithelial ovarian cancer: A prospective randomized trial. Cancer 1989; 63:1074-1078.

20. Le T, Krepart GV, Lotocki RJ, Hewood MS. Does debulking surgery improve survival in biologically aggressive ovarian cancer? Gynecol Oncol 1997; 67:208-14.

21. Adelson MD. Cytoreduction of diaphragmatic metastases using the Cavitron ultrasound surgical aspirator. Gynecologic Oncol 1991; 41: 220-222.

22. Farghaly SA. Surgical techniques for cytoreduction in advanced ovarian malignancy. Am J Obstet Gynecol 1993; 168:736.

23. Fanning J, Hilgers RO. Loop electrical excision procedure for intensified cytoreduction of ovarian cancer. Gynecol Oncol 1995; 57:188-90.

24. Hoskins WJ, Bundy BN, Thigpen JT, Omura GA. The influence of cytoreductive surgery on recurrence-free interval and survival in small-volume stage III epithelial ovarian cancer: A Gynecologic Oncology Group Study. Gynecol Oncol 1992; 47:56-166.

25. Scarabelli C, Gallo A, Zarrellia, Visentin C, Campagnutta E. Systematic pelvic and para-aortic lymphadenectomy during cytoreductive surgery in advanced ovarian cancer: Potential benefit on survival. Gynecol Oncol 1995; 56:328-37.

26. Hacker NF. Systematic pelvic and para-aortic lymphadenectomy for advanced ovarian cancer-therapeutic advance or surgical folly? Gynecol Oncol 1995; 56:325-7.

27. Chambers JT, Merino MJ, Kohorn EI, Schwartz PE. Borderline ovarian tumors. Am J Obstet Gynecol 1988; 159:1088-1094.

28. Kaern J, Trope CG, Abeler V. A retrospective study of 370 borderline tumors of the ovary treated at the Norwegian Radium Hospital 1970-1982. A review of clinico-pathological features and treatment modalities. Cancer 1993; 71:1810-20.

29. Bell DA, Weinstock MA, Scully RE. Peritoneal implants of ovarian serous borderline tumors: Histologic features and prognosis. Cancer 1988; 62:2212-22.

30. Lim-Tan SK, Cajigas HB, Scully RE. Ovarian cystectomy for serous borderline tumors. A follow-up study of 35 cases. Obstet Gynecol 1988; 72:775-80.

31. Bell DA, Scully RE. Ovarian serous borderline tumors with stromal microinvasion: A report of 21 cases. Hum Path 1990; 21:397-403.

32. Ahmed FY, Wiltshaw E, A'Hern RP, et al. Natural history and prognosis of untreated stage I epithelial ovarian cancer. J Clin Oncol 1996; 14:2968-2975.

33. Young RC, Walton LA, Ellenberg SS, et al. Adjuvant therapy in stage I and stage II epithelial ovarian cancer: Results of two prospective randomized trials. N Engl J Med 1990; 322:1021-7.

34. Monga M, Carmichael JA, Shelley WE, et al. Surgery without adjuvant chemotherapy for early epithelial ovarian carcinoma after comprehensive surgical staging. Gynecol Oncol 1991; 43:195-197.

35. Young RC, Brady MF, Nieberg RM, et al. Randomized clinical trial of adjuvant treatment of women with early (FIGO I-IIA high risk) ovarian cancer. Int J. Gynecol Cancer 1997; 7 (suppl 2):17.

36. Bolis G, Colombo N, Pecorelli S, et al. Adjuvant treatment for early epithelial ovarian cancer: results of two randomized clinical trials comparing cisplatin to no further treatment or chromic phosphate. Ann Oncol 1995; 6:887-893.

37. Columbo N, Chiari S, Maggioni A, Bocciolone E, Torri V, Mangioni C. Controversial issues in the management of early ovarian cancer: Conservative surgery and role of adjuvant therapy. Gynecol Oncol 1994; 55:S47-51.

38. Kaufman RJ. Management of advanced ovarian carcinoma. Med Clinics N. Amer 1966; 50:845-856.

39. Wharton JT, Edward CL, Rutledge FN. Long-term survival after chemotherapy for advanced epithelial ovarian carcinoma. AM J Obstet Gynecol 1984; 148:997- .

40. Goodman HM, Harlow BL, Sheets EE, et al. The role of cytoreductive surgery in the management of stage IV epithelial ovarian carcinoma. Gynecol Oncol 1992; 46:367-71.

41. Liu P, Benjamin I, Morgan M, et al. Effect of surgical debulking on survival in Stage IV ovarian cancer. Gynecol Oncol 1997; 64:4-8.

42. Curtin JP, Malik R, Venkatraman ES, Barakat RR, Hoskins WJ. Stage IV ovarian cancer: impact of surgical debulking. Gynecol Oncol 1997; 64:9-12.

43. Munkarah AR, Hallum AV III, Morris M, et al. Prognostic significance of residual disease in patients with Stage IV epithelial ovarian cancer. Gynecol Oncol 1997; 64:13-17.

44. Omura GA, Bundy BN, Berek JS, Curry S, Delgado G, Mortel R. Randomized trial of cyclophosphamide plus cisplatin with or without doxorubicin in ovarian carcinoma: A Gynecologic Group study. 1989; 7:457-65.

45. Alberts DS, Green S, Hannigan EV, et al. Improved therapeutic index of carboplatin plus cyclophosphamide versus cisplatin plus cyclophosphamide: Final report by the Southern Oncology Group of a phase III randomized trial in stage III and IV ovarian cancer. J Clin Oncol 1992;10:706-17.[Erratum, J Clin Oncol 1992; 10:1505.]

46. Swenerton K, Jeffrey J, Stuart G, et al. Cisplatin-cyclophosphamide versus carboplatin-cyclophosphamide in advanced ovarian cancer: A randomized phase III study of the National Cancer Institute of Canada Clinical Trial Group. J Clin Oncol 1992; 10:718-26.

47. Bertelsen K, Jakobsen A, Stroyer I, et al. A prospective randomized comparison of 6 and 12 cycles of cyclophosphamide, adriamycin and cisplatin in advanced epithelial ovarian cancer: A Danish Ovarian Study Group trial (DACOVA). Gynecol Oncol 1993; 49:30-36.

48. Hakes TB, Chalas E, Hoskins WJ, et al. Randomized prospective trial of 5 versus 10 cycles of cyclophosphamide, doxorubicin and cisplatin in advanced ovarian carcinoma. Gynecol Oncol 1992; 42:284-289.

49. McGuire WP, Hoskins WJ, Brady MF, et al. Assessment of dose-intensive therapy in suboptimally debulked ovarian cancer: A Gynecologic Oncology Group study. J Clin Oncol 1995; 13:1589-1599.

50. McGuire WP, Hoskins WJ, Brady MF, et al. Cyclophosphamide and cisplatin compared with paclitaxel and cisplatin in patients with stage III and IV ovarian cancer. N Engl J Med 1996; 334:1-6.

51. Muggia FM. Braly PS, Sutton G, et al. Phase III of cisplatin (P) or paclitaxel (T) versus their combination in suboptimal Stager III and IV epithelial ovarian cancer (EOC). Gynecologic Oncology Group study #132. Proc ASCO 1997; 16:352a.

52. Eisenhauer EE, Ten Bokkel-Huinink WW, Swenerton KD, et al. European-Canadian randomized trial of paclitaxel in relapsed ovarian cancer: High dose versus low-dose and long versus short infusion. J Clin Oncol 1994; 12:2654-2666.

53. Rosman M, Hayden CL, Thiel RP, Chambers S, Chambers J, Kohorn EI, Schwartz PE. Prognostic indicators for poor risk epithelial ovarian cancer. Cancer 1994; 74:1323-28.

54. Schwartz PE, Smith JP. Second-look operations in ovarian cancer. Am J Obstet Gynecol 1980; 138:1124-1130.

55. Stanhope CR, Smith JP, Rutledge F. Second trial drugs in ovarian cancer. Gynecol Oncol 1977; 5:52-8.

56. Chambers SK, Chambers JT, Kohorn EI, Lawrence R, Schwartz PE. Evaluation of the role of second-look surgery in ovarian cancer. Obstet Gynecol 1988; 72:404-408.

57. Rubin SC, Hoskins WJ, Saigo PE, et al. Prognostic factors for recurrence following negative second-look laparotomy in ovarian cancer patients treated with platinum-based chemotherapy. Gynecol Oncol 1991; 42:137-41.

58. Casey AC, Farias-Eisner R, Pisani AL, et al. What is the role of reassessment laparoscopy in the management of gynecologic cancers in 1995? Gynecol Oncol 1996; 60:454-461.

59. Levin L, Hryniuk WM. Dose intensity analysis of chemotherapy regimens in ovarian carcinoma. J. Clin Oncol 1987; 5:756-67.

60. Kaye SB, Paul J, Cassidy CR, et al. Mature results of a randomized trial of two doses of cisplatin for the treatment of ovarian cancer. J Clin Oncol 1996; 14:2113-2119.

61. McGuire WP. Primary treatment of epithelial ovarian malignancies. Cancer 1993; 71:1541-50.

62. Gore M, Mainwaring P, A'Hern R, et al. Randomized trial of dose-intensity with single-agent carboplatin in patients with epithelial ovarian cancer. J Clin Oncol 1998; 16:2426-2434.

63. Sarosy G, Kohn E, Stone DA, et al. Phase I study of Taxol and granulocyte colony-stimulating factor in patients with refractory ovarian cancer. J Clin Oncol 1992; 10:1165-1170.

64. Lund B, Hansen M, Hansen OP, Hansen HH. High-dose platinum consisting of combined carboplatin and cisplatin in previously untreated ovarian cancer patients with residual disease. J Clin Oncol 1989; 7:1469-73.

65. Lund B, Hansen M, Hansen OP, Hansen HH. Combined high-dose carboplatin and cisplatin and ifosfamide in previously untreated ovarian cancer patients with residual disease. J Clin Oncol 1990; 8:1226-30.

66. Legros M, Dauplat J, Fleury J, et al. High-dose chemotherapy with hematopoietic rescue in patients with stage III to IV ovarian cancer: long-term results. J Clin Oncol 1997; 15:1302-8.

67. Aghajanian C, Fennelly D, Shapiro F, et al. Phase II study of "dose-dense" high-dose chemotherapy treatment with peripheral-blood progenitor-cell support as primary treatment for patients with advanced ovarian cancer. J Clin Oncol 1998; 16:1852.

68. Markman M, Rothman R, Hakes T, Reichman B, Hoskins W, Rubin S, Jones W, Almandrone's L, Lewis JL, Jr. Second-line platinum therapy in patients with ovarian cancer previously treated with cisplatin. J Clin Oncol 1991; 9:389-93.

69. Thigpen JT, Vance RB, Khansur T. Second-line chemotherapy for recurrent carcinoma of the ovary. Cancer 1993; 71:1559-64.

70. Stiff PJ, Bayer R, Kerger C, et al. High-dose chemotherapy with autologous transplantation for persistent/relapsed ovarian cancer: a multivariate analysis of survival for 100 consecutively treated patients. J Clin Oncol 1997; 15:1309-17.

71. Kudelka AP, Tresukosol D, Edwards CL, et al. Phase II study of intravenous topotecan as a 5-day infusion for refractory epithelial ovarian carcinoma. J Clin Oncol 1996; 14:1552-1557.

72. ten Bokkel-Huinink W, Gore M. Carmichael J, et al. Topotecan versus paclitaxel for the treatment of recurrent epithelial ovarian cancer. J Clin Oncol 1997; 15:2183-93.

73. Hochster H, Wadler S, Runowitz C, et al. Activity and pharmacodynamics of 21-day topotecan infusion in patients with ovarian cancer previously treated with platinum-based chemotherapy. J Clin Oncol 1999; 17:2553.

74. Bajetta E, DiLeo A, Biganzoli L, et al. Phase II study of vinorelbine in patients with pretreated advanced ovarian cancer: Activity in platinum-resistant disease. J Clin Oncol 1996; 14:2546-2551.

75. DeLena M, Lorusso V, Bottalico C, et al. Revertant and potentiating activity of lonidamine in patients with ovarian cancer previously treated with platinum. J Clin Oncol 1997; 15:3208-3213.

76. Muggia FM, Hainsworth JD, Jeffer S, et al. Phase II study of liposomal doxorubicin in refractory ovarian cancer: anti-tumor activity and toxicity modification by liopsomal encapsulation. J Clin Oncol 1997; 15:987-93.

77. Kaufmann M, von Minckwitz G. Gemcitabine in ovarian cancer: An overview of safety and efficacy. Eur J Cancer 1997; 33:S31-33.

78. Segna RA, Dottino PR, Mandeli SP, Konsker K, Cohen CJ. Secondary cytoreduction for ovarian cancer following cisplatin therapy. J Clin Oncol 1993; 11:434-39.

79. van der Burg MEL, van Lent M, Buyse M, et al. The effect of debulking surgery after induction chemotherapy on the prognosis in advanced epithelial ovarian cancer. N Engl J Med 1995; 332:629-634.

80. van der Burg, MEL, van Lent M, Kobierska A, et al. After 6 years follow-up intervention debulking surgery remains an independent prognostic factor for survival in advanced epithelial ovarian cancer: An EORTC Gynecologic Cancer Cooperative Group study. Int J Gynecol Cancer 1997; 7(suppl 2):28.

81. Howell SB, Zimm S, Markman M, et al. Long-term survival of advanced refractory ovarian carcinoma patients with small-volume disease treated with intraperitoneal chemotherapy. J Clin Oncol 1987; 5:1607-12.

82. Markman M, Berek JS, Blessing JA, McGuire WP, Bell J, Homesley HD. Characteristics of patients with small-volume residual ovarian cancer unresponsive to cisplatin-based ip chemotherapy: Lessons learned from a Gynecologic Oncology Group phase II trial of ip cisplatin and recombinant alpha-interferon. Gynecol Oncol 1992; 45:3-8.

83. Kirmani S, Braly PS, McClay EF, et al. A comparison of intravenous versus intraperitoneal chemotherapy for the initial treatment of ovarian cancer. Gynecol Oncol 1994; 54:338-44.

84. Alberts DS, Liu PY, Hannigan EV, et al. Phase III study of intraperitoneal (IP) cisplatin (CDDP)/intravenous (IV) cyclophosphamide (CPA) vs. IV CDDP/IV CPA in patients (PTS) with optimal disease stage III ovarian cancer: A SWOG-GOG-ECOG intergroup study (int 0051). Proceed ASCO 1995; 14:273.

85. Stewart JA, Belinson JL, Moore AL, et al. Phase I trial of intraperitoneal recombinant interleukin-2/lymphokine-activated killer cells in patients with ovarian cancer. Cancer Res 1990; 50:6302-10.

86. Stewart JSW, Hird V, Snook D, et al. Intraperitoneal yttrium-90-labeled monoclonal antibody in ovarian cancer. J Clin Oncol 1990; 8:1941-50.

87. Hird V, Maraveyas A, Senook D, et al. Adjuvant therapy of ovarian cancer with radioactive monoclonal antibody. Br J Cancer 1993; 68:403-6.

88. Pujade-Lauraine E, Guastalla JP, Colombo N, et al. Intraperitoneal recombinant interferon gamma in ovarian cancer patients with residual disease at second-look laparotomy. J Clin Oncol 1996; 14:343-350.

89. Berek, JS, Markman M, Stonebraker B, et al. Intraperitoneal interferon α in residual ovarian carcinoma: A phase II Gynecologic Oncology Group study. Gynecol Oncol 1999; 75:10-14.

90. Berek JS, Markman M, Blessing JA, et al. Intraperitoneal α interferon alternating with cisplatin in residual ovarian carcinoma: A phase II Gynecologic Oncology Group study. Gynecol 1999; 74:48-52.

91. Nelson BE, Rosenfield AT, Schwartz PE. Preoperative abdominopelvic computed tomography prediction of optimal cytoreduction in epithelial ovarian carcinoma. J Clin Oncol 1993; 11:166-72.

92. Schwartz PE, Rutherford TJ, Chambers JT, et al. Neoadjuvant chemotherapy for advanced ovarian cancer: Long-term survival. Gynecol Oncol 1999; 72:93-99.

93. Surwit E, Childers J, Atlas I, et al. Neoadjuvant chemotherapy for advanced ovarian cancer. Int J Gynecol Cancer 1996; 6:356-366.

94. Dorigo O, Berek JS. Gene therapy for ovarian cancer: development of novel treatment strategies. Int J Gynecol Cancer 1997; 7:1-13.

Chapter 5

ULTRASOUND AND OVARIAN CANCER

Leeber Cohen and David A. Fishman
Department of Obstetrics and Gynecology, Divisions of Ultrasound and Gynecologic Oncology, Northwestern University Medical School, Chicago, IL, 60611

1. INTRODUCTION

The last thirty years have seen rapid technological advances in ultrasound evaluation of the ovaries. These advances include real-time ultrasound in the 1970's, endovaginal probes in the mid 1980's, color Doppler in the early 1990's, and power Doppler imaging and 3-dimensional imaging in the late 1990's. With each of these technologies, investigators have attempted to improve on the diagnostic accuracy of ultrasound in discriminating benign from malignant disease.

Hundreds of papers have been published in the medical literature regarding the role of ultrasound in identifying ovarian cancer. For the sake of analysis these articles can be divided into two broad categories. The first category analyzes the role of diagnostic ultrasound in discriminating between benign and malignant adnexal masses that have been already been identified on pelvic examination or other imaging modalities. The second category of articles looks at the ability of ultrasound to identify ovarian cancer in asymptomatic patients.

2. EPIDEMIOLOGY

To understand the limitations of diagnostic ultrasound as a screening test for ovarian cancer, certain epidemiologic issues must be understood. Ovarian cancer is presently the fifth leading cause of cancer deaths among women in the United States [1]. During a woman's lifetime she has a 1.6% risk of developing ovarian cancer. Ninety percent of women diagnosed with ovarian cancer are above 44 years of age [2]. The prevalence of ovarian cancer in menopausal women is about 50/100,000 [3]. The majority of these cases are epithelial type, and 70-75% are diagnosed at Stage III-IV. Despite advances in chemotherapy and surgical technique, 5-year survival remains approximately

10% for late stage disease [4]. To make an impact on survival, therefore, early-stage disease must be identified, since cure rates for Stage I disease approach 90% [5].

3. SCREENING TESTS

Interpreting the literature can be made difficult by several confusing variables. Many papers fail to distinguish between epithelial ovarian cancer (EOC) and non-epithelial ovarian cancers. Even more significantly, borderline epithelial neoplasms are sometimes included in sensitivity for identifying Stage I disease. Including these neoplasms in screening results can inflate the rate at which Stage I disease is identified; it does not accurately reflect the rate at which Stage I epithelial ovarian cancer can be identified.

Any screening test for a relatively low-prevalence disease must be both very sensitive (a positive test in an individual with the disease) and very specific (a negative test in screened patients without disease). Jacobs *et al* have calculated that to achieve a positive predictive value of 10%, a screening test must have a specificity of 99.6%. Stated differently, at a specificity of 99.6%, one out of every ten patients taken to the operating room will actually have cancer [6].

The sensitivity of a screening test for ovarian cancer is determined by the number of women who develop the disease within a given time interval after the screen. Obviously the longer the interval the lower the sensitivity will be. As reviewed by Bell *et al*, only 6/25 published prospective screening studies provide analyzable data [7]. The study by Jacobs *et al* of 22,000 low-risk menopausal women, using a mult-imodal screen of CA125 followed by ultrasound, reported a sensitivity of 79% (95% CI 49-95%) at one year and 58% (95% CI 34-80%) at 2 years [6].

Van Nagell *et al* have recently published the results of 14,469 asymptomatic women, both low and high-risk scanned annually during a 12 year period [8]. The sensitivity for all stages of disease was 81% (17/21 cases). The sensitivity for detecting Stage I epithelial ovarian cancer (excluding borderline tumors and granulosa cell tumors) was 31% (5/16) [9]. The authors note that ultrasound performed poorly in identifying ovarian cancer in women with normal size ovaries.

False-positive screen rates have varied depending on the screening modality used. Jacobs *et al* used a multimodal screen of CA125 followed by ultrasound and had a .1% false-positive rate. Bourne used transvaginal ultrasound with color Doppler imaging and reported a .2% false positive rate. Van Nagell *e. al* using transvaginal ultrasound alone reported a 1.2% false positive rate [6,8,10]. Bell *et al* estimate that assuming an annual incidence of 40/100,000 for ovarian cancer, 30-60 operations would be performed for every ovarian cancer detected using transvaginal gray-scale ultrasound. This figure is lowered to 7.0-17.5 by the addition of color Doppler. Multimodal screening achieved the lowest rate at 2.5-15 [7].

Any screening test for ovarian cancer must detect a high proportion of ovarian cancers at Stage I. A systematic review of the ovarian cancer screening literature by Bell summarized 8 prospective ultrasound series in 15,834 low-risk women and found that 67% (95% CI 22-96) of the ovarian cancers were detected at Stage I. In 5 series employing multimodal screening with CA-125 followed by ultrasound, the detection rate for Stage I disease among 27,560 low-risk women was 50%(95% CI 19-75). In 6 series of 3,146 high-risk women with a family history of ovarian cancer the detection rate for Stage I disease was 25% (95% CI 3-65)[7].

Cost is also a major consideration in screening for ovarian cancer. To justify screening costs, the University of Kentucky group limited scan costs to $35.00 [11]. Assuming a more standard fee of $150.00 for a screening transvaginal ultrasound, the approximate cost of identifying one case of Stage I ovarian cancer would be approximately $400,000 [9].

4. CLASSIFICATION SYSTEMS FOR ADNEXAL MASSES

Multiple ultrasound classification systems have been described to assess the benign or malignant nature of an adnexal mass. Early ultrasound papers took advantage of the available pathologic literature and attempted to predict the risk for malignancy based on the morphologic appearance of the mass [12-14]. A widely used classification system was proposed by Hermann *et al.* in 1987 using transabdominal ultrasound [15]. The proposed classification system divided masses into cystic masses <10cm or >10cm, complex masses, and solid masses. Masses containing thick septations, internal solid excrescences, irregular borders, or if ascites is present are graded as probably malignant (Figures 1-4). The predictive value for malignant disease was 73.1% and benign disease 95.6%. This system clearly was limited by the resolution of abdominal ultrasound and was very dependent on the expertise of those interpreting the test. Finkler *et al* demonstrated that the specificity of transabdominal ultrasound in predicting malignancy could be improved by the addition of CA125 [16]. The effect was mainly seen in menopausal women.

With the improved resolution of vaginal ultrasound Sassone *et al* described a classification system which required grading of inner wall structure, wall thickness, septations, and echogenicity. The authors found a sensitivity of 100% for predicting malignancy and 37% for predicting benign disease [17]. The authors found that the specificity would have been markedly better except that the pathologically proven benign cystic teratomas had complex echo-architecture and were scored potentially malignant. The scoring system of Sassone was subsequently modified by Lerner et al [18].

Ferazzi et al. in 1997 published a multicenter study of 330 masses and found that the Sassone and Lerner scores were 93% and 90% sensitive for predicting malignancy. The specificity of their scoring systems was markedly improved by allowing for the histologic prediction of hemorrhagic cysts, endometriomas, and cystic teratomas [19]. The transvaginal echo-features of hemorrhagic cysts have been described by Okai et al (Figures 5,6)[20]. The appearance of endometriomas and cystic teratomas has been described by Cohen (Figures 7-11)[21,22]. Papers by Milad and Cohen and Valentin confirm that these histologies can be predicted with 90-95% accuracy [23,24].

Histologic prediction of tumor type from gray-scale ultrasound appearance is fraught with several hazards. Valentin has noted that in only 50% of cases is the ultrasound sufficiently characteristic to predict histology with certainty [24]. There is clearly overlap between the appearance of complex-appearing benign masses and that of some malignant tumors. In premenopausal women advantage is taken of the fact that most hemorrhagic cysts and functional cysts resolve spontaneously in 6-8 weeks. Statistically a large number of the remaining masses will be endometriomas, cystic teratomas, and cyst-adenomas. Endoscopic surgeons have taken advantage of these facts to advocate laparoscopic removal of persistent benign-appearing masses. Large laparoscopic series by Canis et al and Nezhat et al confirm that malignancy can be encountered inadvertently at laparoscopy [25,26]. This happened 2.5% and < 0.5% of the time in the two series, respectively. In the hands of less experienced practitioners this happens more frequently. Maiman and Seltzer have documented that improper staging and treatment can occur in these cases [27].

5. COLOR DOPPLER EVALUATION OF ADNEXAL MASSES

The role of color Doppler in evaluating adnexal masses received a great deal of attention in 1991 with the publication by Kurjak et al of a series of 690 masses in 14,317 women [28]. The authors found that a resistive index $\leq$.4 could be used to discriminate malignant from benign masses. The authors found that 54/55 malignant masses were identified by an RI $\leq$ .4 and 623/624 benign masses by an RI > .4. This yielded a sensitivity of 96.4%, specificity of 99.8%, with an overall diagnostic accuracy of 99.5%. Papers by Timor-Tritsch et al and Fleischer et al showed similar sensitivity but less specificity [29,30]. Timor-Tritsch recommended combining a morphologic classification with color Doppler analysis. Fleisher and Jones III recommended a multiparameter approach with conventional transvaginal sonography as the primary screening technique and color Doppler as an adjunct [31].

Other investigators found that color Doppler performed much less accurately than initially reported. Reports by Tekay and Jouipilla, Valentin *et al*, Bromley *et al* from 1992-1994 did not support the initial enthusiasm for color Doppler screening as significant overlap was noted between the resistive indices seen in benign and malignant ovarian masses [32-34]. A subsequent paper by Tekay and Jouipilla found that low-resistance vessels could be identified in 43% of benign tumors and 25% of the normal ovaries [35]. They also found that scanning in the follicular phase did not improve the ability to discriminate between benign and malignant tumors. The NIH consensus report in 1995 reviewed this subject and concluded that color Doppler as a secondary test may improve specificity but that the test remains investigational [36]. Multiple logistic models have been proposed to combine transvaginal gray scale imaging and with color Doppler as a secondary test. This subject has been reviewed by Alcazar and Jurado [37].

Some authors have reported better diagnostic accuracy by using peak systolic velocity rather than resistive indices. Power Doppler energy (or color Doppler energy) has also been advocated. Tailor *et al* in 1998 did not confirm that the diagnostic accuracy was improved significantly by using either peak systolic velocity measurements or color Doppler energy rather than traditional color Doppler [38]. A paper by Guerriero *et al* reviews color Doppler energy testing and suggests that diagnostic specificity is improved [39]. It remains unknown if either color Doppler or power Doppler will increase the number of Stage I ovarian cancers identified in screening programs. The role of power Doppler 3-dimensional imaging is investigational.(Figures 12-15)[40-42].

6. MANAGEMENT OF CYSTIC OVARIAN MASSES

Cystic masses of the ovary >2.4 cm are quite common in asymptomatic women, occurring in approximately 13% of premenopausal women and 6% of postmenopausal women [43]. Expectant management of cystic masses in the premenopausal patient will result in spontaneous resolution of these masses the great majority of the time. In the series of Osmers *et al*, 90% of follicular cysts resolved spontaneously without intervention [44]. He followed a protocol that included 4-6 weeks of expectant management followed by a trial of birth control pills if resolution had not occurred. The use of birth control pills to involute functional or hemorrhagic physiologic cysts of the ovary was first championed by Spanos [45]. The role of birth control pills for treatment of physiologic cysts has been questioned in a paper by Steinkampf *et al* [46].

It has become clear with the widespread use of CT scans and MRI that simple cystic masses of the ovary are a not an uncommon finding. Multiple different authors have recommended expectant management of simple small menopausal cysts without excresences (Figure 16)[47-49]. Spontaneous resolution occurs up to 30% of the time [43,48]. The ACOG Committee on

Quality Assessment recommends surgery for asymptomatic postmenopausal ovarian tumors if they are solid, complex, or increasing in size; if ascites is noted; or if CA-125 is elevated [50].

7. SUMMARY

From the published studies it would appear that ultrasound is a very sensitive tool for identifying advanced stage ovarian cancer. The identification of Stage I ovarian cancer with ultrasound screening is more problematic since only 25 to 50% of ovarian cancers are identified in low-risk and high-risk respectively using this technique. Due to the low annual prevalence of ovarian cancer routine screening of premenopausal women or low-risk women after the menopause is unlikely to be cost-effective.

The subject of biologic markers to screen for ovarian cancer is addressed elsewhere in this book. It is clear that a primary screening test less expensive than ultrasound is needed. The multicenter National Cancer Institute screening program is designed to evaluate possible new markers. At this time ovarian cancer screening should be done in high-risk groups under careful investigational scrutiny. Patients who are high-risk should be carefully advised of the limitations of diagnostic ultrasound in identifying early stage disease.

Transvaginal ultrasound in expert hands is sensitive but not ideally specific for discriminating benign from malignant disease. The judicious use of color Doppler evaluation may help discriminate with greater specificity.

REFERENCES

1. Greenlee RT, Murray T, Bolden S, Wingo PA. Cancer Statistics, 2000. CA-A Cancer J Clin 2000; 50:7-33.
2. Yancik R. Ovarian Cancer. Age contrasts in incidence, histology, disease stage at diagnosis, and mortality. Cancer 1993; 71:517-528.
3. Yancik R, Ries LG, Yates JW. Ovarian cancer in the elderly: an analysis of surveillance. Am J Obstet Gynecol 1986; 154:639-645.
4. Ozols R, Rubin S, Thomas G, Robboy S, "Epithelial Ovarian Cancer." In Principles and Practice of Gynecologic Oncology, 2d ed. Hoskins WJ, Perez CA, Young RC, eds. Philadelphia, PA: Lippincott-Raven, 1997.
5. Young RC, Walton LA, Ellenberg SS, et al. Adjuvant therapy in Stage I and II epithelial ovarian cancer. Results of two prospective randomized trials. N Engl J Med 1990; 322:1021-1029.
6. Jacobs I, Davies AP, Bridges J, et al., Prevalence screening for ovarian cancer in postmenopausal women by CA 125 measurement and ultrasonography. BMJ 1993; 306:1030-1033.
7. Bell R, Petticrew M, Sheldon T, The performance of screening tests for ovarian cancer: results of a systematic review. B J Obstet Gynecol 1998; 105:1136-1147.

8. van Nagell, J R., DePriest PD, Reedy MB, et al. The efficacy of transvaginal sonographic screening in asymptomatic women at risk for ovarian cancer. Gynecol Oncol, in press.

9. Fishman D, Cohen L. Is transvaginal ultrasound effective for screening asymptomatic women for the detection of early stage epithelial ovarian carcinoma? Gynecol Oncol , in press

10. Bourne TH, Campbell S, Reynolds KM, et al. Screening for early familial ovarian cancer with transvaginal ultrasonography and colour blood flow imaging. BMJ 1993; 306:1025-1029.

11. Pavlik EJ, van Nagell JR, DePriest PD, et al, Participation in transvaginal ovarian cancer screening: compliance, correlation factors, and costs. Gynecol Oncol 1995; 57:395-400.

12. Lawson TL, Albarelli JN. Diagnosis of gynecologic pelvic masses by gray scale ultrasonography: Analysis of specificity and accuracy. Am J Roentgenol 1977; 128:1003-1007.

13. Fleischer AC, James AE, Millis JB, et al. Differential diagnosis of pelvic masses by gray scale sonography. Am J Roentgenol 1978; 131:469-474.

14. Walsh JW, Rosenfield AT, Jaffe CC, et al. Prospective comparison of ultrasound and computed tomography in the evaluation of gynecologic pelvic masses. Am J Roentgenol 1978; 131:955-959.

15. Hermann UJ, Locher GW, Goldhirsch A. Sonographic patterns of ovarian tumors: Prediction of malignancy. Obstet Gynecol 1987; 69:777-781.

16. Finkler NJ, Benacerraf B, Wojciechowski C, et al. Comparison of serum CA 125, clinical impression, and ultrasound in the preoperative evaluation of ovarian masses. Am J Obstet Gynecol 1988; 72:659-663.

17. Sassone AM, Timor-Tritsch IE, Artner A, et al. Transvaginal sonographic characterization of ovarian disease: evaluation of a new scoring system to predict malignancy. Obstet Gynecol 1991; 78:70-76.

18. Lerner JP, Timor-Tritsch IE, Federman A, Abramovich G. Transvaginal ultrasonographic characterization of ovarian masses with an improved,weighted score. Am J Obstet Gynecol 1994; 170:81-85.

19. Ferrazzi E, Zanetta G, Dordoni D, et al. Transvaginal ultrasonographic characterization of ovarian masses: a comparison of five scoring systems in a multicenter trial. Ultrasound Obstet Gynecol 1997; 10:192-197.

20. Okai T, Kobayashi K, Ryo E, et al. Transvaginal sonographic appearance of hemorrhagic functional ovarian cysts and their spontaneous regression. Int J Gynecol Obstet 1994; 44:47-52.

21. Cohen L,Valle R, Sabbagha R. A comparison of preoperative ultrasound images of surgically proven endometriomas scanned by both transabdominal and transvaginal techniques. J Gynecol Surg 1995; 11:27-32.

22. Cohen L, Sabbagha R. Echo patterns of benign cystic teratomas by transvaginal ultrasound. Ultrasound Obstet Gynecol 1993; 3:120-123.

23. Milad M, Cohen L. Preoperative ultrasound assessment of adnexal masses in premenopausal women. Int J Gynecol Obstet 1999; 66:137-141.

24. Valentin L. Pattern recognition of pelvic masses by gray-scale ultrasound imaging: the contribution of Doppler ultrasound. Ultrasound Obstet Gynecol 1999; 14:338-347.

25. Canis M, Mage G, Pouly J, et al., Laparoscopic diagnosis of adnexal cystic masses: a 12-year experience with long-term follow-up. Obstet Gynecol 1994; 83:707-712.

26. Nezhat F, Nezhat C, Welander CE, et al. Four ovarian cancers diagnosed during laparoscopic management of 1011 women with adnexal masses. Am J Obstet Gynecol 1992; 167:790-796.

27. Maiman M, Seltzer V, Boyce J. Laparoscopic excision of ovarian neoplasms subsequently found to be malignant. Obstet Gynecol 1991; 77:563-565.

28. Kurjak A, Zalud I, Alfirevic Z. Evaluation of adnexal masses with transvaginal color ultrasound. J Ultrasound Med 1991; 10:295-297.

126

29. Timor-Tritsh I, Lerner J, Monteagudo A, et al. Transvaginal ultrasonographic characterization of ovarian masses by means of color flow-directed Doppler measurements and a morphologic scoring system. Am J Obstet Gynecol 1993; 168:909-913.

30. Fleischer A, Rodgers W, Rao B, et al. Assessment of ovarian tumor vascularity with transvaginal color doppler sonography. J Ultrasound Med 1991; 10:563-568.

31. Fleischer A, Jones H. Editorial: Color Doppler sonography of ovarian masses: the importance of a multiparameter approach. Gynecol Oncol 1993; 50:1-2.

32. Tekay A, Joupilla P. Validity of pulsatility and resistance indices in classification of adnexal tumors with transvaginal color Doppler ultrasound. Ultrasound Obstet Gynecol 1992; 2:338-344.

33. Valentin L, Sladkevicius P, Marsal K. Limited contribution of Doppler velocimetry to the differential diagnosis of extrauterine pelvic tumors. Obstet Gynecol 1994; 83:425-433.

34. Bromley B, Goodman H, Benaceraff BR. Comparison between sonographic morphology and Doppler waveform for the diagnosis of ovarian malignancy. Obstet Gynecol 1994; 83:125-130.

35. Tekay A, Joupilla P. Blood flow in benign ovarian tumors and normal ovaries during the follicular phase. Obstet Gynecol 1995; 86:55-59.

36. NIH Consensus Development Panel on Ovarian Cancer. J Am Med Assoc 1995; 273:491-497.

37. Alcazar J, Jurado M. Prospective evaluation of a logistic model based on sonographic morphologic and color Doppler findings developed to predict adnexal malignancy. J Ultrasound Med 1999; 18:837-842.

38. Tailor A, Juirkovic D, Bourne T, et al. Comparison of transvaginal color Doppler imaging and color Doppler energy for assessment of intraovarian blood flow. Obstet Gynecol 1998; 91:561-567.

39. Guerrirro S, Ajossa S, Risalvato A, et al. Diagnosis of adnexal malignancies by using color Doppler energy imaging as a secondary test in persistent masses. Ultrasound Obstet Gynecol 1998; 11:277-282.

40. Chan L, Lin S, Uerpairojkit B, et al. Evaluation of adnexal masses using three-dimensional ultrasonographic technology: preliminary report. J Ultrasound Med 1997; 16:349-354.

41. Bonilla-Musoles F, Raga F, Osborne N. Three-dimensional ultrasound evaluation of ovarian masses. Gynecol Oncol 1995; 59:129-135.

42. Kurjak A, Kupesic S, Breyer B, et al. The assessment of ovarian tumor angiogenesis: what does three-dimensional power Doppler add: Ultrasound Obstet Gynecol 1998; 12:136-146.

43. Schulman H, Conway C, Zalud I, et al. Prevalence in a volunteer population of pelvic cancer detected with transvaginal ultrasound and color flow Doppler. Ultrasound Obstet Gynecol 1994; 4:414-420.

44. Osmers R, Osmers M, von Maydell B, et al. Preoperative evaluation of ovarian tumors in the premenopause by transvaginosonography. Am J Obstet Gynecol 1996; 175:428-434.

45. Spanos W. Preoperative hormonal therapy of cystic adnexal masses. Am J Obstet Gynecol 1973; 551-556.

46. Steinkampf M, Hammond K, Blackwell R. Hormonal treatment of functional ovarian cysts: a randomized, prospective study. Fertil Steril 1990; 54:775-777.

47. Bonilla-Musoles F, Ballester J, Simon C, et al. Is avoidance of surgery possible in patients with perimenopausal ovarian tumors using transvaginal ultrasound and duplex color Doppler sonography? J Ultrasound Med 1993; 12:33-39.

48. Bailey C, Ueland F, Land G, et al. The malignant potential of small cystic ovarian tumors in women over 50 years of age. Gynecol Oncol 1998; 69:3-7.

49. Goldstein S, Subramanyam B, Snyder J, et al. The postmenopausal cystic adnexal mass: potential role of ultrasound in conservative management. Obstet Gynecol 1989; 76:8-10.

50. ACOG Committee on Quality Assessment, Criteria set 15 (April 1996).

FIGURE LEGENDS

Figure 1. This transabdominal scan reveals a complex 15 x 10 cm mass with complex internal septations filled with low-level echogenicity. The tumor was a Stage IA borderline mucinous adenocarcinoma.

Figure 2. This transvaginal scan shows an 8 x 3 cm complex cystic and solid mass in the right adnexa. It was a Stage IIIC fallopian tube carcinoma.

Figure 3. This transvaginal image demonstrates a 6 x 5 cm multi-loculated mass with multiple internal excrescences. It represented a Stage IIIC borderline papillary adenocarcinoma.

Figure 4. This complex multi-septated mass, seen transvaginally, reveals the typical appearance of a mucinous cystadenoma. The absence of flow within the septations is noted.

Figure 5. This 5 x 3.5 cm transvaginal image reveals a complex hemorrhagic corpus luteum which had recently occurred. Clot-like echo without vascular flow is noted.

Figure 6. This 5 x 5 cm transvaginal study reveals a resorbing hemorrhagic cyst with complex internal echogenicity in a lace-like pattern.

Figure 7. This 4 x 3 cm biloculated mass was enlarging in a perimenopausal woman. Pathology revealed an endometriotic cyst. Endometriotic cysts frequently are filled with uniform low-level echoes as noted in one of the two cystic locules.

Figure 8. This transabdominal study demonstrates a 6 cm cystic mass filled with low-level echogenicity. Pathology revealed an endometriotic cyst in a premenopausal patient.

Figure 9. This transvaginal study reveals a 2 x 1 cm densely echogenic, well-circumscribed mass within a normal-sized ovary. This echo pattern is suggestive of a benign cystic teratoma. These masses frequently show posterior shadowing. Vascular flow is usually not noted within the areas of dense echogenicity unless struma-ovari or malignant components are present.

Figure 10. This unusual transvaginal study reveals a highly complex 8 x 4 cm mass. Pathology revealed a benign cystic teratoma with carcinoid component. Shadowing is noted. Color Doppler imaging of this mass was negative for flow.

Figure 11. This transvaginal power Doppler study reveals a biloculated complex mass. One of the loculations contains an area of internal excrescence without flow. The preoperative differential diagnosis included benign cystic teratoma, adenofibroma, nnd borderline tumor. Pathology revealed a benign cystic teratoma. Experience in our lab has shown that overlap occurs in the ultrasound appearance of these histologic types.

Figure 12. This large cystic mass, scanned transabdominally, contained areas of lirregular excrescence as labelled by the arrowhead. Due to the size of the tumor, vascularity of the mass, and patient age (in the 20's), malignant germ cell tumor was suspected. A Stage I malignant germ cell tumor was confirmed at surgery.

Figure 13. This figure represents a 3-dimensional study of the tumor excrescence pictured in Fig. 12. The tumor excrescence is very well-defined, and a blood vessel can be seen entering the excrescence.

Figure 14. This transvaginal image reveals an elongated cystic mass with two septations. It was felt to represent a benign hydrosalpinx.

Figure 15. This 3-dimensionally rendered image was performed on the same mass pictured in Fig. 14. It shows the typical appearance of a hydrosalpinx with perpendicular septations noted along the long axis of the mass. The internal wall of the dilated fallopian tube is clearly visualized.

Figure 16. This transvaginal 3-dinensional acquisition reveals a simple thin-walled 4 cm cyst in three orthogonal planes, in a postmenopausal patient. A rendered image of the internal cyst wall is noted in the bottom right corner. This patient has been managed expectantly with scans every six months, with no change in size or architecture of the mass.

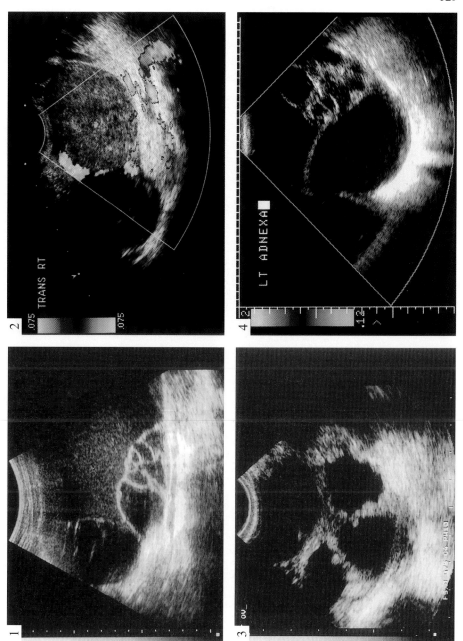

130

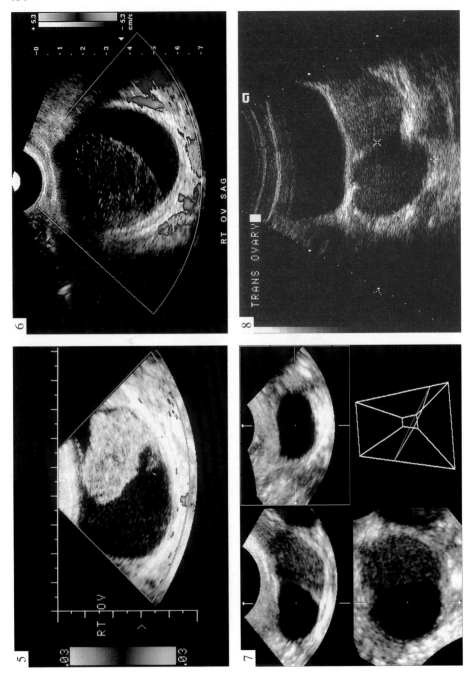

131

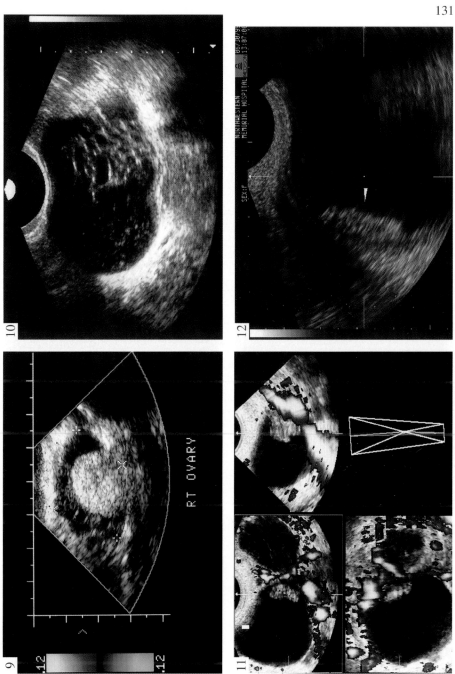

132

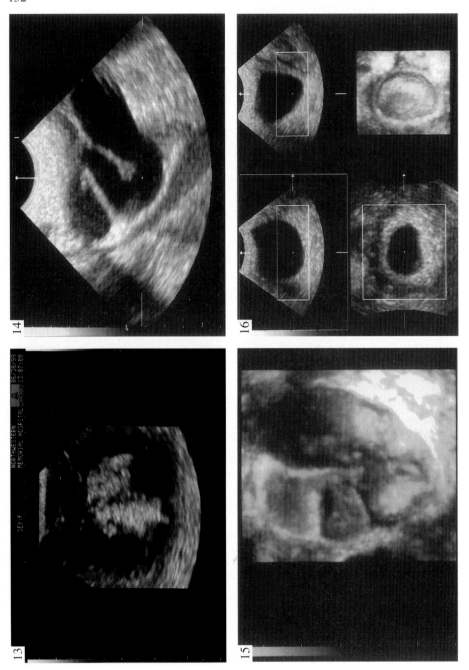

Chapter 6

GENE THERAPY

Warner K. Huh, Mack N. Barnes, F. Joseph Kelly, and Ronald D. Alvarez
Division of Gynecologic Oncology, Department of Obstetrics and Gynecology
University of Alabama at Birmingham,
Birmingham, AL 35233

Ovarian carcinoma continues to be the most common cause of death from gynecologic malignancy in the United States. This high fatality rate can be attributed to a lack of early, effective screening strategies and lack of specific symptoms associated with early stage disease. Thus, approximately 70% of women with ovarian cancer present with advanced stage disease. Although advances in surgical therapy and chemotherapy have improved progression free survival, the long-term 5-year survival rate rarely exceeds 30% for patients diagnosed with this disease (1).

Most human cancers are now recognized to occur as the result of acquired genetic alterations in normal cellular DNA. The initial work of Vogelstein *et al* (2,3) correlated pathologic neoplastic progression with specific genetic alterations in colon cancer, and several investigators have attempted to clarify similar correlations in ovarian cancer. Gene therapy, defined as the modification of the genetic composition of "somatic" cells for therapeutic gains, is a rational new therapy to investigate in the context of ovarian cancer. The numerous molecular changes that occur with the development of ovarian cancer allow for a wide variety of gene therapy approaches.

1. GENE THERAPY TREATMENT STRATEGIES

Current gene therapy strategies are based on our advances and current knowledge in the molecular biology of malignant transformation and progression. Treatments are directly based on specific genetic alterations, oncogenes, and tumor-specific antigens. Gene therapy directed strategies are divided into four categories: molecular chemotherapy, mutation compensation, immunopotentation, and alteration of resistance and sensitivity to conventional therapies. Molecular chemotherapy attempts to enhance the specific delivery of drugs to malignant cells, thereby sparing toxic effects on non-malignant tissues. The principle of mutation compensation is based on

134

either the replacement of tumor suppressor genes, inactivation of dysregulated genes, or direct interference with aberrant signal transduction pathways. The third strategy, immunopotentation, attempts to enhance the body's own natural immune response to tumor cells. The last strategy attempts to decrease tumor cell resistance to chemotherapy and radiotherapy or to limit dose-limiting toxicity associated with these conventional therapies.

1.1. Molecular Chemotherapy

Molecular chemotherapy is based on specific delivery and expression of a gene-encoded toxin in cancer cells in order to achieve tumor killing. Both conventional chemotherapy and molecular chemotherapy are dependent on delivery of a toxin to cells for tumor eradication; however, conventional chemotherapy is largely limited by its non-specificity and thus, its potential amount of toxicity. The therapeutic index is a general measure of differential toxic side effects between malignant and normal cells, and the premise behind molecular chemotherapy based strategies is to improve the therapeutic index by improving the selective delivery or expression of a toxin. Toxin expression can be achieved by both direct and indirect strategies. The direct strategy uses a gene that encodes a specific toxin, and in contrast, the indirect method is based on the delivery of a pro-drug that is subsequently converted into a toxic metabolite that ultimately leads to cellular death (Figure 1).

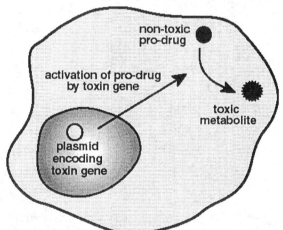

Investigators have primarily focused on indirect approaches of molecular chemotherapy and the two most common strategies utilize genes that encode cytosine deaminase (CD) and the herpes simplex thymidine kinase (HSV-TK) gene. CD is an enzyme that is found in prokaryotic systems that is able to convert 5-fluorocytosine to 5-fluorouracil (4). However, this system is of limited benefit in the setting of ovarian cancer since 5-fluorouracil has not been shown to be an extremely active agent. On the contrary, the thymidine kinase (TK) gene from the herpes simplex virus (HSV) has been frequently used to accomplish molecular chemotherapy in the context of ovarian cancer. TK is an enzyme that specifically functions in the salvage cycle of DNA synthesis. This enzyme is also present in mammalian cells; however, the viral form is significantly more sensitive to anti-viral agents such as acyclovir and ganciclovir (GCV). Preferential monophosphorylation of GCV by HSV-TK is the fundamental mechanism by which TK can be used for a specific cytotoxic effect (5). GCV is further phosphorylated by other cellular factors to a tri-phosphate form that becomes incorporated into cellular DNA. Incorporation of triphosphorylated GCV halts both DNA synthesis and RNA polymerase activity and thus results in cellular death (6). Again, since the mammalian form of TK has a much lower affinity for GCV, normal cells tend to be spared from the toxic effects of this system when GCV is given at low levels. This prodrug/enzyme combination has an improved specificity and therapeutic index by enhancing the cytotoxicity of GCV in cells that have been specifically transduced to express viral TK (7).

Culvert *et al* (8) first described the "bystander effect" associated with HSV-TK mediated cell killing. They noted that a greater number of tumor cells were actually killed than initially transduced by the TK gene. This observation may imply that toxin gene expressing cells exert a noxious effect on surrounding cells. Possible explanations include endocytosis of toxic debris, exposure to soluble toxins, and vascular destruction, but it is important to note that none of these theories have been confirmed (9). Another theory suggested by Mesnil *et al* (10), involves transfer of phosphorylated GCV molecules from HSV-TK positive cells into HSV-TK negative cells through gap junctions. Other studies indicate that CD8[+] lymphocytes mediate an immune response to adjacent cells via the lysis of HSV-TK transfected cells (11,12). One clear advantage of the bystander effect is that it overcomes the need to achieve near total quantitative tumor cell transduction to attain adequate tumor killing.

1.1.1. HSV-TK Based Protocols

Ovarian cancer is an appropriate disease process for gene therapy since 90% of women have disease within the peritoneal cavity at the time of diagnosis. This compartmentalized model allows for easy and uncomplicated delivery of viral vectors to the cavity through an intraperitoneal route and provides a cavity for effective vector concentration, efficient *in vivo* transduction, and an ideal setting for the "bystander effect."

Freeman and others (13) have used the mouse peritoneal cavity as a model of human ovarian carcinoma and also demonstrated that bystander killing effect could be effectively established in a murine fibrosarcoma cell line that expressed as few as 10% HSV-TK-positive cells. Moreover, they were able to show that *ex vivo* mixing of TK-positive and TK-negative cells, before injection into mice, could cause tumor reduction following treatment with ganciclovir. They advanced this model by demonstrating that tumor cells injected into the peritoneal cavity with only 50% TK-positive cells, prolonged survival when compared to untreated animals. Using these important results, Freeman hypothesized that human ovarian carcinoma could potentially be treated in a similar manner since roughly 90% of patients have disease within the peritoneal cavity. Thus, in their clinical protocol, ovarian cancer patients are injected intraperitoneally with irradiated cells from the PA-1 ovarian tumor cell line that are retrovirally transduced to express the HSV-TK gene. The anti-tumor effect was intended to occur solely as the result of a bystander effect. Preliminary results of their phase I trial demonstrated acceptable toxicity (14).

Link *et al* (15) were able to demonstrate the ability to indirectly transfect ovarian cancer cells with retroviral vector producer cells (LTKOSN.2) *in vitro*. When treated with ganciclovir, a significant direct cytotoxic effect in addition to a bystander effect was observed. In an *in vivo* peritoneal adenocarcinoma model using a colon carcinoma cell line, there was a significant therapeutic benefit using this treatment strategy. Based on these findings, Link *et al* (16) have initiated a phase I clinical trial for human ovarian cancer patients. Preliminary results demonstrated acceptable toxicity. Four of 9 patients were reported to have an anti-tumor response, although gene transfer was noted to be low.

Alvarez and Curiel have also proposed a clinical protocol based on adenoviral mediated delivery of HSV-TK. Initial work *in vitro* demonstrated that in a mixed population of ovarian cancer cells with only 10% HSV-TK positive cells, there was greater than 70% cell death following the administration of ganciclovir. Following this, they were able to construct and validate a recombinant adenoviral vector containing the HSV-TK gene (AdHSV-TK) and demonstrate this vector can transfect primary ovarian cancer cells derived from malignant ascites of ovarian cancer patients at 50% efficiency (17). *In vitro* studies demonstrated the selective toxicity of this adenoviral vector in ovarian cancer cell lines in addition to primary cells following treatment with ganciclovir. An *in vivo* model subsequently confirmed the validity of this approach. Specifically, mice were injected intraperitoneally with the ovarian cancer cell lines, SKOV3.ip1 and later injected with the recombinant HSV-TK adenovirus. Treated animals demonstrated enhanced survival and diminished tumor burden when compared to control animals (18). These findings have served as the basis for a Phase I human clinical trial whereby previously treated ovarian cancer patients are administered AdHSV-TK intraperitoneally with intravenous ganciclovir.

At this time, fourteen patients have been treated on this protocol and it appears that AdHSV-TK with ganciclovir is feasible in the setting of human ovarian cancer patients and well tolerated at the doses studied. 38 percent of patients experienced transient Grade1/2 fever and 23% experience fatigue, pain, and nausea which may have been vector related. Furthermore, four patients experienced complications with the Tenckhoff catheter including one obstruction. Thirty eight percent of patients were noted to have stable disease while on the protocol (19).

1.2. Mutation Compensation

Mutation compensation is a strategy that is largely based on the identification of genes and their products that contribute to the development of cancer. Thus, targeted ablation of a dominant oncogene, replacement of an altered tumor suppressor gene, or interference with the function of a growth factor or its receptor are examples of this strategy. Targeting can be directed at multiple different levels including DNA, messenger RNA, or protein. It has been shown that in some cases abrogation of an overexpressed or dysregulated oncogene can result in correction of a malignant phenotype (20,21).

Oligodeoxynucleotides have been used to specifically target a dominant oncogene at the DNA level by creating a triple helix. This triple helix effectively inactivates DNA. This strategy requires the construction of oligodeoxynucleotides that bind to polypurine and polypyrimidine rich typically located in regulatory regions that are located upstream to targeted genes (22). Triplex forming oligonucleotides have been targeted against the c-myc promoter, epidermal growth factor receptor promoter, erbB-2 promoter and the H-ras promoter regions (23-27).

Anti-sense based strategies have been used to target dominant oncogenes at the level of mRNA. Anti-sense oligonucleotides are RNA sequences that are complimentary to the mRNA of the gene of interest and ultimately induce translational arrest, impair transport, or initiate RNase degradation of mRNA (Figure 2). Ideal targets for anti-sense ablation are those in which there is no normal counterpart mRNA. Targets for "knockout" or anti-sense ablation include mutant forms of K-ras, H-ras, c-myb, c-myc, insulin-like growth factor (IGF) 1 receptor, bcr-abl, and p53 genes (28-42).

Another strategy directed toward targeting genes at the RNA level includes ribozymes. Ribozymes are small oligonucleotides that are capable of catalyzing RNA cleavage reactions at sequence-specific sites. The "hammer head" class of ribozymes has the ability to fold into a secondary structure resembling the head of a hammer. This class of ribozymes is able to cleave a target RNA strand after a GUA, GUC, or GUU triplet sequence. Synthetic

138

hammer head ribozymes can be targeted against specific mRNA molecules by including anti-sense sequences that will hybridize with mRNA messages immediately juxtaposed to the selective cleavage site. Oncogenes targeted by ribozymes include H-ras, and bcr-abl (43-46).

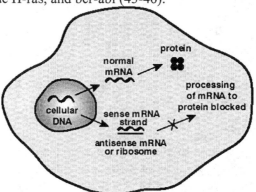

Recent discoveries have uncovered the importance of tumor suppressor genes in the setting of malignant transformation of cells. An intact gene appears to be critical in the repair of DNA damage that might otherwise transform into a malignant phenotype. Moreover, it has been thought that tumor suppressor genes play a role in apoptosis or programmed cellular death. Approximately 45-80% of all primary ovarian cancers have alterations in the tumor suppressor p53 gene (47,48). Santoso *et al* demonstrated that delivery of the wild-type p53 gene to ovarian carcinoma cells that were p53 deficient abrogated the malignant phenotype (49). This concept has been subsequently validated by Mujoo and others. They demonstrated that recombinant adenoviral delivery of wild-type p53 gene prolonged survival in mice growing human ovarian cancer xenografts (50). Janicek *et al*, using antisense oligonucleotides targeted to p53 and c-myc, demonstrated growth inhibitory effects that functioned synergistically in some ovarian carcinoma cell lines (51). Wolf *et al.* demonstrated that ovarian cancer cells are growth inhibited by transfection with adenovirus-mediated p53 regardless of their endogenous p53 status (52). Additional utility of gene therapy may be found in its ability to enhance treatment of ovarian cancer cells with conventional chemotherapeutic agents. To this end, adenoviral mediated delivery of p53 has been demonstrated to sensitize ovarian cancer cells to paclitaxel and cisplatin in both *in vitro* and *in vivo* models of ovarian carcinoma (54,55). Holt *et al* focused on BRCA-1 gene in familial breast and ovarian carcinomas as a specific gene target and showed that retroviral transduction of ovarian cancer cells with wild-type BRCA-1 inhibited tumor growth (53).

PTEN and p16 are cell cycle regulatory genes that have been delivered by adenoviral mediated gene transfer and have resulted in growth inhibition in ovarian cancer cell lines (56,57). Bax represents a member of the pro-apoptotic Bcl gene family. Delivery of adenovirus containing Bax gene constructs have been shown to induce ovarian tumor cell cytotoxicity and apoptosis in *in vitro* cell culture, as well as, nude mouse models of ovarian carcinoma (58,59). Further utility of Bax mediated gene therapy also may lie in its ability to sensitize ovarian cancer cells to the effects of chemotherapy or ionizing radiation (60,61).

Another mutation compensation strategy involves the use of dominant negative mutations. When translated, these sequences produced a non-functional form of the protein of interest (Figure 3). The use of dominant mutations to inactivate proteins involves the heterologous expression of a mutant protein that can inhibit the normal function of the native gene product produced by a cell. Dominant negative mutations are most commonly used to inhibit proteins that must aggregate into multimers in order to exert their function. There are several overexpressed tyrosine kinase growth factor receptor proteins that have oligomeric functional units, which makes them good candidates for inhibition by dominant negative mutations. Multiple investigators have employed dominant negative mutations to inhibit epidermal growth factor receptor, IGF-1 receptor, platelet derived growth factor receptor, and vascular endothelial growth factor receptor (62-66).

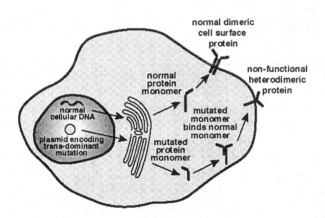

Intracellular single-chain antibodies have also been used as a novel, mutation compensation based strategy. These molecules have been designed to achieve targeted ablation of the protein product of a dominant oncogene. These entities consist of the antigen binding variable light and heavy chains of an immunoglobulin molecule connected by peptide spacer region. The expression of a single chain antibody (sFv) at the endoplasmic reticulum has been shown to result in entrapment of the erbB-2 protein (Figure 4), thus preventing its translocation to the cell membrane. This strategy effectively

140

abrogates the autocrine growth factor loop and ultimately, malignant transformation (67-69). Similar work with intracellular expression of single chain antibodies against epidermal growth factor has been studied as well (70).

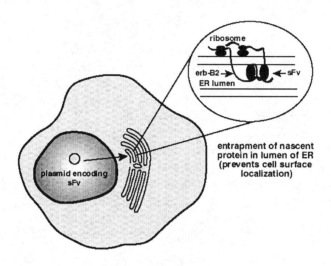

entrapment of nascent protein in lumen of ER (prevents cell surface localization)

1.2.1. Mutation Compensation Protocols Based on Delivery of Tumor Suppressor Genes

Tait *et al.*, in an early phase I trial, examined the utility of intraperitoneal instillation of a retroviral vector encoding the BRCA1 gene in patients with recurrent of progressive ovarian cancer (71). Using Southern blot analysis on samples of tumor recovered from patients, these authors estimated that only 5-10% of tumor cells were transduced with the retroviral vector. Again, no significant toxicity was observed. Preliminary results from a second gene replacement phase I trial were reported by Buller *et al.* using an adenoviral vector encoding p53 in patients with recurrent ovarian carcinoma (72). Acceptable toxicity was observed and, interestingly, no significant adverse effects were observed from repetitive dosing of the adenovirus.

1.2.2. Mutation Compensation Protocols Targeting erbB-2

Curiel *et al* demonstrated the ability of an intracellular single chain immunoglobulin (sFv) in causing selective erbB-2 ablation (67). The intracellular expression of anti-erbB-2 sFv resulted in downregulation of cell surface erbB-2, which is felt to be secondary to entrapment of nascent transmembrane tyrosine kinase receptor at the level of endoplasmic reticulum. These researchers were also able to demonstrate significant cytotoxicity in erbB-2 overexpressing human ovarian cancer cell *in vitro* (67). A replication deficient recombinant adenovirus encoding anti-erbB-2 sFv was created and demonstrated a high level of peritoneal tumor cell transduction in a murine model (69). Furthermore, significant anti-tumor activity and enhanced survival was seen with this anti-erbB2 sFv vector in an intraperitoneal ovarian cancer murine model (69).

These results have led to the development of a clinical phase I protocol whereby advanced stage ovarian cancer patients are treated intraperitoneally with a recombinant adenovirus encoding an anti-erbB-2 sFv. Acute toxicity, vector safety, and efficiency of gene transfer and expression were evaluated in this trial. Fifteen patients have been treated per this protocol and followed for toxicity. Transient Grade 1/2 fever was experience by 60% of patients, and other Grade 1/2 symptoms including nausea, fatigue, and gastrointestinal symptoms were also experienced and again, transient. Of note, there was no dose limited vector related toxicity in this study. Of those patients evaluable for response, 38% had stable disease and 61% had evidence of progressive disease. One of two patients without measurable disease was noted to have normalization of her CA-125 at the eight-week evaluation mark and other has remained without clinical evidence of disease 6 months post treatment.

Zhang *et al* (73) were able to demonstrate that adenovirus type 5 (Ad5) E1a gene products and the SV40 large T antigen inhibit transcription of HER-2/neu (erbB-2) promoter and suppress malignant transformation induced by HER-2/neu. Also, they were able to demonstrate that both cationic liposomes and adenoviral vectors can efficiently deliver E1a or large T antigen into tumor cells in mice and suppress tumor growth and improve survival. These findings have led to a phase I protocol which delivers the E1a gene to advanced ovarian cancer patients using a liposomal vector.

Alternatively, Ueno *et al.* have targeted down regulation of the erbB-2 protein by liposome mediated delivery of the E1A gene (74). These authors have noted significant ovarian tumor cell growth inhibition in vitro and prolonged survival in animal models of ovarian carcinoma. Moreover, these authors have demonstrated that E1a mediated down regulation of erbB-2 can sensitize cells to the toxic effects of paclitaxel chemotherapy. Adenoviral mediated gene transfer of anti-erbB-2 single chain antibodies have been shown to sensitize erbB-2 overexpressing SKOV-3 ovarian cancer cells to the toxic effects of cisplatin (75).

1.3. Immunopotentiation

The recent advances in tumor immunology have stimulated interest in the development of gene therapy strategies based on the induction of the immune response against tumor-associated antigens. Immunopotentiation is largely dependent on the ability of the immune system to recognize and target these molecules to achieve tumor killing. The ability of the immune system to recognize a tumor-specific antigen and mount both a humoral and cellular response has been documented (76); patients with ovarian cancer have been shown to exhibit cytotoxic T lymphocytes (CTLs) specifically against erbB-2 (77,78). Furthermore, CD4[+] and CD8[+] tumor infiltrating lymphocytes (TILs) have been identified as important mediators of the cellular immune response to ovarian cancers (79,80). Gene therapy strategies that are based on immunopotentiation are categorized into two different types: passive and active immunotherapy (Figure 5).

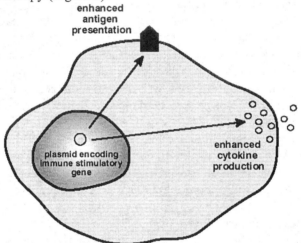

Passive immunotherapy is based on the use of pre-formed immunologic elements to augment the immune system's response to tumor cells. This is accomplished by isolating and expanding tumor infiltrating lymphocytes or tumor-associated lymphocytes *ex vivo* and subsequently re-administering these lymphocytes to the patient. Gene transfer technology has been used to improve the specificity of TILs to tumor cells in order to enhance their anti-tumor effects. For instance, lymphocytes have been transduced with a gene encoding for a chimeric erbB-2 antibody and a T-cell receptor. These genes specifically consist of variable domains from monoclonal antibodies that are joined to T-cell receptor-signaling chains. Once the novel gene product is expressed, the modified lymphocytes targets erbB-2 cells and starts T cell activation (81,82). Hwu *et al* transduced TIL precursors with chimeric genes via retroviruses and was able to show effective recognition of ovarian tumor cells with subsequent T cell activation, lysis of cells, and release of cytokines *in vitro* (83). Others have focused on genetically engineering lymphocytes to manufacture increased concentrations of interleukin-2 (IL-2) and tumor necrosis factor alpha (84), cytokines known to play an important role in chemotaxis and cell-mediated anti-tumor immunity.

Active immunotherapy is based on the initiation or augmentation of the immune system response against unrecognized or poorly immunogenic tumors. Specifically, this form of therapy relies on techniques that increase local concentrations of cytokines and other co-stimulatory molecules or increase expression of known tumor antigens to enhance the immune response against unidentified tumor antigens. For example, investigators have transduced tumors with genes that encode IL-2 and tumor necrosis factor alpha. IL-2 has been shown to directly stimulate $CD8^+$ CTLs (85), and tumor necrosis factor-alpha has been shown to recruit macrophages by chemoattraction (86) and stimulate cytotoxic activity of B cells (87). Interferon-gamma has been shown to stimulate the expression of MHC molecules and to recruit numerous mediators of the immune system (88,89).

It is also known that tumors exhibiting down-regulation of major histocompatibility complex (MHC) genes are poorly immunogenic (90). Efforts have been directed towards increasing MHC expression by genetic manipulation of tumor cells, thus stimulating the native immune response to tumor cells and their respective antigens. Such immunologic help may involve genes encoding cytokines, accessory molecules, or major histocompatibility complex antigens (85,86,91-95). This approach has been often described as "tumor vaccines" and has been shown to have anti-tumor activity *in vivo* against human melanomas (95) and other neoplastic models.

Investigators have attempted to augment the immune response by increasing expression of known tumor antigens through specific delivery of constructs that encode these tumor-associated antigens. Studies based on the use of human carcinoembryonic antigen has shown some promise by demonstrating cellular and humoral responses in addition to providing protection against colon carcinoma cells expressing syngeneic carcinoembryonic antigen (96). Moreover, some ovarian cancer patients have cytotoxic T-lymphocytes directed against the erbB-2 oncoprotein, thus indicating that this protein may also act as tumor-associated antigen (97)

1.3.2. Adoptive Immunotherapy Based Protocol

T-cell based therapies utilizing IL-2 and tumor reactive T-cells have been developed for patients with metastatic melanoma with significant reduction in tumor volume in some patients (98,99). Investigators have attempted to broaden the utility of adoptive cellular immunity in epithelial cancers by creating chimeric antibody/T-cell receptor genes composed of variable domains from monoclonal antibodies joined to T-cell receptor-signaling chains. Hwu *et al* (100) and Rosenberg *et al* (99) have demonstrated that T-cells retrovirally transduced with this gene can recognize antibody-defined antigens of ovarian cancer cells and that this type of recognition ultimately lead to T-cell activation, lysis, and cytokine release *in vitro*. Furthermore, these T-cells can react against tumor antigens defined by monoclonal antibodies in an *in vivo* murine model (101).

Based on these findings, these investigators have proposed a phase I clinical trial for the treatment of patients with advanced ovarian cancer whereby the Mov-γ receptor, a chimeric receptor derived from the monoclonal antibody Mov18 that recognizes a highly expressed antigen in ovarian adenocarcinoma, is introduced into OKT3-stimulated peripheral blood lymphocytes. These modified lymphocytes are subsequently administered to the patient.

1.4. Multi-Drug Resistance (MDR)

Manipulation of the multi-drug resistance gene that encodes for glycoprotein p170 is a strikingly different approach to tumor control from those described previously. It is well known that the response of tumors to chemotherapy is largely dependent on the dose; however, conventional chemotherapy regimens are limited by its inherent toxicity on bone marrow. Also, researchers have identified that some epithelial tumors exhibit resistance to numerous drugs (102-107). Thereafter, investigators identified a drug efflux pump glycoprotein (p170) and the MDR1 cDNA (108,109). By transducing the MDR1 gene into bone marrow, one can effectively protect hematopoietic stem cells and thus, increase the doses of conventional chemotherapeutic agents (108). Essentially, this approach improves tumor toxicity while limiting hematotoxic side effects. Sorrentino *et al* demonstrated its feasibility by showing that bone marrow cells that were transduced with the MDR1 gene were subsequently resistant to paclitaxel chemotherapy (110). However, this approach has been criticized for its short-lived duration and low levels of protein expression by the hematopoietic system *in vivo*. Bienzle *et al* were able to overcome this by using extended cell cultures with multiple exposures to virus before re-implantation (111). As a result, they were able to show significant levels of protein expression in re-implanted stem cells for up to 2 years. One other concern about this approach is the possibility of tumor cells being present within stem cell cultures, which would theoretically increase the risk of relapse on re-implantation. However, this theoretical problem has been avoided by the inherent natural resistance of bone marrow cells to adenoviral transduction. One is able to deliver adenoviral toxins or pro-apoptotic genes to a bone marrow cell culture in order to kill tumor cells yet simultaneously preserve bone marrow cells for future use (112-114).

Given the low levels of amplification of the MDR1 gene in ovarian cancers, manipulation of the MDR1 gene in this setting may prove to be a possible treatment of ovarian cancer (115). Again, one can increase the doses of conventional chemotherapy while protect the bone marrow from untoward effects. In a murine model, researchers were able to demonstrate increased resistance to chemotherapy side effects in hematopoietic stem cells that were transduced by the MDR1 gene (108).

1.4.1. Multi-Drug Resistance Gene-Based Protocol

Studies have indicated that cell lines transduced with the MDR1 gene demonstrate significant resistance to numerous drugs where are commonly used in solid tumors including ovarian cancers such as actinomycin-D, vincristine, adriamycin, and paclitaxel (108). However, some studies indicate that ovarian cancer patients uncommonly expressed elevated levels of MDR1 mRNA (116,117), and some investigators have successfully modified hematopoietic stem cells with retroviral vectors that carry and express the MDR gene in an animal model setting (118-122). Deisseroth and others have created a protocol whereby the bone marrow of refractory ovarian cancer patients is modified with the MDR1 gene. Specifically, early progenitor cells are harvested and then modified with a retroviral vector containing the MDR1 gene. Following treatment of systemic disease with high-does cyclophosphamide and thiotepa, the modified stem cells containing the MDR genes are transplanted back into the recipient and the patient will subsequently receive cyclic chemotherapy with paclitaxel.

2. FUTURE VECTOR DEVELOPMENTS OF OVARIAN CANCER GENE THERAPY APPROACHES

As discussed previously, there has been a tremendous effort toward translating basic research findings in the laboratory to the bedside with respect to human gene therapy trials. As we continue to collect data from these initial trials, further refinements of gene therapy approaches and clinical gene therapy protocols need to be made in order to realistically improve the survival rate of women with ovarian cancer. Central to the realization of the potential of gene therapy approaches is the ability to accomplish efficient and specific gene delivery to cancer cells, and as the Orkin-Motulsky report to the NIH indicates, greater research emphasis on basic areas of gene transfer and expression is needed. Additionally, the importance of correlative studies in gene therapy cannot be overstated. A lesson of major importance in gene therapy trials to date, is the realization that these vector systems are clearly inadequate to achieve a meaningful clinical effect.

For example, one trial demonstrated low efficiencies of tumor cell transduction at standard adenoviral concentrations (124). Moreover, other studies indicate that host inflammatory and immunologic responses to the vector have resulted in limited vector efficiency and treatment toxicity. (125,126). It has been shown that gene therapy vectors may disseminate beyond the tumor compartment (127), and resultant non-tumor transduction could result in significant toxicity (128,129). It is also known that both retroviruses and adenoviruses have limitations as well. Retroviruses are limited by the size of their payloads and carry up to 8 kilobases (kb) of material. Also, they are often inactivated by serum complement, difficult to produce at high titers, and transduce only dividing cells given their stable integration into the host genome. Adenoviruses are limited by their low levels of gene expression, and host inflammatory responses to adenoviruses have been well documented (125).

Addressing this issue, Zwiebel et al (130) have used endothelial cells vehicles to achieve tumor eradications by incorporation into areas of tumor angiogenesis. This type of targeting has been used to achieve localization of anti-tumor products to tumor sites with significant tumor suppression. At the University of Alabama at Birmingham, researchers have attempted to use normal human endothelial cells expressing toxin genes as a vector for achieving delivery to tumor cells in situ. Rancourt et al (131) were able to show that these cellular vehicles can also achieve a bystander effect. Moreover, there was enhanced survival with these vectors in a murine model of ovarian carcinoma. This method of exploited cells as gene delivery vectors may have significant advantages over viral vectors for molecular chemotherapy approaches.

Addressing the issue of limited gene transfer efficiency with standard adenoviruses, Vanderkwaak et al (132) demonstrated significantly improved transduction in both ovarian cancer cell lines and primary ovarian cancer cells derived from malignant ascites in ovarian cancer patients with an RGD-modified adenovirus. By altering the H1 loop of the fiber knob of the adenovirus with a tripeptide insertion, one is able to alter and improve the tropism of adenoviruses through preferential binding to cell membrane integrins. Standard adenoviruses enter cells by binding to the coxsackie-adenovirus receptor (CAR), and it has been shown that primary epithelial tumors including ovarian carcinomas routinely express low levels of CAR. Thus, this modified adenovirus may prove to be useful in improving the transduction of primary ovarian carcinomas cells. Work is currently underway to develop a clinical Phase I protocol employing this modified adenovirus to evaluate specifically tumor targeting and anti-tumor effect.

In other studies, Dmitriev et al were able to fuse a recombinant soluble form of CAR to human epidermal growth factor (EGF) and investigated its ability to target adenoviral infection to the EGF receptor overexpressed in cancer cell lines. They were able to clearly demonstrate that enhancement of gene transfer efficiency in cell lines overexpressing EGF receptor via a non-CAR pathway (data submitted). It is clear that re-targeting mechanisms for gene therapy will need to be further investigated and utilized in order to overcome limitation in gene transfer efficiency and efficacy.

Conditionally replicative viral vectors represent another possible method to address the suboptimal tumor transduction of therapeutic genes *in vivo* (133). A replication-competent virus is able to selectively replicate within tumor cells and leave normal cells unaffected. This improved viral transduction would have two possible therapeutic benefits. First, tumor specific replication of a viral vector encoding an anti-tumor gene would increase the viral concentration at the tumor interface with spread of viral vectors into the tumor mass. This would theoretically improve the tumor transduction efficiency and the efficacy of the vector. Second, the use of lytic viruses would create virus-mediated oncolysis which would occur irrespective of the delivered therapeutic anti-tumor gene. The viral-mediated oncolysis could be further amplified by delivery of an anti-tumor gene. Conditionally replicative adenoviral vectors have been developed which possess an IL-6 autocrine arc resulting in viral mediated tumor cell oncolysis. ONYX Inc. has developed a vector which is an attenuated adenovirus that replicates in cancer cells and causes selective tumor lysis.

Adenoviruses possess a natural lytic life cycle, which can be exploited to make the viral vector specifically replicate in and kill tumor cells. Bischoff et al (134) reported a mutant adenovirus that that replicate within p53-negative cells and mediates specific tumor cell killing. Rancourt et al (135) have shown that an E1A-deleted adenovirus can be rendered replication-competent on induction of the infected cells by IL-6. Thus, in the presence of IL-6, replication of E1A-deleted viruses leads to specific killing of infected tumor cells both *in vitro* and *in vivo*. Moreover, this system is particular useful since ovarian carcinoma cell lines and primary ovarian carcinoma cells express IL-6 in an autocrine fashion. As a result, the adenovirus replicates and destroys tumor cells by using one of the tumor cell's gene products.

Suzuki et al were able to demonstrate enhanced oncolytic potency when incorporating the RGD motif into the adenoviral fiber knob into replication-competent adenoviruses (data submitted). Again, application of tropism modification in replication-competent adenoviruses is significant since there is either an absence or low levels of CAR in primary ovarian cancer cells, which would limit the usefulness of standard replication-competent adenoviruses.

Another limitation of adenoviruses is their inability to integrate into the host genome. The viral recombinant genome is usually located epichromosomally in transduced target cells. These sequences are not transferred to daughter cells after replication of transduced cells. Thus, the duration of transgene expression is limited. In an attempt to overcome this problem, researchers have developed a chimeric viral vector system that employs that advantages of both retroviral and adenoviral vectors. This strategy uses adenoviral vectors to induce target cells to function as producers of retroviral vectors *in vivo*. The progeny retroviral particles are then able to transduce neighboring cells, thus improving the transduction efficiency (136).

Lentiviruses are another class of retroviral vectors, for which the best known virus is the human immunodeficiency virus. Lentiviruses have the advantage of retaining the ability to infect both dividing and non-dividing cells. An attractive aspect of packaging transgenes within the lentiviral genome is the sustained expression (greater than 6 months) that has been observed in experimental systems (137).

Another vector that has attributes similar to lentivirus is the adeno-associated virus (AAV) is a DNA based member of the human parvovirus family that depends on co-infection with a helper adenovirus for growth and replication. In contrast to alternative viral based gene delivery systems, recombinant AAV lack all viral genes, are non-immunogenic, and can infect dividing and quiescent cells (138). The most attractive aspect of AAV vectors is the stable and long term expression of transgenes that has been observed in animal studies. Tropism targeted AAV vectors have been developed for use in hematopoetic malignancies and may offer a means of enhancing therapeutic effect and therapeutic index (139,140).

Safety concerns related to the use of viral particles as gene delivery vehicles in humans has led to research in non-viral delivery systems. In addition, the use of alternatives to viral particles often enables the investigator to package larger amounts of transgene DNA and avoids the immunogenicity inherent in most viral systems. The simplest approach to non-viral delivery of genetic material is administration of naked plasmid DNA (141). Small amounts of naked DNA will be taken up and translated by cells. This approach is probably limited in clinical use secondary to extremely poor gene transfer efficiency when delivered to systemic or regional tumors and the non-specificity of the delivery system. Cationic lipids have been the most extensively studied non-viral based gene delivery system. While these lipids do not appear to attain equivalent gene transfer efficiency as the adenovirus, lipid based systems can accommodate large DNA sequences, can be manufactured in unlimited quantity, and have been safely applied in clinical trials to date (141). Alternative classes of synthetic cationic polymer vector systems have been investigated. Polyethylamines can mediate efficient gene transfer without the use of an endosome disruption component. In addition, bioplymers, such as gelatin and chitosan have been used to develop gene delivery microspheres (142).

3. CONCLUSION

Advances in immunology and virology and characterization of the molecular basis of cancer have brought the genetic treatment of neoplasms to the clinical realm and there is great promise of gene therapy becoming a realistic treatment option. The amount of research and interest in translational studies in gene therapy has increased exponentially in the last five years, and undoubtedly, this will continue to expand and make a significant impact in ovarian cancer treatment

With toxicity data from Phase I trials, Phase II and III studies can be initiated to determine the efficacy of gene therapy in the setting of ovarian cancer and the needed refinements for other gene therapy strategies. Of course, major obstacles and issues still exist and must be resolved before these and future approaches can be applied widely to ovarian cancer patients. However, the rapid advances in molecular technology and gene delivery system will hopefully lead to improved gene-based treatment strategies for women with ovarian cancer.

REFERENCES

1. Crawford R, Shephard J. Management of Epithelial Ovarian Cancer. In: Shingleton H, Fowler W, Jordan J, Lawrence W, eds. Gynecologic Oncology: Current Diagnosis and Treatment. London: W B Saunders, 203-212, 1996.
2. Kinzler KW and Vogelstein B: Lessons from hereditary colorectal cancer. Cell 1996; 87:159-170.
3. Kinzler KW and Vogelstein B: Landscaping the cancer terrain. Science 1998;280:1036-1037.
4. Hirschowitz E, Ohwada A, Pasca W, Russi T, Crystal R. *In vivo* adenovirus-mediated gene transfer of the *Eschrichia Coli* cytosine deaminase gene to human colon carcinoma-derived tumors induces chemosensitivity to 5-fluorocytosine. Human Gene Ther 1995;6:1055-63.
5. Elion G, Furman P, Fyfe J, DeMiranda P, Beauchamp L, Schaeffer H. Selectivity of action of an antiherpetic agent, 9-(2-hydroxyethoxymethyl) guanine. Proc Natl Acad Sci USA 1977;74:5716-20.
6. Furman P, McGujirt P, Keller P, Fyfe J, Elion G. Inhibition by acyclovir of cell growth and DNA synthesis of cells biochemically transformed with herpes virus genetic information. Virology 1980;102:420-30.
7. Abe A, Takeo T, Emi N, Tanimoto M, Ueda R, Yee J, et al. Transduction of a drug-sensitive toxic gene into human leukemia cell lines with a novel retroviral vector. PSEMB 1993;203:354-8.

150

8. Culvert K, Ram Z, Walbridge S, Ishii H, Oldfield E, Blaese R. *In vivo* gene transfer with retroviral vector-producing cells for the treatment of experimental brain tumors. Science 1992;256:1550-52.

9. Vile R, Nelson J, Castleden S,Chong H, Hart I. Systemic gene therapy of murine melanoma using tissue specific expression of the HSV-tk gene involves an immune component. Cancer Res 1994;54:6228-34.

10. Mesnil M, Piccoli C, Tiraby G, Willecke K, Yamasaki H. Bystander killing of cancer cells by herpes simplex virus thymidine kinase gene is mediated by connexins. Proc Natl Acad Sci USA 1996;93:1831-5.

11. Gagandeep S, Brew R, Green B, et al. Prodrug-activated gene therapy: Involvement of an immunological component in the 'bystander' effect. Cancer Gene Therapy 1996;3: 83-88.

12. Consalvo M, Mullen Ca, Modesti A, et al. 5-fluorocyostine induced eradication of murine adenocarcinoma engineered to express the cytosine deaminase suicide gene requires host immune competence and leaves an efficient memory. J Immunology 1995;154: 5302-5312.

13. Freeman S, Abboud C, Whartenby K, Packman C, Koeplin D, Moolten F, et al. The "bystander effect": Tumor regression when a fraction of the tumor mass is genetically modified.Cancer Res 1993;53:5274-83.

14. Robinson W, Adams J, Marrogi A, Freeman S. Vaccine therapy for ovarian cancer using herpes simplex virus thymidine kinase (HSV-TK) suicide gene transfer technique: A phase I study. Gynecol Oncol 1998; 68:88.

15. Link C, Moorman D. Clinical protocols: A phase I trial of in vivo gene therapy with the Herpes Simplex Thymidine Kinase/Ganciclovir system for the treatment of refractory of recurrent ovarian cancer. Cancer Gene Ther 1995;2:230-1.

16. Link C, Eldeman M, Tennant L, et al. LTKOSN.1 murine vector producer cell(VPC) for the in vivo delivery of the herpes simplex thymidine kinase (HSV-TK) gene for ovarian cancer. Am Soc Gene Ther Abstract #915 (1999).

17. Rosenfeld ME, Feng M, Michael SI, et al. Adenoviral-mediated delivery of the herpes simples virus thymidine kinase gene selectively sensitizes human ovarian carcinoma cells to ganciclovir. Clin Cancer Research 1995;1:1571-1580.

18. Rosenfeld ME, Wang M, Siegal GP, et al. Adenoviral-mediated delivery of herpes simplex virus thymidine kinase results in tumor reduction and prolonged survival in a SCID mouse model of human ovarian carcinoma. J Mol Med 1996;74:455-462.

19. Alvarez R, Gomez-Navarro J, Wang M, et al. Adenoviral mediated suicide gene therapy for ovarian cancer (No. 107) Gynecol Oncol 2000; 76:258.

20. Quattrone A, Fibbi G, Anichini E, Pucci M, Zamperini A, Capaccioli S, et al. Reversion of the invasive phenotype of transformed human fibroblasts by anti-messenger oligonucleotide inhibition of urokinase receptor gene expression. Cancer Res 1995;55: 90-5.

21. Shaw Y, Chang S, Chiou S, Chang W, Lai M. Partial reversion of transformed phenotype of B104 cancer cells by antisense nucleic acids. Cancer Letters 1993;69:27-32.

22. Douglas J, Curiel D. Targeted gene therapy. Tumor Targeting 1995;1:67-84.

23. Helm C, Shrestha K, Thomas S, Shingleton H, Miller D. A unique c-myc-targeted triplex-forming oligonucleotide inhibits the growth of ovarian and cervical carcinomas *in vitro*. Gynecol Oncol 1993;49: 339-43.

24. Durland R, Kessler D, Gunnell S, Duvic M, Pettitt B, Hogan M. Binding of triplex helix-forming oligonucleotides to sites in gene promoters. Biochemistry 1991;30:9246-55.

25. Ebbinghouse S, Gee J, Rodu B, Mayfield C, Sanders G, Miller D. Triplex formation inhibits HER-2/*neu* transcription *in vitro* . J Clin Invest 1993;92:2433-9.

26. Mayfield C, Ebbinghouse S, Gee J, Jones D, Rodu B, Squibb M, et al. Triplex formation by the human H-*ras* promoter inhibits Sp1 binding and *in vitro* transcription. J Biol Chem 1994;269:18232-8.

27. Mayfield C, Squibb M, Miller D. Inhibition of nuclear protein binding to the human Ki-*ras* promoter by triplex-forming oligonucleotides. Biochemistry 1994;33:3358-63.
28. Mukhopadhyay T, Tainsky M, Cavender A, RothJ. Specific inhibition of K-*ras* expression and tumorigenicity of lung cancer cells by antisense RNA. Cancer Res 1991;51:1744-8.
29. Georges R, Mukhopadhyay T, Zhang Y, Yen N, Roth J. Prevention of orthotopic human lung cancer growth by intratracheal instillation of a retroviral antisense K-*ras* construct. Cancer Res 1993;53:1743-6.
30. Saison-Behmoaras T, Tocque B, Rey I, Chassignol M, Thuong N, Helene,C. Short modified antisense oligonucleotide directed against Ha-*ras* point mutation induces selective cleavage of the mRNA and inhibits T24 cell proliferation. EMBO J 1991;30: 1111-6.
31. Calabretta B, Sims R, Valtieri M, Caracciolo D, Szczylik C, Venturelli D, et al. Normal and leukemic hematopoietic cells manifest differential sensitivity to inhibitory effects of c-*myb* antisense oligodeoxynucleotides: An *in vitro* study relevant to bone marrow purging. Proc Natl Acad Sci USA 1991;88:2351-5 .
32. Ratajczak M, Kant J, Luger S, Hijiya N, Zhang J, Zon G, et al. *In vivo* treatment of human leukemia in a scid mouse model with c-*myb* antisense oligonucleotides. Proc Natl Acad Sci USA 1992;89:11823-7.\
33. Wickstrom E, Bacon T, Gonzalez A, Freeman D, Lyman G, Wickstrom E. Human promyelocytic leukemia HL-60 cell proliferation and c-*myc* protein expression are inhibited by an antisense pentadecadeoxynucleotide targeted against c-*myc* RNA. Proc Natl Acad Sci USA 1988;85:1028-32.
34. Harel-Ballan A, Ferris D, Vinocour M, Holt J, Farrar W. Specific inhibition of c-myc protein biosynthesis using an antisense synthetic deoxynucleotide in human T lymphocytes. J Immunol 1988;140:2431-5.
35. McManaway M, Neckers L., Loke S., Al-Nasser A, Redner R, Shiramizu B, et al. Tumour-specific inhibition of lymphoma growth by an antisense oligodeoxynucleotide. Lancet 1990;35:808-11.
36. Collins J, Herman P, Schuch C, Bagby G. c-myc antisense oligonucleotides inhibit the colony-forming capacity of Colo 320 colonic carcinoma cells. J Clin Invest 1992;89: 1523-27.
37. Janicek M, Sevin B, Nguyen H, Averette H. Combination anti-gene therapy targeting c-myc and p53 in ovarian cancer cell lines. Gynecol Oncol 1995;59:87-92.
38. Neuenschwander S, Roberts C, LeRoith D. Growth inhibition of MCF-7 breast cancer cells by stable expression of an insulin-like growth factor 1 receptor antisense ribonucleic acid. Endocrinology 1995;136:4298-303.
39. Resnicoff M, Abraham D, Yutanawiboonachi W, Rotman H, Kajstura J, Rubin R, et al. The insulin-like growth factor 1 receptor protects tumor cells from apoptosis *in vivo* . Cancer Res 1995;55:2463-9.
40. Resnicoff M, Ambrose D, Coppola D, Rubin R. Insulin-like growth factor-1 and its receptor mediate autocrine proliferation of human ovarian carcinoma cell lines. Lab Invest 1993;69: 756-60.
41. Szczylik T, Skorski T, Nicolaides N, Manzella L., Malaguarnera L., Venturelli D, et al. Selective inhibition of leukemia cell proliferation by BCR-ABL antisense oligodeoxynucleotides. Science 1991;253:562-5.
42. Skorski T, Nieborowska-Skorska M, Nicolaides N, Szczylik C, Iversen P, Iozzo R, et al. Suppression of Philadelphia leukemia cell proliferation in mice by BCR-ABL antisense oligodeoxynucleotide. Proc Natl Acad Sci USA 1994;91:4504-8.
43. Kashani-Sabet M, Funato T, Florenes V, Fodstad O, Scanlon K. Suppression of the neoplastic phenotype *in vivo* by an anti-*ras* ribozyme. Cancer Res 1994;54:900-2.
44. Kashani-Sabet M, Funato T, Tone T, Jiao L, Wang W, Yashida E, et al. Reversal of the malignant phenotype by an anti-*ras* ribozyme. Antisense Res Dev 1992;2:3-15.

152

45.   Lange W, Cantin E, Finke J, Dolken G. *In vitro* and *in vivo* effects of synthetic ribozymes targeted against BCR/ABL mRNA. Leukemia 1993;7:1786-94.
46.   Snyder D, Wu Y, Wang J, Rossi J, Swiderski P, Kaplan B, et al. Ribozyme mediated inhibition of bcr-abl gene expression in a Philadelphia chromosome-positive cell line. Blood 1993;82:600-5.
47.   Milner B, Allan L, Eccles D,et al. p53 mutation is a common genetic event in ovarian carcinoma. Cancer Res 1993;53:2128-2132.
48.   Porter P, gown A, Kramp S, et al. Widespread p53 overexpression in human malignant tumors. Am J Pathol 1992; 140: 145-153.
49.   Santoso JT, Tang DC, Lane SB, et al. Adenovirus-based p53 gene therapy in ovarian cancer. Gynecol Oncol 1995;59:171-178.
50.   Mujoo K, Maneval DC, Anderson SC, et al. Adenoviral-mediated p53 tumor suppressor gene therapy of human ovarian carcinoma. Oncogene 1996;12:1617-1623.
51.   Janicek M, Sevin B, Nguyen H, Averette H. Combination anti-gene therapy targeting c-myc and p53 in ovarian cancer cell lines. Gynecol Oncol 59:87,1995
52.   Wolf J, Mills G, Bazzet L et al. Adenovirus mediated p53 growth inhibition of ovarian cancer cells is independent of endogenous p53 status. Gynecol Oncol 75:261,1999.
53.   Holt JT, Thompson Me, Szabo C, et al. Growth retardation and tumour inhibition by BRCA1. Nature Genetics 1996;12:223-225.
54.   Song K, Cowan K, Sinha B. In vivo studies of adenovirus-mediated p53 gene therapy for cis-platin resistant human ovarian tumor xenografts. Oncology Res 1999;11:153.
55.   Nielsen L, Lipari P, Dell J, et al. Adenovirus mediated p53 gene therapy and paclitaxel have synergistic efficacy in models of human head and neck, ovarian, prostate, and breast cancer. Clin Cancer Res 1998;4:835.
56.   Minaguchi T, Mori T, Kanamori Y, et al. Growth suppression of human ovarian cancer cells by adenovirus mediated transfer of the PTEN gene. Cancer Res 1999 59:6063.
57.   Wolf J, Kim T, Fightmaster D, et al. Growth suppression of human ovarian cancer cell lines by the introduction of a p16 gene via a recombinant adenovirus. Gynecol Oncol 1999; 73:27.
58.   Xiang J, Piche A, Gomez-Navarro J, Siegal, GP, Alvarez RD, Curiel DT: An inducible recombinant adenoviral vector encoding bax selectively induces apoptosis in ovarian cancer cells. Tumor Targeting 4:1-9, 1999.
59.   Tai Y, Strobel T, Kufe D, Cannistra S. In vivo cytotoxicity of ovarian cancer cells through tumor-selective expression of the BAX gene. Cancer Res 59:2121,1999.
60.   Xiang J, Gomez-Navarro J, Arafat W, Liu B, Parker S, Alvarez R, Siegal G, Curiel D: Pro-apoptotic treatment with an adenovirus encoding bax enhances the effect of chemotherapy in ovarian cancer: J Gene Medicine 2:97-106, 2000.
61.   Arafat WO, Gomez-Navarro J, Xiang J, Barnes M, Mahareshti P, Alvarez RD, Siegal, GP, Badib AO, Buchsbaum D, Curiel DT, Stackhouse MA: An adenovirus encoding proapoptotic bax induces apoptosis and enhances the radiation effect in human ovarian cancer. Molecular Therapy 1:1-7, 2000.
62.   Redemann N, Holzmann B, von Ruden T, Wagner E, Schlessinger J, Ullrich A. Anti-oncogenic activity of signalling-defective epidermal growth factor receptor mutants. Mol Cell Biol 1992;12:491-8.
63.   Ueno H, Colbert H, Escobedo J, Williams L. Inhibition of PDGF beta receptor signal transduction by coexpression of a truncated receptor. Science 1991:252:844-8.
64.   Prager D, Li H, Asa S, Melmed S. Dominant-negative inhibition of tumorigenesis *in vivo* by human insulin-like growth factor I receptor mutant. Proc Natl Acad Sci USA 1994;91:2181-5.
65.   Millauer B, Shawver L, Plate K, Risau W, Ullrich A. Glioblastoma growth inhibited *in vivo* by a dominant-negative *flk* -1 mutant. Nature 1994;367:576-9.

66. Shamah S, Stiles C, Guha A. Dominant-negative mutants of platelet-derived growth factor revert the transformed phenotype of human astrocytoma cells. Mol Cell Biol 1993; 12:1674-9.

67. Deshane J, Loechel F, Conry R, Siegal G, King C, Curiel D. Intracellular single-chain antibody directed against erbB-2 down-regulates cell surface erbB-2 and exhibits a selective antiproliferative effect in erbB-2 overexpressing cancer cell lines. Gene Ther 1994;3:332-7.

68. Beerli R, Winfried W, Hynes N. Intracellular expression of single chain antibodies reverts erbB-2 transformation. J Biol Chem 1994;269:23931-6.

69. Deshane J, Grim J, Loechel S, Siegal G, Alvarez R, King C, et al. Intracellular antibody directed against erbB-2 mediates targeted tumor cell eradication by inducing apoptosis.Cancer Gene Ther 1996;3:89-98.

70. Beerli R, Wels W, Hynes N. Autocrine inhibition of the epidermal growth factor receptor by intracellular expression of a single-chain antibody. Biochem and Biophys Res Comm 1994;204:666-72.

71. Tait D, Obermiller P, Frazier S, et al. A Phase I trial of retroviral BRCA1sv gene therapy in ovarian cancer. Clin Cancer Res 1997; 3:1959.

72. Buller R, Pegram M, Runnebaum I, A Phase I/II trial of recombinant adenovrial human p53 intraperitoneal gene therapy in recurrent ovarian cancer (No. 37) Gynecol Oncol 1999;72:452.

73. Zhang Y, Yu D, Xia W, Hung M. HER-2/neu targeting cancer therapy via adenovirus-mediated E1A delivery in an animal model. Oncogene 1995;10:1947-54.

74. Ueno N, Bartholomeusz C, Herrmann J, et al. E1A mediated paclitaxel sensitization in HER-2/neu overexpressing ovarian cancer SKOV-3.ip1 through apoptosis involving the caspase-3 pathway. Clin Cancer Res 2000; 6:250.

75. Barnes M, Deshane J, Siegal G, et al. Novel gene therapy strategies to accomplish growth factor modulation induces enhanced tumor cell chemosensitivity. Clin Cancer Res 1996; 2:1089.

76. Sahin U, Tureci O, Schmitt H et al. Human neoplasms elicit multiple specific immune responses in the autologous host. Proc Natl Acad Sci USA 1995;92:11810-11813.

77. Peoples GE, Goedegeguure PS, Smith R, et al. Breast and ovarian cancer-specific cytotoxic T lymphocytes recognize the same HER-2/neu-derived peptide. Proc Natl Acad Sci USA 1995;92:432-436.

78. Ionnaides CG, Fisk B, Fan D, et al. Cytotoxic T cells isolated from ovarian malignant ascites recognize a peptide derived from the HER-2/neu protooncogene. Cell Immunol 1993;151:225-234.

79. Merogi AJ, Marrogi AJ, Ramesh R, et al. Tumor-host interation: Analysis of cytokines, growth factors, and tumor-infiltrating lymphocytes in ovarian carcinoma. Hum Pathol 1997;38:321-331.

80. Kooi S, zhang HZ, Patenia R, et al. HLA class I expression on human ovarian carcinoma cells correlates with T-cell infiltration in vivo and T-cell expansion in vitro in low concentrations of recombinant interleukin-2. Cell Immunol 1996;174:116-118.

81. Stancovski I, Schinder DG, Waks T, et al. Targeting of T lymphocytes to neu/HER-2-expressing cells using chimeric single chain Fv receptors. J Immunol 1993;151:6577-6582.

82. Eshhar Z, Waks T, Gross G, et al. Specific activation and targeting of cytotoxic lymphocytes through chimeric single chains consisting of antibody-binding domains and the and subunits of the immunoglobulin and T-cell receptors. Proc Natl Acad Sci USA 1993;90:720-724.

83. Hwu P, Shafer GE, Treisman J, et al. Lysis of ovarian cancer cells by human lymphocytes redirected with a chimeric gene composed of an antibody variable region and Fc receptor gamma chain. J Exp Med 1993;178:361-366.

84. Yannelli J, Hyatt C, Johnston S, Hwu P, Rosenberg S. Characterization of human tumour cell lines transduced with the cDNA encoding either tumor necrosis factor a (TNF-a or interleukin-2 (IL-2). J Immunol Methods 1993;161:77-90.

85. Fearon ER, Pardoll DM, Itaya T, et al Interluekin –2 production by tumor cells bypasses T helper function in the generation of an antitumor response. Cell 1990;60:397-403.

86. Blankenstein T, Qin Z, Uberla K et al. Tumor suppression after tumor cell-targetedd tumor necrosis factor a gene transfer. J Exp Med 1991;173:1047-1052.

87. Lopez-Cepero M, Garcia-Sanz JA, Herbert L, et al. Soluble and membrane-bound TNF-alpha are involved in the cytotoxic activity of B cells from tumor-bearing mice against tumor targets. J Immunol 1994;152:3333-3341.

88. Lu Y, Ussery DG, Muncaster MM, et al. Evidence for retinoblastoma protein (Rb) dependent and independent IFN-gamma responses: RB coordinately rescues IFN-gamma induction of MHC class II gene transcription in noninducible breast carcinoma cells. Oncogene 1994;9:1015-1019.

89. Matory YL, Chen M, Dorfman DM, et al. Antitumor activity of three mouse mammary cancer cell lines after interferon-gamma gene transfection. Surgery 1995;118:251-256.

90. Tanaka K, Isselbacher KJ, Khoury G, et al. Reversal of oncogenesis by the expression of a major histocompatibility comples class I gene. Science 1985;228:26-30.

91. Asher A, Mule J, Kasid A, Restifo N, Salo J, Reichart C, et al. Murine tumor cells transduced with the gene for tumor necrosis factor-alpha. Evidence for paracrine immune effects of tumor necrosis factor against tumors. J Immunol 1991;146:3227-34.

92. Golumbek P, Lazenby A, Levitzky H, Jafee L, Karasuyama H, Baker M, et al. Treatment of established renal cancer by tumor cells engineered to secrete interleukin-4. Science 1991;254:713-6.

93.. Gansbacher B, Bannerji R, Daniels B, Zier K, Cronin K, Gilboa E. Retroviral vector-mediated gamma-interferon gene transfer into tumor cells generates potent and long lasting antitumor immunity. Cancer Res 1990;50:7820-5.

94. Tahara H, Lotze M. Antitumor effects of interleukin-12 (IL-12): applications for the immunotherapy and gene therapy of cancer. Gene Ther 1995;2:96-106.

95. Nabel G, Nabel E, Yang Z, Fox B, Plautz G, Gao X, et al. Direct gene transfer with DNA-liposome complexes in melanoma: expression, biological activity, and lack of toxicity in humans. Proc Natl Acad Sci USA 1993;90:11307-11.

96. Conry R, Lobuglio A, Loechel F, Moore S, Sumerel L, Barlow D, et al. A carcinoembryonic antigen polynucleotide vaccine has *in vivo* antitumor activity. Gene Ther 1995;2:59-65.

97. Disis M, Smith J, Murphy A, Chen W, Cheever M. *In vitro* generation of human cytolytic T-cells specific for peptides derived from the HER-2/neu protooncogene protein. Cancer Res 1994;54:1071-6.

98. Rosenberg S, Packard B, Aebersold P, Solomon D, Topalian S, Toy S, et al. Use of tumor infiltrating lymphocytes and interleukin-2 in the immunotherapy of patients with metastatic melanoma. Preliminary report. N Engl J Med 1988;319:1676-80.

99. Rosenberg S, Yannelli J, Yang J, Topalian S, Schwartzentruber D, Weber J, et al. Treatment of patients with metastatic melanoma with autologous tumor-infiltrating lymphocytes and interleukin 2. J Natl Cancer Inst 1994;86:1159-66.

100. Hwu P, Shafer G, Treisman J, Schindler D, Gross G, Cowherd R, et al. Lysis of ovarian cancer cells by human lymphocytes redirected with a chimeric gene composed of an antibody variable region and the Fc receptor chain. J Exp Med 1993;178:361-6.

101. Hwu P, Yang J, Cowherd R, Treisman J, Shafer J, Eshhar Z, Rosenberg S. *In vivo* antitumor activity of T cells redirected with chimeric antibody/T-cell receptor genes. Cancer Res 1995;55:3369-73

102. Biedler J, Riehm H. Cellular resistance to actinomycin D in chinese hamster cells in vitro: cross resistance, radioautographic, and cytogenetic studies. Cancer Res 1970;30:1174-84.

103. van der Zee A, Hollema H, Suurmeijer A, Krans M, Sluiter W, Willemse P, et al. Value of p-glycoprotein, glutathione S-tranferase pi, c-erbB-2, and p53 as prognostic factors in ovarian cancer. J Clin Oncol 1995;13:70-8.

104. Chin K, Tanaka S, Darlington G, Pastan I, Gottesman M. Heat-shock and arsenic increase expression of the multi-drug resistance (MDR1) gene in human renal carcinoma cells. J Biol Chem 1990;265:221- 6.

105. Chan H, Haddad G, Thorner P, Deboer G, Lin Y, Ondrusek N, Yeger H, Ling V. P-gycoprotein expression as a predictor of the outcome of therapy for neuroblastoma. N Eng J Med 1991;325:1608-14.

106. Holtzmayer T, Hilsenbeck S, Van Hoff D, RoninsonI. Clinical correlates of MDR-1 (P-glycoprotein) gene expression in ovarian and small cell lung carcinomas. J Natl Cancer Inst 1992;84:1486-91.

107. Verrelle P, Meissonnier F, Fonck Y, Feillel V, Dionet C, Kwiatkowski F, et al. Clinical relevance of immunohistochemical detection of multidrug resistance p-glycoprotein in breast cancer. J Natl Cancer Inst 1991;83:111-6.

108. Champlin R, Kavanagh J, Deisseroth A. Use of safety-modified retrovirus to introduce chemotherapy resistance sequences into normal hematopoietic cells for chemoprotection during the therapy of ovarian cancer: A pilot trial. Hum Gene Ther 1994;5:1507-22.

109. Endicott J, Ling V. The biochemistry of P-glycoprotein mediated drug resistance. Annu Rev Biochem 1989;58:137-71.

110. Sorrentino BP, Brandt SJ, Bodine D, et al. Selection of drug-resistant bone marrow cells in vivo after retroviral transfer of human MDR1. Science 1992;257:99-103.

111. Bienzle D, Abrams-Ogg AC, Kruth SA, et al. Gene transfer into hematopoetic stem cells: Long term maintenance of in vitro activated progenitors without marrow ablation. Proc Natl Acad Sci USA 1994;91:350-354.

112. Clarke MF, Apel IJ, Benedict MA, et al. A recombinant bcl-xs adenovirus selectively induces apoptosis in cancer cells but not in normal bone marrow. Proc Natl Acad Sci USA 1995;92:11024-11028.

113. Kim M, Wright M, DeShane J, et al. A novel gene therapy strategy for elimination of prostate carcinoma cells from human bone marrow. Hum Gene Therapy 1997;8:157-170.

114. Seth P, Brinkmann U, Schwartz GN, et al. Adenovirus-mediated gene transfer to human breast tumor cells: An approach for cancer gene therapy and bone marrow purging. Cancer Res 1996;56:1346-1351.

115. Goldstein LJ, Galski H, Fogo A, et al. Expression of a multidrug resistance gene in human cancers. J Natl Cancer Inst 1989;81:116-124.

116. Schurs E, Raymond M, Bell J, Gros P. Characterization of the multidrug resistance protein expressed in cell clones stably transfected with the mouse mdr1 cDNA. Cancer Res 1989;49:2729-34.

117. Devault A, Gros P. Two members of the mouse mdr gene family confer multidrug resistance with overlapping but distinct drug specifities. Mol Cell Biol 1990;10:1652-63.

118. Ueda K, Cardarelli C, Gottesman M, Pastan I. Expression of a full-length cDNA for the human "MDR1" gene confers resistance to colchicine, doxrubicin, and vinblastine. Proc Natl Acad Sci USA 1987;84:3004-8.

119. Goldstein L, Galski H, Fojo A, Willingham M, Lai S, Gadzar A, et al. Expression of a multidrug resistance gene in human cancers. J Natl Cancer Inst 1989;81:116-24.

120. Pastan I, Gottesman M, Ueda K, Lovelace E, Rutherford A, Willingham M. A retrovirus carrying an MDR1 cDNA confers multidrug resistance and polarized expression of p-glycoprotein in MDCK cells. Proc Natl Acad Sci USA 1988;85:4486-90.

156

121. Hanania E, Deisseroth A. Serial transplantation shows that early hematopoietic precursor cells are transduced by MDR-1 retroviral vector in mouse gene therapy model. Cancer Gene Ther 1994;1:21-5.

122. Sorrentino B, Brandt S, Bodine D, Gottesman M, Pastan I, Cline A, et al. Selection of drug-resistant bone marrow cells *in vivo* after retroviral transfer of human MDR1. Science 1992;257:99-103.

123. Orkin SH, Motulsky AG: Report and Recommendations of the Panel to Assess the NIH Investment in Research on Gene Therapy. http://www.nih.gov/od/orda/panelrep.htm

124. Sterman DH, Treat J, Elshami AA, et al. A phase I clinical trial of adenoviral-mediated herpes simplex virus thymidine kinase gene therapy for malignant mesothelioma. Preliminary Results, in Gene Therapy for Cancer V, San Diego, CA, 1996 P29 (abstr).

125. Yang Y, Nunes FA, Berencsi K, et al. Cellular immunity to viral antigens limits E1-deleted adenoviruses for gene therapy. Proc Natl Acad Sci USA 1994;91:4407-4411.

126. Yang Y, Li Q, Ertl HC, et al. Cellular and humoral immune responses to viral antigens create barriers to lung-directed gene therapy with recombinant adenoviruses. J Virol 1995;69:2004-2015.

127. Goodman JC, Trask TW, Chen SH, et al. Adenoviral-mediated thymidine kinase gene transfer into the primate brain followed by systemic ganciclovir: Pathologic, radiologic, and molecular studies. Human Gene Therapy 1996;7:1241-1250.

128. Yee D, McGuire Se, Brunner N et al. Adenovirus-mediated gene transfer of herpes simplex virus thymidine kinase in an ascites model of human breast cancer. Human Gene Therapy 1996;7:1251-1257.

129. Brand K, Arnold W, Bartels T, et al. Liver-associated toxicity of the HSV-tk/GCV approach and adenoviral vectors. Cancer Gene Therapy 1997;4:9-16.

130. Ojeifo JO, Forough R, Paik S, et al. Angiogensis-directed implantation of genetically modified endothelial cells in mice. Cancer Res 1995;55:2240-2244.

131. Rancourt C, Robertson MW, Wang M, et al. Endothelial cell vehicles for delivery of cytotoxic genes as a gene therapy approach for carcinoma of the ovary. Clin Cancer Res 1998;4:265-270.

132. Vanderkwaak T, Wang M, Gomez-Navarro J, et al: An advanced generation of adenoviral vectors selectively enhances gene transfer for ovarian cancer gene therapy approaches. Gynecol Oncol 1999;74:227.

133. Rancourt C, Curiel DT: Conditionally replicative adenoviruses for cancer therapy. Advanced Drug Delivery Rev 1997;27:67-81.

134. Bischoff JR, Kirn DH, Williams A, et al. An adenovirus mutant that replicates selectively in p53-deficient human tumor cells. Science 1996;274:373-376.

135. Rancourt C, Piche A, Gomez-Navarro J, et al. Interleukin-6 modulated conditionally replicative adenovirus as an antitumor/cytotoxic agent for cancer therapy. Clinical Cancer Research 1999;5:43-50.

136. Bilbao G, Feng M, Rancourt C, et al. Adenoviral/retroviral vector chimeras-A novel strategy to achieve high efficiency stable transduction in vivo. FASEB J 1997;11:624-634.

137. Miyoshi H, Takahashi M, Gage F, Verma I. Stable and efficient gene tranfer into the retina using an HIV based lentiviral vector. Proc Natl Acad Sci USA 1997;94:10319.

138. Bueler H. Adeno-associated viral vectors for gene transfer and gene therapy. Biol Chem 1999; 380:613.

139. Bartlett J, Kleinschmidt J, Boucher R, Samulski R. Targeted adeno-associated virus vector transduction of nonpermissive cells mediated by a bispecific F(ab' gamma)2 antibody. Nature Biotech 1999 ;17:181.

140. Yang Q, Mamounas M, Kennedy S, et al. Development of novel cells surface CD34 targeted recombinant adeno-associated virus vectors for gene therapy. Hum Gene Ther 1998; 9:1929.

141. Li S, Huang L. Nonviral gene therapy: Promises and challenges. Gene Therapy 2000; 7:31.

142. Roy K, Mao H, Huang S, Leong K. Oral gene delivery with chitosan-DNA nanoparticles generates immunologic protection in a murine model of peanut allergy. Nat Med 1999; 5:387

II.   RESEARCH

A. Malignant Transformation

Chapter 7

NORMAL OVARIAN SURFACE EPITHELIUM

Alice S.T. Wong and Nelly Auersperg
Department of Obstetrics and Gynaecology, University of British Columbia,
Vancouver B.C., V6H 3V5, Canada

1.   INTRODUCTION

The ovarian surface epithelium (OSE) is the part of the pelvic mesothelium that covers the ovary. It is also referred to in the literature as ovarian mesothelium (OM) (1, 2) or normal ovarian epithelium (NOE) (3), and it used to be called 'germinal epithelium' because it was mistakenly believed to give rise to germ cells. Because of its inconspicuous appearance and apparent lack of significant functions, the OSE remained among the least known components of the ovary until the last few decades, when increasing histopathologic and immunocytochemical evidence from clinical specimens suggested that the OSE might be the source of the most common and lethal of ovarian cancers, i.e. the epithelial ovarian carcinomas (1, 4-6). However, until relatively recently, there were no experimental systems for the study of the origin of these neoplasms. Animal models of epithelial ovarian cancer are not available because, except in aging hens (7), ovarian tumors in other animal species do not arise in OSE but in follicular, stromal or germ cells, and the biology of these tumors is fundamentally different from that of epithelial ovarian cancer. The establishment of culture systems posed problems because of the minute size and limited growth potential *in vitro* of OSE. In the 1980ties, the first tissue culture systems for OSE from different species (4, 8-13), including human (12, 13), were developed. Subsequently, information about the normal functions of OSE and its relationship to ovarian cancer expanded rapidly. The results of these studies showed that OSE is physiologically much more complex than would be predicted from its inconspicuous appearance, and they support the hypothesis that the ovarian epithelial cancers arise in this simple epithelium. Recently, the capacity of OSE to give rise to ovarian adenocarcinomas was demonstrated experimentally for the first time. This was achieved by introducing SV40 large T antigen and constitutively expressed E-cadherin into normal OSE in culture. The resulting phenotype closely resembled neoplastic OSE, and the cells formed adenocarcinomas in SCID mice (14, 15).

This review summarizes the main characteristics of OSE, with emphasis on those properties that might contribute to its propensity to undergo neoplastic progression.

2. EMBRYONIC DEVELOPMENT

In the early embryo, the future OSE is that part of the coelomic epithelium that overlies the presumptive gonadal area. By periodic proliferation and differentiation, which may be regulated by steroid hormones, the OSE gives rise to portions of the gonadal blastema. These include ingrowths of fetal OSE cells into the future ovarian cortex which are thought to take part in the development of the granulosa cells by direct differentiation and/or by inductive interactions (16-20). In addition to the role of the coelomic epithelium as a progenitor of granulosa cells via the fetal OSE, this epithelium invaginates in the vicinity of the presumptive gonads to give rise to the Mullerian (paramesonephric) ducts, i.e. the primordia for the epithelia of the oviduct, endometrium and endocervix. Thus, the coelomic epithelium in and near the gonadal area has the capacity to differentiate along many different pathways, and the close developmental relationship between the Mullerian ducts and the OSE is considered to contribute significantly to the propensity of metaplastic and neoplastic adult OSE to assume Mullerian characteristics.

Although the future OSE and the extraovarian coelomic epithelium resemble one another in their embryonic origin, histologic composition and their anatomical relationship to the pelvic cavity, they are not identical. One of the most interesting differences between these two parts of the pelvic mesothelium is the expression of CA125, a cell surface glycoprotein of unknown function, which, in the adult, is both an epithelial differentiation marker and a tumor marker for ovarian and Mullerian duct-derived neoplasms (21). CA125 is expressed by the oviductal, endometrial and endocervical epithelia, as well as by the pleura, pericardium and peritoneum of first and second trimester human fetuses and of adult women, but not by OSE. OSE is therefore the only one of these coelomic epithelial derivatives that either never acquired this differentiation marker or lost it early in development (22). The former interpretation would support the idea that OSE is less differentiated and less committed to a mature mesothelial phenotype than the rest of the pelvic peritoneum. The expression of CA125 in OSE-derived epithelial carcinomas indicates that the adult OSE has retained the competence of the embryonic coelomic epithelium for Mullerian differentiation, at least under pathological conditions.

3. OSE IN THE ADULT
3.1.   Structure

In the mature woman, OSE is an inconspicuous monolayered flat-to cuboidal epithelium with few distinguishing features (1, 23, 24). It is characterized by apical microvilli, a basal lamina, and the keratin types 7, 8, 18 and 19 which are typical for simple epithelia (Fig. 1). The lack of CA125 (22) and the presence of mucin, 17β-hydroxysteroid dehydrogenase, cilia and several antigenic markers (4, 13, 24-30) distinguish OSE from extraovarian mesothelium. Intercellular contact and epithelial integrity of OSE are maintained by simple desmosomes, incomplete tight junctions (4, 13), integrins (31, 32) and N-cadherin (33-36).

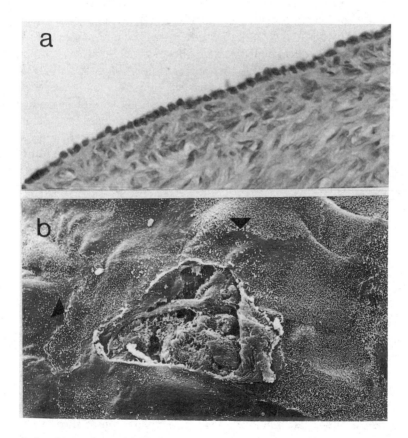

Figure 1. Ovarian surface epithelium. (a), cross section through the ovarian surface, which is covered by the cuboidal, monolayered normal OSE. Hematoxylin and eosin. (b), scanning electron micrograph of a normal ovarian surface. The cells are covered with microvilli and occasional cilia. In the center of the figure, part of the OSE has been accidentally detached, revealing the underlying tunica albuginea. Arrowheads indicate cell boundaries.

The OSE is separated from the ovarian stroma by a basement membrane which overlies a collagenous connective tissue layer, the tunica albuginea. This layer is responsible for the whitish color of the ovary. It is thinner and less resilient than the tunica albuginea in the testis, but likely provides a partial barrier to the diffusion of nutrients and bioactive agents between the ovarian stroma and the OSE. The OSE differs from all other epithelia, including the extraovarian pelvic peritoneum, by its tenuous attachment to underlying structures, including its basement membrane from which it is easily detached by mechanical means. The absence of OSE in many surgical specimens, which is almost certainly caused by handling and drying during surgical procedures, was responsible for the widely held opinion that OSE is frequently absent in ovaries of older women (37). Whether the loose attachment of OSE has any physiological consequences is not known. However, in combination with the barrier to interactions with underlying tissues formed by the tunica albuginea, it is tempting to speculate that the normal OSE is less dependent on epithelio-mesenchymal interactions and more autonomous than other epithelia. Such autonomy could, conceivably, be related to its propensity to undergo neoplastic changes.

With age, the human ovary assumes increasingly irregular contours and forms OSE-lined surface invaginations (clefts) and epithelial inclusion cysts in the ovarian cortex. It has been suggested that the squamous and cuboidal forms of OSE cells on the ovarian surface represent cell groups that, respectively, have or have not undergone postovulatory proliferation (37). In addition, OSE cells tend to be flat to cuboidal on free surfaces but assume columnar shapes within clefts and inclusion cysts. Whether these shape changes are the result of crowding secondary to localized mitogenic stimuli or whether they reflect genetically determined metaplastic changes is not clear, but they might be derived by either process. The importance of surface invaginations and inclusion cysts lies in the propensity of the OSE in these regions to undergo metaplastic changes, i.e. to take on phenotypic characteristics of Mullerian (usually tubal) epithelia, which include columnar cell shapes and several markers found in ovarian neoplasms, including CA125 and E-cadherin (4, 25, 27, 33, 35, 38). (Fig. 2). Furthermore, OSE-lined clefts and inclusion cysts, rather than surface OSE, are common sites of neoplastic progression. (39-41). It has been suggested that the inclusion cysts form from OSE fragments that are trapped in ruptured follicles at the time of ovulation (42, 43). However, inclusion cysts are more numerous in ovaries of multiparous women than in nulliparous women who ovulate more frequently, and the cysts are particularly numerous in women with polycystic ovarian disease, a condition which is characterized by anovulation or infrequent ovulation (41). Scully (41) proposed as an alternative that inclusion cysts arise through inflammatory adhesions of OSE at apposed sites of surface invaginations, in combination with localized stromal proliferation. The predilection of the OSE lining epithelial inclusion cysts to undergo neoplastic progression strongly suggests the presence of tumor-promoting micro-

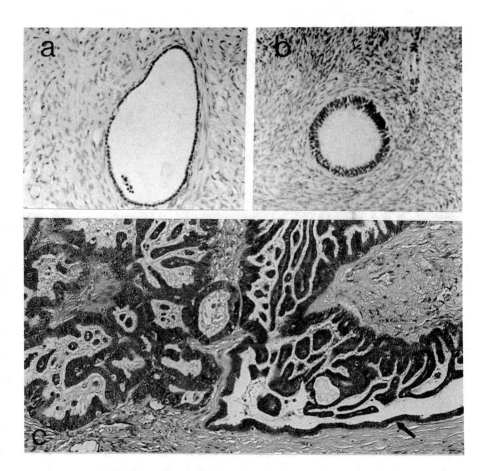

Figure 2. Neoplastic progression of OSE. (a) epithelial inclusion cyst lined with normal, cuboidal epithelium. (b) epithelial inclusion cyst lined with columnar, ciliated metaplastic epithelium. (c) low grade serous adenocarcinoma characterized by complex gland-like spaces and papillae, arising from OSE (arrow). Hematoxylin and eosin.

environmental factors in these sites. Their nature has not been defined but several factors could play a role: (1) The OSE in epithelial inclusion cysts may be exposed to autocrine stimuli which promote neoplastic progression through OSE-derived cytokines and hormones, since these agents could accumulate to bioactive levels in such confined sites but diffuse into the pelvic when secreted by OSE on the ovarian surface. In support of this hypothesis, it has been shown that normal OSE secretes bioactive cytokines including IL-1 and IL-6 (44), that IL-1 and IL-6 enhance the proliferation of ovarian carcinomas (45), that IL-1 causes changes in gene expression including the induction of tumor necrosis factor (TNFα) which is a mitogen for OSE (46, 47), and that human chorionic gonadotrophin (hCG) is produced by normal and neoplastic OSE (25) and is also mitogenic for OSE (48). (2) OSE within inclusion cysts is not separated from underlying stroma by the tunica albuginea, and, therefore has more access to stromally derived and blood-borne growth factors and cytokines that may promote neoplastic progression. Important in this regard is the observation that, in inclusion cysts located near the ovarian surface, metaplastic and dysplastic changes tend to be more pronounced on the side near the stroma than on the side adjacent to the tunica albuginea (40, 41).

3.2.   Differentiation

In vivo and in culture, normal adult OSE has both epithelial and mesenchymal characteristics which reflect its close developmental relationship to ovarian stromal cells and support the concept that this epithelium is relatively uncommitted and closer to a pleuripotential precursor form than other derivatives of the embryonic coelomic epithelium (29). The epithelial features of OSE include desmosomes, tight junctions, basement membrane, keratin and apical microvilli and cilia. However, the epithelial differentiation markers E-cadherin and CA125, which characterize most female reproductive epithelia, are rare in human OSE and essentially limited to papillae and inclusion cysts. Instead of E-cadherin, the dominant intercellular adhesion molecule of OSE is N-cadherin, which is more characteristic of mesenchymally derived tissues, including the embryologically related granulosa cells and extraovarian mesothelium (36). Furthermore, OSE cells constitutively coexpress keratin with vimentin which is a mesenchymal intermediate filament (49, 50) and, in addition to the epithelial collagen type IV they produce the connective tissue collagens types I and III (29).

OSE cells have the ability to modulate to a fibroblast-like form. This modulation encompasses shape changes, decreases in intercellular contact and loss of epithelial differentiation markers including keratin (29, 51, 52). Similar modulations occur *in vivo* in mesodermally derived cell types closely related to OSE, such as pleural mesothelial cells responding to injury (53), and the cells of the developing Mullerian duct during regression in response to Mullerian inhibiting substance (54). This capacity of OSE to undergo epithelio-mesenchymal conversion may confer advantages during the post-ovulatory repair of the ovarian surface: it likely increases motilty, alters proliferative responses and the deposition of extracellular matrix, and renders the cells contractile which contributes to wound healing (31). Epithelio-mesenchymal conversion might also function as a homeostatic mechanism to accommodate OSE cells that became trapped within the ovary at ovulation, by allowing them to become incorporated into the ovarian stroma as stromal fibroblasts. In culture, the degree and time sequence of this conversion appear to be influenced by undefined serum factors. It is accelerated by growing the cells on rat tail-derived collagen-coated plastic (Fig. 3), and it is particularly prominent in three-dimensional culture systems including collagen gels (31) and collagen sponge matrices (52).

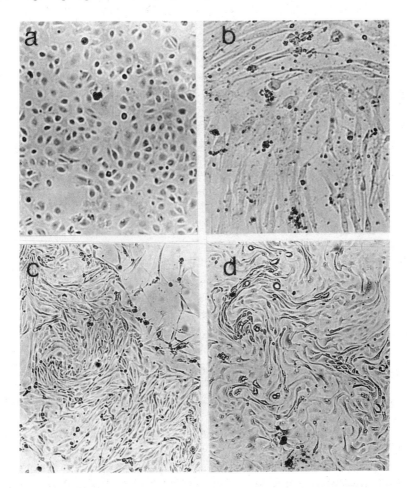

Figure 3. Morphology and growth pattern of normal, metaplastic and neoplastic OSE cultures. (a) Normal OSE forms monolayers of epithelial cells on plastic but (b) becomes atypical and fibroblastic-like on rat tail-derived collagen coated plastic. (c) elongated cells that sometimes formed colonies appearing as whirls, signifying metaplastic OSE (36). (d) such colonies are also observed in cultures derived from ovarian serous adenocarcinomas.

One of the most unusual aspects of ovarian carcinogenesis are the changes in differentiation that accompany neoplastic progression. This aberrant differentiation occurs in such a high proportion of ovarian carcinomas that it serves as the basis for the classification of a high proportion of these cancers as serous (Fallopian tube-like), endometrioid (endometrium-like) and mucinous (endocervical-like) adenocarcinomas. The high frequency of these differentiation-associated changes suggests that they might confer a selective advantage on the transforming OSE. At the cellular level, these changes are expressed by the appearance of altered cell shapes, E-cadherin, junctional complexes, epithelial membrane antigens and secretory products including mucins and CA125 (4, 33, 35, 55, 56). Histologically, the tumors form polarized epithelia, papillae, cysts and glandular structures. Thus, unlike carcinomas in most other organs where epithelial cells become less differentiated in the course of neoplastic progression than the epithelium from which they arise, the differentiation of ovarian carcinomas is more complex that that of OSE. Only in the late stages do these specialized epithelial features diminish though they can persist even when the tumors are metastatic or in the ascites form (35). Tissue culture studies have shown that OSE cells undergoing neoplastic progression not only develop complex epithelial phenotypes, but become firmly committed to these phenotypes and unresponsive to signals causing mesenchymal conversion (52).

3.3.   Functions

The OSE transports materials to and from the peritoneal cavity and takes part in the cyclical ovulatory ruptures and repair. Most of these functions vary with the reproductive cycle and are therefore likely hormone dependent (1, 4, 48). There is convincing evidence that nulliparity and, probably, hyperovulation treatment for infertility, increase the risk of ovarian cancer, while oral contraceptives and pregnancies are protective. These observations support the hypothesis, first proposed by Fathalla in 1971 and subsequently supported by epidemiologic and experimental data (6, 57, 58), that frequent ovulation contributes to increased risk. The most generally accepted explanation of this relationship is that the repeated rupture and repair of the OSE at the sites of ovulation provides an opportunity for genetic aberrations. OSE cells are profoundly influenced by the extracellular matrix (ECM) and they, in turn, modulate ECM synthesis, lysis and physical restructuring (31). The OSE contains lysosome-like inclusions and produces proteolytic enzymes which may contribute to follicular rupture (31, 59). However, this concept has been questioned because of inconsistencies in the timing within the ovulatory cycle of the appearance of lysosomes in the OSE, and the observation that follicles denuded of overlying OSE can also rupture (60). The cyclic, localized loss of OSE near the time of ovulation may be due to apoptosis which is induced by prostaglandins (61, 62) and mediated by Fas (63, 64). In view of these discrepancies, it is possible that the proteolytic capacity of the OSE contributes to the remodeling, rather than the breakdown, of the periovulatory ovarian cortex. OSE likely also takes part in the restoration of the ovarian cortex by the synthesis of both epithelial and connective tissue-type components of the extracellular matrix (29, 31, 65). OSE also expresses integrins which bind to laminin, collagens, fibronectin and vitronectin and vary in type and amount with the substratum (31, 32). These properties are likely important in the roles of OSE in ovulation and postovulatory repair, and may also influence the phenotypes of OSE-derived malignancies.

Normal OSE cells secrete, and have receptors for agents with growth- and differentiation regulatory capabilities. Human OSE cells have receptors for follicle stimulating hormone (FSH) (66), which supports the hypothesis that the high FSH levels in peri- and postmenopausal women may play a promoting role in ovarian carcinogenesis (67). hCG, which is secreted by normal and neoplastic human OSE (25) and luteinizing hormone (LH) stimulate the proliferation of human and rabbit OSE, indicating that these cells express LH receptors (48, 68, 69).

Receptors for estrogen, progesterone and androgen were found at the mRNA and/or protein level in human OSE (70, 71). No direct effects of these steroids on OSE proliferation have been demonstrated (70) but there is increasing evidence for indirect actions: expression by OSE of the receptor for gonadotropin releasing hormone (GnRH) is reduced by estrogen (72) and estrogen also modulates levels of hepatocyte growth factor (HGF) (73) and epidermal growth factor (EGF), both of which stimulate OSE growth. In contrast to normal OSE, estrogen and prolactin stimulate proliferation of ovarian and breast carcinoma cells and concurrently upregulate BRCA1 mRNA and protein (74, 75). Although there is no evidence for a direct mitogenic effect of ovarian steroids on OSE, corticosteroids enhance OSE proliferation, and combinations of EGF and hydrocortisone are among the most potent mitogens for cultured OSE (13, 45, 76, 77).

EGF has numerous functions in the ovary, which include inhibition of FSH effects and induction of LH receptor (78), inhibition of estrogen production (79) and of theca differentiation (80) and stimulation of progestin biosynthesis (81). OSE cells express receptors for EGF and respond to EGF stimulation by increased proliferation. EGF also affects the differentiation of human OSE cells: within few days of EGF treatment in culture, the cells convert from an epithelial to the spindle-shaped morphology and lose epithelial differentiation markers such as keratin (13). EGF is   not present in large amounts in the plasma (82) but is released from platelets during the clotting process. It is likely, therefore, that high levels of EGF are present due to the hemorrhage that occurs during follicular rupture (83). The resulting localized stimulation of the OSE likely contributes to its rapid postovulatory proliferation and perhaps also to epithelio-mesenchymal conversion of OSE cells trapped within the ruptured follicle. Transforming growth factorα (TGFα) is a structural homologue of EGF and also binds to the EGF receptor (84). TGFα has been demonstrated immunohistochemically in human theca cells and in OSE, and stimulates DNA synthesis by cultured human OSE cells (85). TGFα levels in the normal ovary increase after menopause, i.e. at the peak incidence of ovarian neoplasms (86, 87). Amphiregulin, another EGF homologue, is also a potent mitogen for OSE cells and appears to control OSE and ovarian cancer cell proliferation in a complex manner (88). Of particular interest for ovarian cancer is the type I receptor tyrosine kinase family (RTK I), also known as ErbB family of epithelial growth factor receptors (89), which includes HER1 (synonymous with EGF receptor), HER2, HER3 and HER4. These receptors interact in multiple ways, which modify their influence on various cell types (89). Normal OSE cells express EGF receptors but little or no HER-2 (Her2/neu). In contrast, HER2 is amplified and overexpressed in 25-30% of ovarian and breast cancers. This overexpression, as well as overexpressed EGF receptor, are associated with a poor prognosis (86, 89-92). The HER2 receptor is activated by heregulins which are a family of ligands that includes the heregulin/neu differentiation factor (92). Other factors that stimulate OSE growth include basic fibroblast growth factor (bFGF) (77), platelet derived growth factor (PDGF) (93) and tumor necrosis factorα (TNFα) (46, 47, 94).

A number of agents inhibit OSE growth. These include GnRH which is an autocrine growth inhibitor for normal OSE (95) and several members of the TGFβ family of growth factors (96). TGFβ itself acts as an autocrine growth inhibitor for cultured human OSE (97) and also counteracts the growth-stimulatory effect of EGF (98). Interestingly, 5α-dihydrotestosterone downregulates the expression of mRNA for the TGFβ receptors I and II in ovarian carcinoma lines (99), suggesting that it might also counteract growth inhibitory effects of TGFβ) in normal OSE. Another member of the TGFβ family, anti-Mullerian hormone (AMH), which causes regression of the Mullerian ducts in male fetuses, is produced by granulosa cells throughout the reproductive life of women (100), but no information of its effects on OSE seems to be available. Steroidogenic factor 1 (SF1), a transcription factor which regulates the differentiation of granulosa cells and inhibits their proliferation, is also growth-inhibitory in rat OSE cells (101). Responses by normal OSE that are retained by ovarian carcinomas include growth inhibition by TGFβ (97) and growth stimulation by bFGF (102), EGF and TGFα (91). The responses to other factors change with neoplastic progression. Thus, in contrast to its growth stimulatory effect on OSE, TNFα inhibits the growth of ovarian cancer cells (94) and, while PDGF stimulates growth of OSE, many ovarian carcinomas lose the PDGF receptors (93).

A growth factor which has attracted increasing attention is HGF. HGF is produced primarily by mesenchymal and stromal cells, and acts on epithelial cells by a paracrine mechanism through its receptor tyrosine kinase encoded by the *c-met* protooncogene. In the adult ovary, the expression of Met persists in the OSE, granulosa cells, and Mullerian epithelia (103-106) while theca cells produce HGF (105). Extraovarian mesothelial cells, which share a common embryological origin and anatomical environment with OSE, lack HGF and Met (107). This suggests that expression of the Met receptor might be a feature characteristic of coelomic epithelial derivatives at the urogenital ridge through local differentiation receptor on OSE. The interaction between HGF and its receptor Met represents an important example of multifunctional growth factor-receptor signaling that modulates the proliferation, shape, movement, adhesion, differentiation and synthetic functions of normal epithelia. The physiological influence of HGF on OSE depends on the presence or absence of basement membrane components. For example, induces apoptosis *in vitro* if these cells are cultured on plastic (108), but it is mitogenic when OSE cells are plated on a fibronectin-like extracellular matrix (69). *In vivo*, these modulations may regulate the contributions of OSE to follicular rupture before ovulation, and to postovulatory repair. HGF also affects, and is affected by, the action of various hormones (69, 73, 104). In culture, HGF is mitogenic for both bovine (109) and human (110) OSE.

Cultured human OSE also secretes bioactive cytokines, including interleukin-1 (IL-1), interleukin- (IL-6), macrophage colony-stimulating factor (M-CSF), granulocyte colony-stimulating factor (G-CSF) and granulocyte-macrophage colony-stimulating factor (GM-CSF). Except for a report that IL-1 enhances OSE proliferation (94), little is known about the role and regulation of these cytokines in OSE. While the secretion of cytokines is a normal OSE function (44), their recruitment into autocrine loops may be important during neoplastic progression. For example, M-CSF is secreted by normal and malignant OSE (44, 111). Levels of M-CSF in blood and ascitic fluid correlate with a poor prognosis in ovarian cancer, as does overexpression of the M-CSF receptor *fms* (111). Interestingly, *fms* is expressed by many ovarian cancers but not by benign ovarian tumors (111) or normal OSE (45). Thus, M-CSF, when secreted by normal OSE, acts in a paracrine manner but becomes an autocrine regulatory factor with malignant progression.

4. OSE IN WOMEN WITH HISTORIES OF FAMILIAL OVARIAN CANCER

One of the pressing problems in ovarian cancer management is the lack of markers for the detection of preneoplastic or early neoplastic changes in the OSE. We and other laboratories have investigated this problem by studying the properties of overtly normal OSE from women with histories of familial ovarian cancer. At present, a strong family history of ovarian cancer is the most important and best defined risk factor to develop this disease, and it is associated with 5-10% of ovarian epithelial carcinomas. The risk increases from 1.4% in the general population to 5% for women with one first degree relative and to 8% for women with two first degree relatives affected (first-degree relatives include parents, siblings and children, while second-degree relatives include grandparents, uncles, aunts, cousins and grandchildren). There is also a strong association with familial breast cancer, and a lesser association with familial cancers of the colon and endometrium (3). Three hereditary ovarian cancer syndromes with autosomal dominance have been described (112). These are: 1. Hereditary site-specific ovarian cancer, where a family history of ovarian cancer only is associated with an overall 3.6-fold increase in risk. No specific gene responsible for this syndrome has been indentified. 2. Hereditary nonpolyposis colon cancer/ovarian cancer (Lynch Syndrome II or HNPCC), where ovarian cancer occurs in families that also have a high incidence of carcinomas of the colon and endometrium. It is associated with mutations in the DNA mismatch repair genes hMSH1, hMSH2, hPMS1 and hPMS2 (113). In this syndrome, the increase in risk has not been defined. 3. Hereditary breast/ovarian cancer. There is a 50% increase in ovarian cancer risk among women with family histories of breast cancer, and a similar increase in breast cancer risk among women with family histories of ovarian cancer. Mutations in two genes involved in this syndrome, BRCA1 and BRCA2, appear to be responsible for a high proportion of cancers in women with familial cancer histories. The BRCA1 and BRCA2 proteins regulate DNA damage responses (114) and have been defined as tumor suppressor genes. BRCA1, in particular, plays a major role in ovarian cancer susceptibility. Intensive screening for BRCA1 mutations is going on but the large size of the gene and the great variety of different mutations that have been found complicate screening and risk predictions. The observation that BRCA1 and BRCA2 germ line mutations cause increases in cancer incidence predominantly in the breast, ovary and prostate, although they are present in all tissues, points to interrelationships with hormonal influences. Interactions between BRCA1 and estrogen as well as prolactin have indeed been reported in cancer cells (74, 75, 115), but there seems to be no information available on similar interactions in normal OSE.

There have been several contradictory reports on the occurrence of histologic changes in the OSE of overtly normal ovaries that were removed by prophylactic oophorectomy from healthy women with histories of familial ovarian cancer. A non-blind study (116) demonstrated increased papillomatosis and pseudostratification of the OSE, as well as an increase in inclusion cysts and invaginations in ovaries from women with familial ovarian cancer. In another blind study, only nuclear changes were observed in the OSE of such women (117), while in two other reports no significant differences were observed (118, 119). On the other hand, there is increasing evidence that OSE from women with family histories of ovarian cancer expresses an altered phenotype in culture which might reveal early changes and, perhaps, predictive markers for ovarian carcinogenesis (36, 52, 110, 120). The first indication to suggest that overtly normal OSE from women with family histories of ovarian cancer (FH-OSE) differs from the OSE of women with no family history (NFH-OSE) not only genetically but also phenotypically came in 1995, when CA125 was found to be expressed in more cells and for longer duration in cultured FH-OSE than in NFH-OSE (121). Furthermore, as discussed earlier in this review, normal OSE cells have a tendency to undergo epithelio-mesenchymal conversion in culture. In contrast, ovarian carcinoma cells are nonresponsive to the environmental signals which induce this conversion and remain epithelial indefinitely. FH-OSE cells were found to have a significantly diminished tendency for epithelio-mesenchymal conversion, as indicated by cellular morphology and growth patterns in two- and three-dimensional culture, the expression of CA125, keratin and E-cadherin as epithelial markers, and sponge contraction and collagen type III as mesenchymal markers (36, 52).

Although the factors controlling the aberrant epithelial differentiation in epithelial ovarian carcinogenesis are unknown, these phenotypic modulations depend critically on specific intercellular and cell-extracellular matrix inter-relationships, which in turn modify intracellular signal transduction proteins. One of the most interesting factors is E-cadherin, which is an epithelial adhesion molecule in most adult epithelia, including human oviductal, endometrial and endocervical epithelia. In contrast, E-cadherin expression is rare in human OSE. Normal OSE cells are connected by N-cadherin, which characterizes adhesive mechanisms of mesodermally derived tissues. E-cadherin expression in the human OSE is conditional and related to genotype, stage of neoplastic progression and growth pattern. The expression of E-cadherin increases significantly in metaplastic and dysplastic OSE and in epithelial ovarian carcinomas and diminishes in some, but not all, highly invasive and ascitic carcinomas (33-36). Interestingly, E-cadherin is also enhanced and stabilized in cultures of FH-OSE compared to NFH-OSE (36). The altered expression of E-cadherin in overtly normal OSE of women with hereditary ovarian cancer syndromes, in conjunction with the known capacity of E-cadherin to induce epithelial differentiation (122) implicates this adhesion molecule as a possible inducer of the aberrant Mullerian differentiation that characterizes epithelial ovarian carcinomas. We recently created an epithelial tumorigenic OSE-derived cell line closely resembling ovarian serous adenocarcinoma cells by transfecting the gene for mouse E-cadherin into a non-tumorigenic, SV40 large T-immortalized OSE line (14, 15). These results support the hypothesis that E-cadherin has an inductive influence in the aberrant epithelial differentiation of OSE in ovarian carcinogenesis. Factors regulating E-cadherin expression in female reproductive tissues appear to involve hormonal controls, since estrogen and progesterone were reported to increase E-cadherin mRNA levels in the immature mouse ovary *in vivo* (123). Evidence on the colocalization of both receptor tyrosine kinases and phosphatases with cadherin-catenin complexes suggests that these interactions may be important in the orchestration of different functions of OSE in various physiological and pathological circumstances.

In the human ovary, Met is expressed in normal OSE but becomes upregulated in well-differentiated ovarian carcinomas (103, 106), suggesting that changes in Met expression might coincide with the stage of neoplastic progression when aberrant differentiation is induced. In culture, Met expression is stabilized in FH-OSE cultures and in ovarian carcinoma lines, but not in NFH-OSE cultures (110). Therefore, some of the factors that alter Met levels in the malignant progression of ovarian surface epithelial tumors (103, 106) may already be found in FH-OSE. As Met is characteristically expressed by epithelial cells, the presence of this receptor in FH-OSE represents yet another epithelial differentiation marker (110). Our data revealed concomitant expression of HGF and Met in most cases of FH-OSE and in ovarian cancer lines, but rarely in NFH-OSE. Constitutive tyrosine-phosphorylation of the Met receptor in FH-OSE and ovarian cancer cells, in the absence of exogenous HGF, indicates the presence of a functional autocrine regulatory system in these cultured cells, and suggests that, perhaps, a similar system exists *in vivo*. Therefore, while the expression of Met by OSE is in keeping with the presence of this receptor in most epithelia, the presence of HGF may represent a very early or predisposing step in ovarian surface epithelial neoplastic transformation. Since HGF has the capacity to induce epithelial morphogenesis in a variety of Met expressing epithelia, the interaction between HGF and Met in FH-OSE may contribute to the aberrant Mullerian differentiation that accompanies ovarian carcinogenesis. Exogenous HGF is mitogenic in normal OSE (109, 110). It also stimulates proliferation and motility in ovarian cancer cells, and these properties may contribute to the peritoneal dissemination during ovarian tumor progression (109, 124). HGF is found at high levels in malignant ovarian cystic and ascitic fluid from women with ovarian carcinomas compared to the peritoneal fluid of normal women (124). Since OSE and ovarian cancer cells synthesized only small amounts of HGF, the high levels found in malignancies may be primarily derived from stromal cells and cells of the immune system which are the normal sources of this factor. HGF activates several signaling molecules of the phosphatidyinositol 3-kinase (PI3K) pathway, which has been implicated in cell survival and growth, in normal and neoplastic OSE cells. In contrast to NFH-OSE, some of these molecules, including Akt2 and p70 S6 kinase are constitutively activated in FH-OSE and ovarian cancer cell lines, perhaps through an autocrine HGF-Met loop (125). This increased autonomy of the epithelial phenotype may indicate an early step or predisposition to neoplastic progression by FH-OSE.

Additional differences were observed in SV-40 large T antigen-immortalized FH-OSE cultures compared to immortalized NFH-OSE. The FH-OSE cells were found to exhibit increased telomeric instability and a reduced growth potential indicative of greater proximity to replicative senescence (120). These observations are particularly relevant to the unexplained earlier age of onset which characterizes ovarian cancer in women with family histories (126). The distinguishing features of FH-OSE are summarized in Table 1.

Table 1. Phenotypic alterations in FH-OSE[a] compared to NFH-OSE[b] in vivo and in vitro

Phenotypic alterations in FH-OSE	Reference
In vivo	
Pseudostratification and papillomatosis of the OSE	116
More epithelial inclusion cysts in ovaries	116
Nuclear atypia	117
In culture	
Increased CA125 production	121
Reduced epithelio-mesenchymal conversion	52
Reduced growth potential	52, 120
Telomeric instability	120
Increased E-cadherin expression	36
Autocrine activation of the HGF-Met pathway	110

[a] apparently normal OSE from women with a strong family history of ovarian/breast cancer (at least two first degree relatives who had breast/ovarian cancer), and/or are known to carry a mutation which predisposes to developing ovarian cancer.
[b] no family history of ovarian cancer.

5. CONCLUDING REMARKS

The normal OSE in adult women is a dynamic epithelium which exhibits a high degree of plasticity as shown by morphologic variability, localized changes in adhesive mechanisms, varying proliferative activity and a wide repertoire of secretory functions with products that include extracellular matrix components, cytokines and growth factors. This plasticity permits the OSE to continuously adapt to the complex changes in its environment which range from gross alterations in the contours of the ovary to cyclical endocrine and paracrine influences. The OSE has retained properties of relatively immature, uncommitted pleuripotential cells as reflected by its high growth potential compared to extraovarian mesothelium, its capacity to modulate phenotypically and its ability to differentiate along several pathways. While this immature state may be necessary to provide the OSE with the phenotypic plasticity required by its normal functions, it might also contribute to the propensity of OSE to undergo neoplastic transformation. Changes in overtly normal OSE from women with histories of hereditary ovarian cancer indicate that an increased commitment to epithelial phenotypes, a reduced responsiveness to environmental signals, and the acquisition of autocrine regulatory mechanisms may be among the earliest changes in the process of ovarian carcinogenesis. There is an urgent need for a better understanding of these very early changes in the normal regulation of OSE biology, and for attempts to use this information for cancer prevention and for the identification of new clinical diagnostic and prognostic markers.

ACKNOWLEDGEMENTS

We wish to thank members of the Department of Obstetrics and Gynecology, University of British Columbia, for their cooperation in providing surgical specimens of normal and neoplastic OSE, and Dr. Steven Pelech, University of British Columbia, for his collaboration in the kinase activation studies. Work described in this review was supported by grants from the National Cancer Institute of Canada with funds from the Terry Fox Run.

REFERENCES

1.   Nicosia SV, Saunders BO, Acevedo-Duncan ME, Setrakian S, Degregorio R Biopathology of ovarian mesothelium. In: Ultrastructure of the ovary. Familiari G, Makabe S, Motta PM, eds. Kluwer Academic Publishers, 287-310, 1991.
2.   Nicosia SV, Ku Ni Ni K, Oliveros-Saunders B, Giacomini G, Pierro E, Mayer J, Nicosia RF Ovarian mesothelium (surface epithelium) in normal, pathological and experimental conditions In: Recent advances in microscopy of cells, tissues and organs Motta PM ed. pp. 509-517, 1997.

3. Bast RC Jr, Xu F, Yu Y, Fang XJ, Wiener J, Mills GB Overview: the molecular biology of ovarian cancer. In: Ovarian Cancer 5, Sharp F, Backett T, Berek J, Bast R eds. Isis Medical Media Publishers, Oxford, United Kingdom, pp.87-97, 1998.
4. Nicosia SV, Nicosia RF. Neoplasms of the ovarian mesothelium. In: Pathology of human neoplasms. Azar, HA ed. Raven Press, New York, pp.435-486, 1998.
5. Herbst AL The epidemiology of ovarian carcinoma and the current status of tumor markers to detect disease. [Review]. Am J Obstet & Gynecol 1994; 170:1099-105.
6. Auersperg N, Edelson MI, Mok SC, Johnson SW, Hamilton TC. The biology of ovarian cancer. Semin Oncol 1998; 25:281-304.
7. Fredrickson TN. Ovarian tumors of the hen. Environmental Health Perspectives 1987; 73:35-51.
8. Hamilton TC, Henderson WT, Eaton C. In: Tissue clture in medical Res. (II). Proceedings of 2nd Internl. Symp. Richards RJ and Rajan KT eds. Pergamon press New York, 1980.
9. Adams AT, Auersperg N . Transformation of cultured rat ovarian surface epithelial cells by Kirsten murine sarcoma virus. Cancer Res 1981; 41:2063-2072.
10. Adams AT, Auersperg N. Autoradiographic investigation of estrogen binding in cultured rat ovarian surface epithelial cells. J Histochem & Cytochem 1983; 31:1321-1325.
11. Nicosia SV, Narconis RJ, Saunders BO. Regulation and temporal sequence of surface epithelium morphogenesis in the postovulatory rabbit ovary. In: Developments in Ultrastructure of Reproduction. Alan R Liss, Inc., 1989; 296:111-119.
12. Auersperg N, Siemens CH, Myrdal SE. Human ovarian surface epithelium in primary culture. In Vitro Cell Dev Biol 1984; 20:743-755.
13. Siemens CH, Auersperg N . Serial propagation of human ovarian surface epithelium in tissue culture. J Cell Physiol 1998; 134:347-356.
14. Auersperg N, Pan J, Grove BD, Peterson T, Fisher J, Maines-Bandiera S, Somasiri A, Roskelley CD. E-cadherin induces mesenchymal-to-epithelial transition in human ovarian surface epithelium. Proc Natl Acad Sci USA 1999; 96:6249-6254.
15. Ong A, Maines-Bandiera SL, Roskelley CD, Auersperg N. An ovarian adenocarcinoma line derived from SV40/E-cadherin transfected normal human ovarian surface epithelium. Int J Cancer 2000;85:430-437.
16. Byskov AR, Skakkebaek NE, Stafanger G, Peters H. Influence of ovarian surface epithelium and rete ovarii on follicle formation. J Anat 1977; 123:77-86.
17. Stein LE, Anderson CH. A qualitative and quantitative study of rete ovarii development in the fetal rat: correlation with the onset of meiosis and follicle cell appearance. Anat Rec 1979; 193:197-212
18. Yoshinaga K, Hess DL, Hendrickx AG, Zamboni L The development of the sexually indifferent gonad in the prosimian, *Galago crassicaudatus crassicaudatus*. Am J Anat 1988; 181:89-105
19. Hirshfield AN. Development of follicles in the mammalian ovary. Int Rev Cytol 1991; 124:43-101.
20. Pan J, Auersperg N . Spatiotemporal changes in cytokeratin expression I the neonatal rat ovary. Biochem Cell Biol 1997; 76:27-35.
21. Jacobs, Bast Jr RC. The CA 125 tumour-associated antigen: a review of the literature. [Review] Human Reproduction 1989; 4:1-12.
22. Kabawat SE, Bast RC Jr, Bhan AK, Welch WR, Knapp RC, Colvin RB. Tissue distribution of a coelomic-epithelium-related antigen recognized by the monoclonal antibody OC-125. Int J Gynecol Pathol 1983; 2:275-85.
23. Van Blerkom J, Motta PM. In: The Cellular Basis of Mammalian Reproduction. Urban and Scharzenberg, Baltimore 1979.
24. Blaustein A, Lee H. Surface Cells of the Ovary and Pelvic Peritoneum: A Histochemical and Ultrastructure Comparison. Gynecol Oncol 1979; 8:34-43.

25. Blaustein A, Kaganowicz A, Wells J. Tumor markers in inclusion cysts of the ovary. Cancer 1982; 49:722-726.
26. Nicosia SV, Johnson JH. Surface Morphology of Ovarian Mesothelium (Surface Epithelium) and of Other Pelvic and Extrapelvic Mesothelial Sites in the Rabbit. Int J Gynecol Pathol 1984; 3:249-260.
27. van Niekerk CC, Boerman OC, Ramaekers FCS, Poels LG. Marker profile of different phases in the transition of normal human ovarian epithelium to ovarian carcinomas. Am J Pathol 1991; 138:455-463.
28. van Niekerk CC, Jap PHK, Thomas CMG, Smeets DFCM, Ramaekers FCS, Poels LG. Marker profile of mesothelial cells versus ovarian carcinoma cells. Int J Cancer 1989; 43:1065-1071.
29. Auersperg N, Maines-Bandiera SL, Dyck HG, Kruk PA. Characterization of cultured human ovarian surface epithelial cells: phenotypic plasticity and premalignant changes. Lab Invest 1994; 71:510-518.
30. Zeimet AG, Offner FA, Muller-Holzner E, Widschwendter M, Abendstein B, Fuith LC, Daxenbichler G, Marth C . Peritoneum and Tissues of the Female Reproductive Tract as Physiological Sources of CA-125. Tumor Biol 1998; 19:275-282.
31. Kruk PA, Uitto VJ, Firth JD, Dedhar S, Auersperg N. Reciprocal interactions between human ovarian surface epithelial cells and adjacent extracellular matrix. Exp Cell Res 1994; 215:97-108.
32. Cruet S, Salamanca C, Staedel C, Auersperg N $\alpha v \beta 3$ / vitronectin expression by normal ovarian surface epithelial cells : role in cell adhesion and cell proliferation. Gynecol Oncol 1999; 75:254-260.
33. Maines-Bandiera SL, Auersperg N. Increased E-cadherin expression in ovarian surface epithelium: an early step in metaplasia and dysplasia?. Int J Gynecol Pathol 1997; 16:250-255.
34. Peralta Soler A, Knudsen KA, Tecson-Miguel A, McBreaty FX, Han AC, Salazar H. Expression of E-cadherin and N-cadherin in surface epithelial-stromal tumors of the ovary distinguishes mucinous from serous and endometrioid tumors. Hum Pathol 1997; 28:734-739.
35. Sundfeldt K, Piontkewitz Y, Ivarsson K, Nilsson O, Hellberg P, Brannstrom M, Janson P-O, Enerback S, Hedin L. E-Cadherin Expression in Human Epithelial Ovarian Cancer and the Normal Ovary. Int J Cancer 1997; 74:275-280.
36. Wong AST, Maines-Bandiera SL, Rosen B, Wheelock MJ, Johnson KR, Leung PCK, Roskelley CD, Auersperg N. Constitutive and conditional cadherin expression in cultured human ovarian surface epithelium: Influence of family history of ovarian cancer. Int J Cancer 1999; 81:180-188.
37. Gillett WR, Mitchell A, Hurst PR. A scanning electron microscopic study of the human ovarian surface epithelium: characterization of two cell types. Hum Reprod 1991; 6:645-650.
38. Mittal KR, Goswami S, Demopoulos RI. Immunohistochemical profile of ovarian inclusion cysts in patients with and without ovarian carcinoma. Histochemical J 1995; 27:119-122.
39. Deligdisch L, Einstein A, Guera D, Gil J. Ovarian dysplasia in epithelial inclusion cysts. Cancer 1995; 76:1027-1034.
40. Scully RE Early de novo ovarian cancer and cancer developing in benign ovarian lesions. Int J Gynecol Obstet 1995; 49 Suppl:S9-S15.
41. Scully RE . Pathology of Ovarian Cancer Precursors. J Cell Biochem Suppl 1995; 23:208-218.
42. Radisavljevic S. The pathogenesis of ovarian inclusion cysts and cystomas. Obstet Gynecol 1976; 49:424-429.

43. Murdoch WJ. Ovarian Surface Epithelium During Ovulatory and Anovulatory Ovine Estrous Cycles. Anat Rec 1994; 240:322-326.
44. Ziltener HJ, Maines-Bandiera S, Schrader JW, Auersperg N. Secretion of bioactive interleukin-1, interleukin-6, and colony-stimulating factors by human ovarian surface epithelium. Biol Reprod 1993; 49:635-641.
45. Berchuck A, Kohler MF, Boente MP, Rodriguez GC, Whitaker RS, Bast Jr RC. Growth regulation and transformation of ovarian epithelium. [Review]. Cancer 1993; 71:545-551.
46. Wu S, Rodabaugh K, Martinez-Maza O, Watson JM, Silberstein DS, Boyer CM, Peters WP, Weinberg JB, Berek JS, Bast RC Jr. Stimulation of ovarian tumor cell proliferation with monocyte products including interleukin-1, interleukin-6, and tumor necrosis factor-alpha. Am J Obstet Gynecol 1992; 166:997-1007.
47. Wu S, Boyer CM, Whitaker RS, Berchuck A, Wiener JR, Weinberg JB, Bast Jr RC. Tumor necrosis factor alpha as an autocrine and paracrine growth factor for ovarian cancer: monokine induction of tumor cell proliferation and tumor necrosis factor alpha expression. Cancer Res 1993; 53:1939-1944.
48. Osterholzer H.. Streibel EJ, Nicosia SV. Growth effects of protein hormones on cultured rabbit ovarian surface epithelial cells. Biol Reprod 1985; 33:247-258.
49. Czernobilsky B. Co-expression of cytokeratin and vimentin filaments in mesothelial, granulosa and rete ovarii cells of the human ovary. Eur J Cell Biol 1985; 37:175-190.
50. Hornby AE, Pan J, Auersperg N. Intermediate filaments in rat ovarian surface epithelial cells: changes with neoplastic progression in culture. Biochem Cell Biol 1992; 70:16-25.
51. Nakamura M, Katabuchi H, Ohba T, Fukumatsu Y, Okamura H. Isolation, Growth and Characteristics of human ovarian surface epithelium. Virchows Archiv 1994; 424:59-67.
52. Dyck HG, Hamilton TC, Godwin AK Lynch HT, Maines-Bandiera SL, Auersperg N. Autonomy of the epithelial phenotype in human ovarian surface epithelium: changes with neoplastic progression and with a family history of ovarian cancer. Int J Cancer 1996; 69:429-436.
53. Davila RM, Crouch EC. Role of mesothelial and submesothelial stromal cells in matrix remodeling following pleural injury. Am J Pathol 1993; 142:547-555.
54. Trelstad RL, Hayashi A, Hayashi K, Donahoe PK. The epithelial-mesenchymal interface of the male rat mullerian duct: loss of basement membrane integrity and ductal regression. Devel Biol 1982; 92:27-40.
55. Young RH, Clement PB, Scully RE. The Ovarian. In: Diagnostic surgical pathology. Sternberg SS, ed. Raven Press, New York pp.1655-1734, 1898.
56. van Niekerk CC, Ramaekers FCS, Hanselaar AGJM, Aldeweireldt J, Poels LG. Changes in expression of differentiation markers between normal ovarian cells and derived tumors. Am J of Pathol 1993; 142:157-177.
57. Godwin AK, Testa J, Handel LM, Liu Z, Vanderveer LA, Tracey PA, Hamilton TC. Spontaneous transformation of rat ovarian surface epithelial cells implicates repeated ovulation in ovarian cancer etiology and is associated with clonal cytogenetic changes. J Natl Cancer Inst 1992; 84:592-601.
58. Testa J, Getts L, Salazar H, Liu Z, Handel LM, Godwin AK, Hamilton TC. Spontaneous transformation of rat ovarian surface epithelial cells results in well to poorly differentiated tumors with a parallel range of cytogenetic complexity. Cancer Res 1994; 54:2788-2784.
59. Bjersing L, Cajander S. Ovulation and the role of the ovarian surface epithelium. Experientia 1975; 15:605-608.
60. Espey LL, Lipner H. Ovulation In: The Physiology of Reproduction. Raven Press, Ltd, New York, Chapter 194; 13:725-780.
61. Ackerman RC, Murdoch WJ. Prostaglandin-induced apoptosis of ovarian surface epithelial cells. Prostaglandins 1993; 45:475-485.
62. Murdoch WJ. Programmed cell death in preovulatory ovine follicles. Biol Reprod 1995; 53:8-12.

180

63. Quirk SM, Cowan RG, Huber SH. Fas antigen-mediated apoptosis of ovarian surface epithelial cells. Endocrinol 1997; 138:4558-4566.
64. Baldwin RL, Tran H, Karlan BY. Primary ovarian cancer cultures are resistant to Fas-mediated apoptosis. Gynecol Oncol 1999; 74:265-271.
65. Kruk PA, Auersperg N. A line of rat ovarian surface epithelium provides a continuous source of complex extracellular matrix. In Vitro Cell Dev Biol 1994; 30A:217-225.
66. Zheng W, Magid MS, Kramer EE, Chen YT. Follicle-stimulating hormone receptor is expressed in human ovarian surface epitheliu and Fallopian tube. Am J Pathol 1996; 148:47.53.
67. te Velde ER, Scheffer GJ, Dorland M, Broekmans FJ, Fauser BCJM. Developmental and endocrine aspects of normal ovarian aging. Mol Cell Endocrinol 1998; 145:67-73.
68. Elliott WM, Auersperg N. Growth of normal ovarian surface epithelial cells (HOSE) in reduced serum and defined media. J Cell Biol 1990; 111:58a.
69. Hess S, Gulati R, Peluso JJ. Hepatocyte growth factor induces rat ovarian surface epithelial cell mitosis or apoptosis depending on the presence or absence of an extracellular matrix. Endocrinol 1999; 140:2908-2916.
70. Karlan BY, Jones JL, Greenwald M, Lagasse LD. Steroid hormone effects on the proliferation of human ovarian surface epithelium in vitro. Am J Obstet Gynecol 1995; 173:97-104.
71. Lau K-M, Mok SC, Ho S-M. Expression of human estrogen receptor-α and -β, progesterone receptor, and androgen receptor mRNA in normal and malignant ovarian epithelial cells. Proc Natl Acad Sci USA 1999; 96:5722-5727.
72. Kang SK, Choi K-C, Tai C-J, Auersperg N, Leung PCK Estradiol regulates gonadotropin-releasing hormone (GnRH) and its receptor gene expression and modulates the growth inhibitory effects of GnRH in human ovarian surface epithelial and ovarian cancer cells (submitted).
73. Liu Y, Lin L, Zarnegar R. Modulation of hepatocyte growth factor gene expression by estrogen in mouse ovary. Mol Cell Endocrinol 1994; 104:173-181.
74. Romagnolo D, Annab LA, Thompson TE, Risinger JI, Terry LA, Barrett JC, Afshari CA. Estrogen Upregulation of BRCA1 expression with no effect on localization. Mol Carcinogenesis 1998; 22:102-109.
75. Favy DA, Maurizis J-C, Bignon Y-J, Bernard-Gallon DJ. Prolactin-Dependent Up-Regulation of BRCA1 Expression in Human Breast Cancer Cell Lines. Biochem Biophys Res Commun 1999; 158:284-291.
76. Rodriguez GC, Berchuck A, Whitaker RS, Schlossman D, Clarke-Pearson DL, Bast Jr RC. Epidermal growth factor receptor expression in normal ovarian epithelium and ovarian cancer. II. Relationship between receptor expression and response to epidermal growth factor. Am J Obs & Gyn 1661; 164:745-750.
77. Pierro E, Nicosia SV, Saunders B, Fultz CB, Nicosia RF, Mancuso S. Influence of growth factors on proliferation and morphogenesis of rabbit ovarian mesothelial cells in vitro. Biol of Reprod 1996; 54:660-669.
78. Mondshein JS, Schomberg DW. Growth factors modulate gonadotropin receptor induction in granulosa cell cultures. Science 1981; 211:1179-1180.
79. Hsueh AJW, Welsh TH, Jones PBC. Inhibition of ovarian and testicular steroidogensis by epidermal growth factor. Endocrinol 1981; 108:2002-2004.
80. Erickson GF, Case E. Epidermal growth factor antagonizes ovarian theca-interstitial cytodifferentiation. Mol Cell Endocrinol 1983; 31:71-76.
81. Knecht M, Catt KJ. Modulation of cAMP-mediated differentiation in ovarian granulosa cell by epidermal growth factor and platelet-derived growth factor. J Biol Chem 1983; 258:2789-2794.
82. Oka Y, Orth DN. Human plasma epidermal growth factor/B-urogastrone is associated with blood platelets. J Clin Invest 1983; 72:249-259.

83. Gillet JY, Maillet R, Gautier C. Blood supply and lymph supply of the ovary. In: Biology of the ovary, Motta PM and Makabe ESE, eds. Martinus Nijhoff Publishers, Boston, pp.86-98,1980.

84. Berchuck A, Rodriguez GC, Kamel A, Dodge RK, Soper JT, Clarke-Pearson DL, Bast Jr RC. Epidermal growth factor receptor expression in normal ovarian epithelium and ovarian cancer. I. Correlation of receptor expression with prognostic factors in patients with ovarian cancer. Am J Obstet Gynecol 1991; 164:669-674.

85. Jindal SK, Snoey DM, Lobb DK, Dorrington JH. Transforming Growth Factor α Localization and Role in Surface epithelium of Normal Human Ovaries and in Ovarian Carcinoma Cells. Gynecol Oncol 1994; 53:17-23.

86. Owens OJ, Stewart C, Brown I, Leake RE. Epidermal growth factor receptors (EGFR) in human ovarian cancer. Br J Cancer 1991; 64:907-910.

87. Owens OJ, Leake RE Growth factor content in normal and benign ovarian tumours. European J Obstet Gynecol Reprod Biol 1992; 47:223-228.

88. Johnson GR, Saeki T, Auersperg N, Gordon AW, Shoyab M, Salomon DS, Stromberg K. Response to and expression of amphiregulin by ovarian carcinoma and normal ovarian surface epithelial cells: nuclear localization of endogenous amphiregulin. Biochemical & Biophysical Research Communications 1991; 180:481-488.

89. Klapper LN, Kirschbaum MH, Sela M, Yarden Y. Biochemical and clinical implications of the ErbB.HER signaling network of growth factor receptors. In: Advances in Cancer Research, Academic Press, pp.25-79, 2000.

90. Berchuck A, Kamel A, Whitaker R, Kerns B, Olt G, Kinney R, Soper JT, Dodge R, Clarke-Pearson DL, Marks P et al. Overexpression of HER-2/neu is associated with poor survival in advanced epithelial ovarian cancer. Cancer Res 1990; 50:4087-4091.

91. Kohler M, Bauknecht T, Grimm M, Birmelin G, Kommoss F, Wagner E. Epidermal growth factor receptor and transforming growth factor alpha expression in human ovarian carcinomas. Eur J Cancer 1992; 28A:1432-1437.

92. Aguilar Z, Akita RW, Finn RS, Ramos BL, Pegram MD, Kabbinavar FF, Pietras RJ, Pisacane P, Sliwkowski MX, Slamon DJ. Biologic effects of heregulin/neu differentiation factor on normal and malignant human breast and ovarian epithelial cells. Oncogene 1999; 18:6050-6062.

93. Dabrow MB, Francesco MR, McBrearty FX, Caradonna S. The effects of platelet-derived growth factor and receptor on normal ad neoplastic human ovarian surface epithelium. Gynecol Oncol 1998; 71:29-37.

94. Marth C, Zeimet AG, Herold M, Brumm C, Windbichler G, Muller-Holzner E, Offner F, Feichtinger H, Zwierzina H, Daxenbichler G. Different effects of interferons, interleukin-1β and tumor necrosis factor-α in normal (OSE) and malignant human ovarian epithelial cells. Int J Cancer 1996; 67:826-830.

95. Kang SS, Choi K-C, Cheng KW, Nathwani PS, Auersperg N, Leung PCK 2000 Role of gonadotropin-releasing hormone as an autocrine growth factor in human ovarian surface epithelium. Endocrinol 141:72-80.

96. Taipale J, Saharinen J, Keski-Oja J. Extracellular matrix-associated transforming growth factor-β: Role in cancer cell growth and invasion. In: Advances in Cancer Research, Academic Press, pp.87-134, 1998.

97. Berchuck A, Rodriguez G, Olt G, Whitaker R, Boente MP, Arrick BA, Clarke-Pearson DL, Bast RC Jr. Regulation of growth of normal ovarian epithelial cells and ovarian cancer cell lines by transforming growth factor-beta. Am J Obstet Gynecol 1992; 166:676-684.

98. Vigne J-L, Halburnt LL, Skinner MK. Characterization of bovine ovarian surface epithelium and stromal cells: Identification of Secreted Proteins. Biol Reprod 1994; 51:1213-1221.

99. Evangelou A, Jindal SK, Brown TJ, Letarte M. Down-regulationof transforming growth factor β receptors by androgen in ovarian cancer cells. Cancer Res 2000; 60:929-935.

100. Josso N, Racine C, di Clemente N, Rey R, Xavier F. The role of anti-Mullerian hormone in gonadal develoment. Mol Cell Endocrinol 1998; 145:3-7.

101. Nash DM, Hess SA, White BA, Peluso JJ. Steroidogenic factor-1 regulates the rate of proliferation of normal and neoplastic rat ovarian surface epithelial cells *in vitro*. Endocrinol 1998; 139:4663-4671.

102. Di Blasio AM, Cremonesi L, Vigano P, Ferrari M, Gospodarowicz D, Vignali M, Jaffe RB. Basic fibroblast growth factor and its receptor messenger ribonucleic acids are expressed in human ovarian epithelial neoplasms. Am J Obstet Gynecol 1993; 169:1517-1523.

103. Di Renzo MF, Olivero M, Katsaros D, Crepald T, Gaglia P, Zola P, Sismondi P, Comoglio PM. Overexpression of the Met/HGF receptor in ovarian cancer. Int J Cancer 1994; 58:658-662.

104. Negami AI, Sasaki H, Kawakami Y, Kamitani N, Kotsuji F, Tominaga T, Nakamura T. Serum human hepatocyte growth factor in human menstrual cycle and pregnancy: a novel serum marker of regeneration and reconstruction of human endometrium. Homone Res 1995; 44(suppl 2):42-46.

105. Parrott JA, Vigne J-L, Chu BZ, Skinner MK. Mesenchymal-epithelial interactions in the ovarian follicle involve keratinocyte and hepatocyte growth factor production by thecal cells and their action on granulosa cells. Endocrinol 1994; 135:569-575.

106. Huntsman D, Resau JH, Klineberg E, Auersperg N. Comparison of c-met expression in ovarian epithelial tumors and normal epithelia of the female reproductive tract by quantitative laser scan microscopy. Am J Pathol 1999; 155:343-348.

107. Klominek J, Baskin B, Liu Z, Hauzenberger D. Hepatocyte growth factor/scatter factor stimulates chemotaxis and growth of malignant mesothelioma cells through c-met receptor. Int J Cancer 1998; 76:240-249.

108. Gulati R, Peluso JJ. Opposing actions of hepatocyte growth factor and basic fibroblast growth factor on cell contact, intracellular free calcium levels, and rat ovarian surface epithelial cell viability. Endocrinol 1997; 138:1847-1856.

109. Parrott JA, Skinner M. Expression and action of hepatocyte growth factor in human and bovine normal ovarian surface epithelium and ovarian cancer. Biol Reprod 2000; 62:491-500.

110. Wong AST, Leung PCK, Auersperg N. Hepatocyte growth factor/scatter factor and its receptor c-MET in cultured human ovarian surface epithelium : influence of family history of ovarian cancer. Proc Soc Study Reprod 1999; 32:95-96.

111. Kacinski BM, Carter D, Mittal K, Yee LD, Scata KA, Donofrio L, Chambers SK, Wang KI, Yang-Fent T, Rohrschneider LR et al. Ovarian adenocarcinomas express fms-complementary transcripts and fms antigen, often with coexpression of CSF-1. Am J Pathol 1990; 137:135-147.

112. Auersperg N, Maines-Bandiera SL, Dyck HG. Ovarian carcinogenesis and the biology of ovarian surface epithelium. [Review] J Cell Physiol 1997; 173, 261-265.

113. Nicholaides NC, Papadopoulos N, Liu B et al. Mutations of two PMS homologues in herediatry nonpolyposis colon cancer. Nature 1994; 37:75-80.

114. Kote-Jarai Z, Eeles RA. BRCA1, BRCA2 and their possible function in DNA damage response. Br J Cancer 1999; 81:1099-1102.

115. Fan S, Wang JA, Yuan R, Ma Y, Meng Q, Erdos MR, Pestell RG, Fang Yuan, Auborn KJ, Goldberg ID, Rosen EM. BRCA1 inhibition of estrogen receptor signaling in transfected cells. Science 1999; 284:1354-1356.

116. Salazar H, Godwin AK, Daly MD, Laub PB, Hogan M, Rosenblum N, Boente MP, Lunch HT, Hamilton T. Microscopic benign and invasive malignant neoplasms and a cancer-prone phenotype in prophylactic oophorectomies. J Nat Cancer Inst 1996; 88:1810-1820.

117. Werness BA, Afify AM, Bielat KL, Eltabbakh GH, Piver MS, Paterson JM. Altered surface and cyst epithelium of ovaries removed prophylactically from women with a family history of ovarian cancer. Hum Pathol 1999; 30:151-157.

118. Sherman ME, Lee JS, Burks RT, Struewing JP, Durman RJ, Hartge P. Histopathologic features of ovaries at increased risk for carcinoma. Int J Gynecol Pathol 1999; 18:151-157.

119. Stratton JF, Buckley CH, Lowe D, Ponder BAJ and the United Kingdom Coordinating Committee of Cancer Research (UKCCCR), Familial Ovarian Cancer Study Group. Comparison of prophylactic oophorectomy specimens from carriers and noncarriers of a BRCA1 or BRCA2 gene mutation. J Natl Cancer Inst 1999; 91:626-628.

120. Kruk PA, Godwin AK, Hamilton TC, Auersperg N. Telomeric instability and reduced proliferative potential in ovarian surface epithelial cells from women with a family history of ovarian cancer. Gynecol Oncol 1999; 73:229-236.

121. Auersperg N, Maines-Bandiera S, Booth JH, Lynch HT, Godwin AK, Hamilton TC. Expression of two mucin antigens in cultured human ovarian surface epithelium: Influence of a family history of ovarian cancer. Am J Obstet Gynecol 1995; 173:558-565.

122. Marrs JA, Nelson J. Cadherin cell adhesion molecules in differentiation and embryogenesis. Int Rev Cytol 1996; 165:159-205.

123. MacCalman CD, Farooki R, Blaschuk OW. Estradiol regulates E-cadherin mRNA levels in the surface epithelium of the mouse ovary. Clin Exp Metastasis 1994; 12:276-282.

124. Sowter HM, Corps AN, Smith SK. Hepatocyte growth factor (HGF) in ovarian epithelial tumour fluids stimulates the migration of ovarian carcinoma cells. Int J Cancer 1999; 83:476-480.

125. Wong AST, Pelech SL, Ehlen T, Leung PCK, Auersperg N Autocrine regulation of hepatocyte growth factor-Met: an early step in ovarian carcinogenesis? (submitted).

126. Goldberg JM, Piver SM, Jishi MF, Blumenson L. Age at onset of ovarian cancer in women with a strong family history of ovarian cancer. Gynecol Oncol 1997; 66:3-9.

Chapter 8

CYTOPATHOLOGY OF THE OVARY

DeFrias D.V.S., Okonkwo A.M., Keh P.C., Nayar R.
Department of Pathology, Northwestern University Medical School, Chicago, Illinois 60611

1. NORMAL OVARIAN STRUCTURES

The ovaries are pelvic organs located bilaterally and attached to the uterine cornua and fallopian tubes by several ligaments that maintain their lateral location. There are various components of a normal ovary that are important to recognize. Many of these components undergo cyclical changes secondary to hormonal manifestations.

1.1. Surface Epithelium

The surface epithelium consists of modified peritoneal epithelium similar to the epithelium that lines other extrapelvic structures(Clement 1996). It varies from flat, cuboidal to columnar and may show ciliated cellular structures(Clement 1996). Cells taken during washings or scrapes of the ovarian surfaces are arranged in monolayers. These cells have limited amount of delicate cytoplasm and contain centrally located oval nuclei with small nucleoli that can occasionally be doubled. (Figure 1). Occasionally, the nuclei may have longitudinal clefting or irregularities, but the chromatin consistently appears fine and regularly distributed. It is important to note that mesothelial proliferations resulting from pelvic inflammatory disease may be quite atypical and can be a source of pitfall since they may be mistaken for metastatic adenocarcinoma in peritoneal washings(Clement 1996). Clinical history and pre-operative surgical impression are mandatory in avoiding misinterpretation.

1.2. BRCA1, BRCA2 and Hereditary Breast-Ovarian Cancer
1.2.1. General

Approximately 10% of ovarian cancers are thought to have a hereditary basis. The strongest risk factor for the development of disease is a family history of ovarian cancer. Germline mutations in the BRCA1 and BRCA2 breast-ovarian cancer susceptibility genes appear to account for most hereditary ovarian cancers. A much smaller fraction occur as a result of DNA repair gene mutations (Berchuck et al. 1999). BRCA1 is a phosphoprotein located in the cell nucleus that functions as a negative regulator of the cell cycle (Zhang et al. 1997; Ruffner and Verma 1997; Wang et al., 1997). It is considered an active inhibitor for development of neoplasia (tumor suppressor gene). BRCA1 is located in chromosome 17q21. Gene mutations of BRCA1 have been implicated in 80% of familial breast and ovarian cancers(Hall et al. 1992; Castilla et al. 1994). These mutations are inherited through the germ cell line. The risk of the BRCA1 carrier developing breast carcinoma is between 33% and 50% in contrast to 2% in young patients without inherited mutations(Frank and Braverman 1999). The risk for the development of ovarian carcinoma in these women is also increased (Frank and Braverman 1999; Smith 1996; Futreal et al. 1994) and estimated to be between 28% and 44%(Ford et al. 1994; Easton et al. 1995). Germline mutations in the BRCA2 gene, which is located on chromosome 13q12, may account for as much as 10-35% of ovarian cancers (Berchuck et al. 1999).

1.2.2. Pathologic Findings

The cells scraped from ovarian surface of patients with BRCA1 and BRCA2 mutations show a complex arrangement of cells with florid papillary fronds and large sheets (Figure 2). Some clusters may contain cells with slightly enlarged nuclei and infoldings of the nuclear envelopes are often noticeable (Figure 3). These findings contrast with the cytological features of cells from normal ovaries, which show small monolayers of cuboidal cells with minimal cytoplasm, and occasionally clusters of columnar cells with maintained polarity may be seen. The cytological features seen in BRAC1 and BRCA2 ovaries correlate well with the histological findings, in which complex micropapillary excrescences are seen in foci of the ovarian surface epithelium with multiple clefts deep in the ovarian stroma (Figure 4).

1.2.3. Future Directions

Surveillance and management of young patients with the propensity to develop ovarian carcinoma may include prophylactic surgery, preventive chemotherapy(Frank and Braverman 1999) and most recently a new approach of studying cells obtained by scrapping the ovarian surface during laparoscopy (Fishman, personal communication). Several laboratory techniques may be employed to identify patients that carry this type of abnormality. In the surgical pathology setting, immunohistochemical staining using avidin-biotin-peroxidase complex method is feasible (Lee et al. 1999).

The immunoreactivity is graded by the proportion of malignant cells showing distinctive nuclear staining as well as the aberrant cytoplasmic staining in these cells (Lee et al. 1999; Shen and Vadgama 1997). However, utilization of this methodology is still controversial (Smith 1996; Lee et al. 1999).

1.3. Ovarian Stroma

The ovarian stroma is composed of spindle shaped cells arranged in whorls associated with dense collagen and reticulum components, which becomes more collagenous in older women (Clement 1996). Fragments of cellular stroma are rarely seen in washings. However, forceful scrapes of the ovarian surface may dislodge fragments of cellular stroma and fusiform cells similar to fibroblasts may be identified. Occasionally, stromal projections from the ovarian surface lined by surface epithelium are prominent in perimenopausal and menopausal patients (Clement 1996). In cytological samples these collagen-epithelial structures are named "collagen balls" and are encountered frequently in peritoneal washings (Wojcik and Naylor 1992). The ovarian stroma reacts to a variety of hormonal influences. When decidual changes occur, the cells appear large with variable shape containing ample cytoplasm. The nuclei are oval or rounded and single or multiple enlarged nucleoli are often present. Bizarre forms of decidual cells as well as cells derived from gestational origin, such as syncytial and cytotrophoblasts in patients with tubal pregnancy may be seen in washings, mimicking neoplastic cells.

1.4. Ovarian Follicles

Follicles are rarely seen in washings and are identified only when the ovarian surface epithelium is dislodged and the stroma exposed. A firm scrape however, may yield portions of a follicle particularly as the follicle reaches maturity. In rare instances, an oocyte surrounded by the zona pellucida may be displaced and thus sampled. The granulosa cells that surround the oocyte are oval or cuboidal and have limited amounts of cytoplasm. The chromatin is granular and in cytological samples shows a "neuroendocrine-like" appearance. Call-Exner structures can be seen in cytological samples either as part of a benign follicle or in neoplasms of granulosa cells (Clement 1996). These structures are composed of granulosa cells surrounding small cavities filled with PAS-positive material (Figure 5) A frequent source of false positives are granulosa cells depicting several mitotic figures being mistaken for a malignant process. Theca cells are larger than granulosa cells and have abundant vacuolated cytoplasm, especially noticeable in specimens stained by the giemsa technique. The nuclei are oval

188

or rounded, centrally located with a single prominent nucleoli (Figure 6). Mitotic figures can also be encountered.

1.5. Corpus Luteum

In the absence of fertilization, the follicle structure collapses and the corpus luteum is formed. Macroscopically, the corpus luteum has a bright yellow, convoluted border and a central hemorrhagic coagulum. The periphery of the corpus luteum is composed of polygonal cells with abundant delicate cytoplasm containing vacuolated spaces left by lipid dissolved during processing. The rounded nuclei depict a single or double prominent nucleolus. As the corpus luteum involutes, it undergoes dissolution and is phagocytized (Clement 1996). Fibrosis ensues and corpus albicans replaces the degenerating corpus luteum (Kay et al. 1961) which may contain hemosiderin and ceroid laden macrophages in addition to other elements (Reagan 1950). Cytology samples may show arborization of dense connective tissue with cells containing blunt ended nuclei.

1.6. Benign Ovarian Cysts
1.6.1. Inclusion Cysts

Surface inclusions and cysts are invaginations of the cortical epithelium that may be encountered at any stage of life (Figure 7). They can be single but most frequently are multiple and distributed on the surface of the cortical subepithelial area. Often, a single layer of columnar epithelium lines these cysts (Figure 8). In post-menopausal patients, tubal-like epithelium may be found associated with psammoma bodies(Clement 1996). In peritoneal washings, these calcified structures with the presence of columnar epithelium may be the source of false positive diagnosis of adenocarcinoma (Figure 9). Though surface inclusion cysts are not regularly seen in cytological samples except during scrapes of the ovarian surface, when present should be evaluated with caution

1.6.2. Follicle and Corpus Luteum Cysts

Follicle and corpus luteum cysts are rarely seen at menopause. Nevertheless, solitary or multiple cysts can occur during all other stages of life. Follicle cysts are usually unilocular and lined by granulosa cells and an outer layer of theca cells. Aspiration of follicle cysts yields clear fluid in which small cell clusters and isolated cells with "neuroendocrine-like" chromatin structures are present (Figure 10). Numerous mitotic figures may be identified. In addition, pleomorphism and atypia may be a frequent finding during puerperium, which may be a source of false positive diagnosis in cytological samples. In corpus luteum cysts, the cyst fluid is yellow containing large cells with abundant vacuolated cytoplasm, round nuclei and prominent nucleoli showing similarities with histiocytic cells.

1.6.3. Endometriotic Cyst

These cysts arise secondary to cystic degeneration in foci of endometriosis. They are filled with dark brown fluid, hence the term "chocolate cyst", and are lined by cuboidal/columnar epithelium resembling endometrial cells with many hemosiderin-laden macrophages. Long-standing endometriosis, due to a process of bleeding and regeneration, may depict severe epithelial atypia similar to that seen in neoplasia leading to the possibility of an occasional false positive diagnosis. To compound the problem, there is a documented association of endometriosis with endometrioid and clear cell carcinoma of the ovary. Each case should be diagnosed with care, taking into account the clinical and radiologic information.

2. OVARIAN TUMORS

A large variety of tumors are encountered in the ovary. The great majority (60%) arise from the surface epithelium and are classified according to the histologic differentiation of the epithelium(Gompel and Silverberg 1994). Surface epithelial tumors are further subclassfied into benign, borderline and carcinoma depending on the degree of epithelial proliferation and the presence or absence of stromal invasion(Scully et al. 1998). The latter classification correlates more closely with prognosis than the classification by histologic type. A number of different histologic tumor types, derive from the primitive cells of the embryonic gonad and are designated as germ cell tumors. In adults, they are the second largest group of ovarian neoplasms after epithelial tumors, approximately 30%, and about 95% of them are benign, mature cystic teratomas. In children, 60% of ovarian tumors are of germ cell origin and one third of them are malignant (Scully et al. 1998). A minority of ovarian neoplasms (approximately 10%) originate from the sex cords, stroma or both(Gompel and Silverberg 1994). These tumors are usually benign (fibroma-thecoma), while the granulosa cell tumors are malignant. The remainder of the tumors in this group are rare. Small cell carcinoma is a very rare, aggressive tumor that occurs in young women and is associated with hypercalcemia(Scully et al. 1998). Microscopically, follicle-like structures composed of cells with fine nuclear chromatin may be seen. This tumor must be differentiated from small cell carcinoma of pulmonary type which occurs in older women. Tumors with more than one pattern of epithelium are classified as mixed epithelial tumors(Scully et al. 1998). Undifferentiated carcinomas are tumors in which the surface epithelium cannot be classified into a specific histological type(Russell and Farnsworth 1997). Carcinomas of the ovary spread by direct invasion of adjacent organs and disseminate by peritoneal fluid (Gompel and Silverberg 1994). Many patients present with ascites and the initial diagnosis can be made from peritoneal fluid.

BASIC WHO HISTOLOGIC CLASSIFICATION OF OVARIAN NEOPLASMS

SURFACE EPITHELIAL TUMORS	SEX-CORD STROMAL TUMORS	GERM CELL TUMORS
1. **Serous tumors**	1. **Granulosa-stromal tumors**	1. **Dysgerminoma**
Benign, borderline, malignant	Granulosa cell tumor	2. **Yolk sac tumor**
2. **Mucinous tumors**	Adult and Juvenile	3. **Embryonal**
Endocervical and intestinal	Thecoma-Fibroma group	4. **Polyembryoma**
Benign, borderline, malignant	2. **Sertoli-stromal tumors**	5. **Choriocarcinoma**
3. **Endometrioid tumors**	a. Well differentiated	6. **Teratomas**
Benign, borderline, malignant	b. Moderately differentiated	Immature
4. **Clear cell tumors**	c. Poorly differentiated	Mature
Benign, borderline, malignant	d. Retiform	Monodermal
5. **Transitional cell tumors**	e. Heterologous elements	7.**Mixed germ cell tumors**
Brenner tumor	3. **Sex cord, annular tubules**	**OTHER**
Benign, borderline, malignant	4. **Gynandroblastoma**	**GONADOBLASTOMA**
6. **Squamous cell tumors**	5. **Unclassified**	**GERMCELL/SEX CORD**
7. **Mixed epithelial tumors**	6. **Steroid (lipid) cell tumors**	**TUMOR OF RETE OVARII**
Benign, borderline, malignant	Stromal luteoma	**MESOTHELIAL TUMOR**
8. **Undifferentiated carcinoma**	Leydig cell tumor	**MISCELLANEOUS**

3. SURFACE EPITHELIAL TUMORS
3.1. Serous Tumors
3.1.1. General

Most ovarian neoplasms of surface epithelial origin are serous tumors. These tumors comprise nearly 50% of all surface epithelial tumors with approximately 50% being benign, 15% borderline, and 35% of serous tumors representing invasive cancer(Russell and Farnsworth 1997).

3.1.2. Pathologic findings

Serous neoplasms present as predominantly unilocular, cystic masses containing clear serous fluid and occasionally, thin, mucoid material (Hendrickson 1992). They are frequently bilateral. Borderline and invasive serous tumors are multilocular with a solid and cystic gross appearance, the latter containing soft, friable, papillary projections filling the cyst lumen (Russell and Farnsworth 1997). Histological examination of serous neoplasms show flattened epithelium in benign tumors (Figure 11) and well-formed complex papillary structures in borderline (Figure 12) and carcinomatous tumors(Russell 1996). Glandular and solid areas may also be present in less well-differentiated tumors (Figure 13). The epithelium encountered shows flat, cuboidal to columnar and ciliated cellular structures (Figure 14) akin to the modified peritoneum surrounding the ovary and fallopian tube(Hendrickson 1992). Psammoma bodies, which are concentric, laminated, calcified structures, which occur secondary to cellular degeneration and are present in these tumors (Figure 15). Psammoma bodies do not differentiate between benign and malignant tumors since they may be observed in both (Scully et al. 1998). Histological sections (Figure 16) are necessary to establish the presence of invasion, abnormal architectural findings and evidence of carcinomatous nuclear features(Russell 1996). Aspirated material from borderline tumors show delicate papillary clusters, large sheets and balls of cells with small, round nuclei, inconspicuous nucleoli and scant cytoplasm (Figure 17). However, in the great majority of cases, the cells from borderline serous tumors have the same morphological characteristics as the invasive tumors and it is impossible to define their biological behavior in cytologic samples (Figure 18). In these cases, the diagnostic presence or absence of invasion has to be made on the excised specimen in surgical pathology by evaluating the interphase of the epithelial portion of the tumor and its stroma. If the diagnosis rendered by cytology is adenocarcinoma, (Figure 19) and histologic samples indicate a borderline lesion, the management of the patient follows the histologic diagnosis, unless additional molecular biology studies truly establish the biological behavior of the tumor to be malignant. Markedly atypical cells with vacuolated cytoplasm and very bizarre tumor giant cells with irregular nuclear outlines are seen in invasive tumors (Figure 20). Immunohistochemical stains may be necessary on the cellblock to differentiate poorly differentiated serous carcinomas from other primary or metastatic malignancies in pelvic washings.

3.1.3. Differential diagnosis

Other surface epithelial tumors, specifically endometrioid carcinoma and epithelial mesothelioma are considered in the evaluation of serous neoplasms.

3.2. Mucinous Tumors
3.2.1. General

A great majority of mucinous tumors encountered in the ovary are benign processes with approximately 75% being benign, 10% borderline and 15% carcinomatous(Katsube et al. 1982; Koonings et al. 1989).

3.2.2. Pathologic findings

Multilocular neoplasms are more frequent than unilocular mucinous cystadenomas. Borderline and invasive mucinous neoplasms may contain solid areas as well as papillary fronds protruding into the lumen. The lumens are filled with thick mucinous fluid and single epithelial cells lining the cysts usually float in the fluid giving the cells a rounded appearance mimicking histiocytic cells. In aspirates, the epithelial cells are usually diagnosed as histiocytes and special stains do not solve the problem since histiocytes being phagocytic cells, contain cytoplasmic mucin are also present in the fluid. Only when cellblock and aspirates show true cell clusters can a diagnosis of mucinous neoplasm be accurately issued (Figure 21). Cells identified in aspirates include clusters of small groups of tall columnar cells with round or oval basally located nuclei. The neoplastic cells in mucinous neoplasms are of variable morphology resembling endocervical, gastric or intestinal epithelium (Figure 22). The cell cytoplasm is filled with mucus and the cell arrangement is in a palisading fashion or arranged on end depicting exaggerated honeycombing (Figure 23). Rarely, intestinal type epithelium is present showing small papillae or large monolayers formed by goblet cells with distinctive cytoplasmic spaces. The borderline tumors are formed by thick, rounded and small papillary fronds with some degree of nuclear atypia and abundant cytoplasmic mucin (Figure 24). The background observed in borderline tumors is quite characteristic depicting pools of mucin and histiocytes as well as single rounded epithelial cells. Numerous histological sections are necessary to establish the presence of invasion and/or neoplastic cell stratification of four or greater cell thickness(Hart and Norris 1973), abnormal architectural findings and evidence of carcinomatous nuclear features. Unfortunately, the cellular features in benign cytological samples are in most instances indistinguishable from their borderline counterpart. The invasive type of mucinous tumors may or may not show increased atypical changes making the diagnosis of an invasive tumor difficult. Cytologic specimens of known invasive mucinous tumors do not pose this problem, since the nature of the tumor is already established.

3.2.3. Differential diagnosis

These include other surface epithelial tumors and metastatic carcinoma from gastrointestinal tract, pancreas and cervix.

3.3. Endometrioid Tumors
3.3.1. General

Endometrioid neoplasms are composed of epithelial elements and stroma that resemble the normal endometrium and account for 2-4% of all ovarian tumors. Less than 1% of benign ovarian neoplasms are endometrioid, and almost all of them are adenofibromas(Scully et al. 1998). Only 2-3% of ovarian borderline tumors are endometrioid. Endometrioid carcinomas account for 10- 20% of all ovarian carcinomas(Katsube et al. 1982; Kline et al. 1990; Koonings et al. 1989; Peterson 1991; Russell 1979). These neoplasms occur in older reproductive and postmenopausal women and are frequently associated with endometriosis, ranging in frequency from 11% to 42 %, either in the same ovary or other site in the pelvis. This association can be seen in benign, borderline and malignant endometrioid tumors(Bell and Scully 1985;Snyder et al. 1988; DePriest et al. 1992; Fukunnaga et al. 1997; Mostoufizadeh and Sculley 1980).

3.3.2. Pathologic Findings

Foci of endometriosis or endometriotic cyst may be identified grossly (Scully et al. 1998). Histological types include glandular, cribriform and villoglandular (Scully et al. 1998). Cytological samples are usually obtained from metastasis of invasive carcinoma to a variety of body sites. The cell morphology observed depends primarily on the degree of differentiation. When cells obtained from a metastasis of well-differentiated endometrioid carcinoma are analyzed, a cytopathologist can elaborate on the histological type. However, moderately and poorly differentiated carcinomas yield cells that may mimic a variety of tumors. The borderline lesions present the same difficulties as the serous neoplasms and management of patients is based on the surgical pathology diagnosis, since very few cases can be diagnosed as borderline in cytology samples. A frequent area of pitfall occurs in samples obtained from foci of endometriosis. Cells of long-standing endometriosis and endometrioid cysts may have cellular features identical to malignant cells. Clinical correlation and the presence of only scant cellular components of atypical cells must be evaluated with caution to rule out false positive diagnoses.

3.3.3. Differential Diagnosis

When assessing these tumors, other surface epithelial tumors, and sex cord stromal tumors should be considered.

3.4. Clear Cell Tumors
3.4.1. General

Adenocarcinomas of the clear cell variety comprise approximately 6% of all ovarian cancers and show variable cell patterns(Scully et al. 1998). The most common cellular components are the clear and hobnail cell types. Less frequently, cuboidal, oxyphilic and rarely signet-ring components can be encountered(Scully et al. 1998).

3.4.2. Pathologic Findings

These tumors appear sponge-like and mostly cystic. Histologically, clear cell adenocarcinoma has a variety of architectural patterns including solid, papillary and tubulocystic(Scully et al. 1998). Special stains depict abundant cytoplasmic glycogen and lipid. Mucin is prominent in the luminal surface and apex of the cells, and is abundant in the signet ring cell type(Scully et al. 1998). The cytoplasm of clear cells is abundant, cyanophilic and transparent. The nuclei are enlarged and atypical and macro nucleoli are a frequent feature. The hobnail and cuboidal types have limited amount of cytoplasm, round or oval nuclei and inconspicuous nucleoli seen against a background of granular chromatin (Figure 25). The cells of this tumor type can be easily overlooked if not accompanied by other more atypical cell components. The oxyphilic cells of clear cell adenocarcinoma have similar nuclear features as the clear cell with dense cytoplasm and well-defined borders. It is not always possible to establish the specific histological type of the clear cell neoplasms in aspirates and peritoneal washings. Necrosis may induce pseudoeosinophilia of the cytoplasm precluding a correct assessment of the cell type. Also, the other histological subtypes, resemble a variety of epithelial neoplasms in cytology samples. Occasionally, an admixture of the classic clear cells can be encountered and diagnosed accurately (Figure 26). Clear cell adeno-carcinoma of signet ring cell variety can be diagnosed correctly in cytology samples. However, it cannot be established if it is from primary or metastatic disease of the ovary.

3.4.3. Differential Diagnosis

It is important to differentiate this tumor from other surface epithelial tumors, dysgerminomas and yolk sac tumors.

3.5. Brenner Tumors
3.5.1. General

This group of neoplasms comprises tumors whose epithelium resembles the urothelial lining(Arey 1961) and are thought to arise from metaplastic ovarian surface epithelium(Erlich and Roth 1971). They are uncommon tumors and may be associated with mucinous cystadenomas or other benign epithelial tumors(Scully et al. 1998).

3.5.2. Pathologic Findings

Most Brenner tumors are benign, solid masses, with occasional tumors being solid and cystic borderline or carcinomatous(Scully et al. 1998). Tumors in which malignant transitional epithelium are identified with no benign counterpart are termed transitional cell carcinomas(Austin and Norris 1987). Conversely, tumors in which benign elements are identified adjacent to malignant epithelium are classified as Brenner tumors. Benign Brenner tumors are characterized by variably sized epithelial nests and cystic spaces containing elongate cells with ovoid, longitudinal, grooved nuclei and clear cytoplasm in a fibrotic stroma. Mucinous epithelium may also be present. The malignant variant, show solid and cystic areas lined by stratified epithelium consisting of markedly pleomorphic cells. Squamoid and glandular areas are often present and this finding may disguise the true nature of the tumor(Scully et al. 1998). However, the finding of more typical transitional type epithelium will lead to the correct diagnosis. Destructive stromal invasion is required for diagnosis of malignancy similar to other surface epithelial tumors(Austin and Norris 1987). It may be impossible to differentiate between primary transitional cell carcinoma of the ovary and metastatic transitional cell carcinoma from the urinary bladder without careful clinical evaluation(Scully et al. 1998).

3.5.3. Differential Diagnosis

Endometrioid tumors with squamous differentiation, granulosa cell tumor, carcinoid and metastatic transitional cell carcinoma of bladder are considered in the differential diagnosis of these tumors.

4. SEX CORD STROMAL TUMORS
4.1. Granulosa Cell Tumors
4.1.1. General

This tumor is by far the most frequently encountered sex cord stromal tumor and represents 1-2% of all ovarian tumors(Russell and Farnsworth

1997). There are two histologic types, the adult granulosa cell tumors which most commonly arise in women >20 years (middle aged and older women) and the juvenile granulosa cell tumor which develops in women <20 years of age (children and younger women)(Russell and Farnsworth 1997). They are the most common ovarian tumors with estrogenic manifestations and occasionally produce androgenic hormones(Scully et al. 1998). They are unilateral in 95% of cases and 10- 15% are ruptured when removed.

4.1.2. Pathologic Findings

These tumors are variable in size, often large and solid, occasionally cystic and display a variety of patterns including macrocystic and microcystic morphology(Scully et al. 1998). Common histologic growth patterns are diffuse, trabecular and insular. The best differentiated is the follicular pattern and the microfollicular morphology is the most frequent pattern. The adult type typically has microfollicles, cells with scant cytoplasm and pale angulated nuclei (Figure 27), and the juvenile form has large follicles, cells with moderate to abundant cytoplasm and darker nuclei. When the tumor is functional, the typical endometrial effect is cystic hyperplasia and well differentiated carcinoma develops in less than 5% of cases. On FNA, the neoplastic cells are arranged in rows of cells traversed by prominent vessels. The individual cells show evidence of nuclear molding with moderate pleomorphism, finely granular nuclear chromatin containing prominent longitudinal grooves and scant delicate cytoplasm (Figure 28). Call-Exner bodies can also be seen (Figure 29). Prominent nucleoli may be present in luteinized granulosa cells. In 2% cases, bizarre, enlarged hyperchromatic nuclei including multinucleated cells are seen focally and a search for characteristic areas is warranted in order to make the correct diagnosis. Immunohistochemical stains for inhibin can help classify these cells as being sex cord stromal when performed on cellblocks obtained from washings.

4.1.3. Differential Diagnosis

Tumors to consider in this category include undifferentiated carcinoma, malignant lymphoma, primary or metastatic carcinoid and possibly small cell carcinoma.

4.2. Sertoli-Leydig Cell Tumors
4.2.1. General
This is an uncommon tumor seen in young women and may be hormonally active. Many patients show signs of virilization (Russell and Farnsworth 1997).

4.2.1. Pathologic Findings

They appear grossly as solid and cystic neoplasms. Microscopically, they are composed of tubular structures lined by Sertoli cells admixed with polygonal Leydig cells containing abundant eosinophilic cytoplasm in a variety of architectural patterns. Crystals of Reinke may be present in leydig cells. Heterologous elements may occasionally be present. These elements include mucinous epithelium, cartilage, striated muscle and rarely neuroblasts(Scully et al. 1998).

4.2.3. Differential Diagnosis

Important differential diagnoses include granulosa cell tumor, endometrioid carcinoma, metastatic carcinoma and yolk sac tumor.

4.3. Fibroma-Thecoma Tumors
4.3.1. General

Fibroma-thecomas account for approximately 6% of all primary ovarian tumors and usually occur in middle-aged patients(Gompel and Silverberg 1994). These tumors are mostly benign and are considered a histologic spectrum from fibroma, with spindle cells forming collagen, to specialized theca cells. Thecomas are stromal tumors containing cells with lipid rich cytoplasm resembling theca cells(Gompel and Silverberg 1994).

4.3.2.   Pathologic Findings

Fibromas are large white solid masses and appear histologically as cellular tumors with intersecting bundles of spindle cells in a storiform pattern. Only rare mitotic figures are seen. Fibrosarcomas are considered when > 4 mitosis per 10 high-power fields associated with moderate to severe nuclear atypia is encountered(Scully et al. 1998). Thecomas contain sheets of theca-like cells, which may be luteinized(Scully et al. 1998).

4.3.3. Differential Diagnosis

These tumors are differentiated histologically from other benign tumors including myxoma, sclerosing stromal tumors and massive edema of the ovary.

4.4. Other Tumors of Sex-Cord Stromal Origin

Additional tumors in this group include leydig cell tumors, stromal luteomas, unclassified sex cord-stromal tumors, sex cord tumors with annular tubules (SCTAT), lipid cell tumors, and gynandroblastoma. These tumors are rarely encountered and are often detected because of hormonally induced symptoms. SCTAT is characterized by the presence of simple and complex ring-shaped tubules, often exhibiting focal differentiation towards typical Sertoli cell tumor, granulosa cell tumor or both. It often occurs in Peutz-Jeghers syndrome (PJS) and clinical features depend on presence or absence of this syndrome(Scully et al. 1998). Most of these neoplasms are clinically benign but up to one fifth of those not associated with PJS are clinically malignant. In PJS patients, the tumors are bilateral in two thirds, solid and yellow, whereas they are almost always unilateral in patients without PJS. The histology is similar in both patient types. Extensive hyalinization, micro-follicular granulosa cell areas and well-differentiated Sertoli cell tumor are often present. Ultrastructure often shows Charcot-Bottcher filaments in cells of the annular tubules, consistent with Sertoli cell differentiation. Cytologic samples depict cells with great similarities to granulosa cell tumors including cellular arrangements mimicking Call-Exner bodies.

5. OVARIAN GERM CELL TUMORS
5.1. Dysgerminoma (Ovarian Seminoma)
5.1.1. General

Dysgerminomas are uncommon tumors, which occur mostly in adolescents and young adults. They account for 1-2% of ovarian neoplasms and 3-5% of ovarian malignancies. This neoplasm is the most commonly detected tumor during pregnancy, (the other being serous cystadenoma). They usually present clinically as unilateral masses, right greater than left side, but bilateral in 10-15%. The tumor cells in this lesion are germ cells in an early and sexually indifferent stage of differentiation and are not usually associated with endocrine manifestations. Elevated serum levels of LDH is seen in up to 95% cases at presentation while elevated levels of chorionic gonadotropin (HCG) occurs in approximately 3% of cases. Dysgerminomas are capable of metastatic and local spread and presence of other germ cell components confers a poorer prognosis(Kurman and Norris 1976).

5.1.2. Pathologic Findings

Grossly, dysgerminomas are firm, rubbery, solid masses of variable shape and size. Huge tumor masses (greater than 10 cm) is a poor prognostic feature in these neoplasms. Capsular rupture may lead to adhesions with surrounding structures. Also, hemorrhage and necrosis can lead to secondary cystic change. These areas should be extensively sampled to exclude other neoplastic germ cell elements. The histologic appearance of dysgerminoma is identical to that of testicular seminoma with aggregates of oval to round glycogen-rich tumor cells separated by stroma containing lymphocytes, occasional giant cells and granulomas (Figure 30). The germ cells are large, with discrete cell borders, centrally located nucleus with fine chromatin, 1-2 prominent eosinophilic nucleoli and brisk mitotic activity. While hemorrhage and necrosis are frequently seen, calcifications are unusual and may indicate a burnt out gonadoblastoma. Fine needle aspiration (FNA) shows a dual population of large germ cells and lymphoid cells (Figure 31) and a classic "tigroid" background consisting of lacy PAS-positive cytoplasmic glycogen that dissociates in the smear. Immunohistochemically, placental alkaline phosphatase (PLAP) cytoplasmic positivity is seen in germ cell tumors (Beckstead 1983). Syncytiotrophoblastic giant cells, positive for HCG, are seen in 3 % cases(Zaloudek et al. 1981).

5.1.3. Differential Diagnosis

This tumor is considered with solid yolk sac tumor, embryonal carcinoma, and clear cell carcinoma.

5.2. Yolk Sac (Endodermal Sinus) Tumor
5.2.1. General

This neoplasm is a malignant germ cell tumor thought to arise from undifferentiated embryonal carcinoma by selective differentiation toward yolk sac or vitelline structures(Telium 1959). It is the second most common malignant ovarian germ cell neoplasm after dysgerminoma, accounting for 20% of cases. Majority of patients are under 30 years. There are no endocrine manifestations. Elevated serum AFP level is a useful marker for the primary tumor, metastasis and recurrence.

5.2.2. Pathologic Findings

Yolk sac tumors are almost always large, 3-30 cm, unilateral tumors with predilection for the right ovary. They are usually encapsulated, firm, lobulated with extensive hemorrhage and necrosis and may have adhesions to surrounding structures. The cut surface is mainly solid with frequent gelatinous areas and cystic spaces however; the presence of other neoplastic elements can alter this appearance. Concurrent dermoid cyst is present in 15%. Histologically, a wide spectrum of patterns may be present in the same tumor(Sasaki et al. 1994). Most tumors have, at least focally, a reticular pattern with a loose meshwork of communicating spaces. Schiller-Duval bodies are characteristic, being present in 75% of cases, and consist of a papilla with a central fibrovascular core. Three histologic variants are recognized: (1) polyvesicular vitelline - cysts lined by columnar epithelium, separated by dense stroma (2) hepatoid - large polygonal cells with prominent cell borders, eosinophilic cytoplasm, round central nuclei and prominent nucleoli, growth is in compact masses with intervening thin fibrous bands and hyaline globules are prominent (3) glandular - glands lined by simple or pseudostratified columnar epithelium with intracytoplasmic vacuoles; may show intestinal or endometrioid features. Nonspecific solid and papillary patterns can also occur. A loose stromal component, believed to recapitulate the appearance of extra-embryonic mesenchyme can be striking. FNA biopsy shows papillary and ball-like clusters of large cells with bubbly cytoplasm; Schiller-Duval bodies (seen in cellblock, difficult to appreciate on aspirate smears) and hyaline globules are useful cytomorphologic features.

5.2.3. Differential Diagnosis

Differential diagnosis is extensive and immunohistochemistry can be helpful; AFP, alpha-1-antitrypsin (A1AT), cytokeratin are positive. Mucin is present in yolk sac tumors and adenocarcinomas but is absent in other germ cell tumors.

5.3. Embryonal Carcinoma
5.3.1. General

Embryonal carcinoma is rarer in the ovary than in testis, accounting for 3% of germ cell tumors. It occurs in young patients (4-28 years with a median of 12 years) and about half have endocrine manifestations. Serum HCG and AFP are often elevated in these patients(Kurman and Norris 1976).

5.3.2. Pathologic Findings

These tumors are large and unilateral, have a mean diameter of 17 cm and grossly, a smooth external surface and variegated cut surface is observed. Histologically, large primitive cells with amphophilic/clear cytoplasm, well-defined cell membranes and nuclei with irregular contours, prominent nucleoli, and numerous mitosis are present. The cells resemble those of the embryonic germ disc and grow in solid, papillary and glandular patterns. Eosinophilic hyaline globules and syncytiotrophoblastic giant cells are seen and single cell necrosis is frequently present. FNA biopsy specimens are cellular with poorly differentiated epithelial-like tumor cells in sheets or papillary groupings. Cells resemble those described above and necrosis is commonly seen. Immunohistochemical stains are positive for cytokeratin, PLAP, CD30 and negative for epithelial membrane antigen (EMA). AFP positivity is present in 30% of cases.

5.3.3. Differential Diagnosis

Differential diagnosis includes dysgerminoma (keratin negative) and yolk sac tumors as well as juvenile granulosa cell tumor and rarely poorly differentiated adenocarcinoma (PLAP negative) of surface epithelial type.

5.4. Polyembryoma
5.4.1. General

Polyembryomas are exceedingly rare tumors, with less than 10 cases reported in the last 40 years(Simard 1957). Elevated serum HCG or AFP have been described in these tumors.

5.4.2. Pathologic Findings

These neoplasms are bulky with cut surface being spongy or multicystic, red-brown and hemorrhagic. Exclusive or preponderant content of embryoid bodies that resemble normal early embryos in various stages of development containing germ discks, amniotic cavities, yolk sacs, chorionic elements, and extra-embryonic mesenchyme are encountered. Teratomatous elements, predominantly endodermal, are usually present. The embryoid bodies are often contiguous with intestinal glands, adult hepatic embryonal tissue or yolk sac differentiation. The latter elements if present will be immunoreactive for AFP and / or HCG.

5.4.3. Differential Diagnosis

This entity is considered with other tumors of germ cell origin.

5.5. Choriocarcinoma
5.5.1. General

Pure, non-gestational choriocarcinoma accounts for less than 1% of primitive germ cell tumors of the ovary. It is seen more commonly as a component of mixed germ cell tumor. Gestational choriocarcinomas in the

202

ovary are virtually always metastatic from the uterus or rarely from the fallopian tube. Ovarian choriocarcinomas typically occur in children and young adults. Serum HCG levels are elevated in these patients, leading to precocious puberty.

5.5.2. Pathologic Findings

Pure choriocarcinomas are unilateral, solid, hemorrhagic and friable. They are composed of an intimate admixture of either cytotrophoblast, intermediate trophoblast or both and syncytiotrophoblast. Uninucleate trophoblastic cells with scanty or abundant clear cytoplasm represent either cytotrophoblast (cytokeratin positive) or intermediate trophoblast (cytokeratin, HPL and inhibin positive)(Shih and Kurman 1999). These are seen associated with multinucleated syncytiotrophoblastic giant cells (positive for cytokeratin, HCG, HPL and inhibin and the cells are present in plexiform pattern, often adjacent to vascular sinusoids, which are the cause of massive hemorrhage seen in these tumors. Vascular invasion can be prominent. FNA biopsy reflects this characteristic biphasic pattern of trophoblasts. Both elements must be present to make the diagnosis of choriocarcinoma(Oliva et al. 1993).

5.5.3. Differential Diagnosis

This includes other germ cell tumors in which syncytiotrophoblasts are found such as embryonal carcinoma and dysgerminoma. Yolk sac tumor and poorly differentiated carcinoma should also be considered.

5.6. Teratoma
5.6.1. General

Teratomas are germ cell tumors composed of a variety of tissues usually representing two or three embryonic layers (endoderm, mesoderm, ectoderm) but can occasionally be monodermal. If the neoplastic tissue is uniformly mature, the teratoma is termed mature, and is most often a dermoid cyst. If any fetal or immature tissue is present, a diagnosis of immature teratoma (about 3% of cases) is given. The only exception is when minute foci of immature tissue are identified in a dermoid cyst. These cases behave benignly and are not given this designation. About 65% of teratomas are derived from a single germ cell after the first meiotic division. Almost all dermoid cysts are of post-meiotic origin; they are the most common ovarian tumor, accounting for 30- 45% of all ovarian tumors and 35- 58% of the benign tumors. Over 80% occur during the reproductive years.

5.6.2. Pathologic Findings

Immature teratomas are large (median diameter 18 cm) with a cut surface that is predominantly solid with small cysts containing mucus, blood or hair. The solid areas are usually neural tissue. The contralateral ovary shows a dermoid cyst or other benign tumor in 10% of cases. Immature teratomas are graded on the basis of the amount of immature tissue that they contain and this is usually dependent on neuroectodermal tissue(Nogales et al.1976; O'Connor and Norris 1994). The components of these tumors varies from rare immature foci to predominant largely neuroectodermal tissue with rosettes and tubules. Other elements seen include cartilage, skeletal muscle, and hepatic tissue. A dermoid cyst is a mature teratoma composed predominantly of a cyst lined wholly or partially by epithelium resembling the epidermis with its appendages. Dermoid cysts are ovoid tumors, less than 15 cm in diameter, bilateral in 15% of cases, occasionally multiple in one ovary and contain brown gummous material. Teeth or hair may be seen. Secondary malignant tumors of adult types arise from a constituent of dermoid cysts in 1-2% of cases. A mature solid teratoma is predominantly solid and composed exclusively of mature elements. In this entity, mature tissues representing all three germ cell layers, fetal and adult, are present (Figure 32). Mesodermal, endodermal and ectodermal mature components are present in most cases(Commerci et al. 1994). Ectodermal components usually predominate and include neuroectodermal elements, glia and peripheral nervous tissue. Mesodermal derivatives seen include smooth muscle, bone, teeth, cartilage, and fat. Common endodermal components are respiratory and gastrointestinal epithelia and thyroid tissue. Less commonly seen are retina, pancreas, adrenal, thymus, kidney, lung, breast and prostate. The tissues are often arranged in an "organoid" fashion. A foreign body giant cell reaction can be seen if there is rupture of the cyst. Rarely, mature and immature teratomas are associated with peritoneal implants composed exclusively or mainly of mature glial tissue (grade 0) (Gliomatosis peritonii). Extensive sampling to rule out higher grade implants is necessary.

Monodermal teratomas include struma ovarii, strumal carcinoid, carcinoid, goblet cell carcinoid, neuroectodermal tumors and sebaceous tumors. Focal thyroid tissue is found in up to 20% of dermoids. In struma ovarii however, thyroid is the predominant or sole component. They can be solid or cystic, microscopically resemble normal or rarely neoplastic thyroid tissue. Thyroglobulin positivity confirms the diagnosis of thyroid tissue. Primary carcinoids of the ovary are associated with other teratomatous components, such as dermoid, struma, mature teratoma or cystic mucinous tumor, in 85-90% of cases. The tumor is usually a solid firm nodule that contains discrete masses of "neuroendocrine cells" that show neuron specific enolase (NSE), serotonin and chromogranin immunohistochemically. Rare monodermal teratomas include neuroectodermal, sebaceous tumors and retinal anlage tumors arising in pituitary tissue in dermoid cysts. FNA biopsy of teratomas needs appropriate sampling to ensure representation of all components. Calcification is common and the cysts often contain keratinous debris. Sampling of epithelial, mesenchymal and endodermal components is more likely from the solid areas (Figure 33).

5.6.3. Differential Diagnosis

Differential diagnosis of immature teratomas includes heterologous malignant mesodermal mixed tumors and primitive neuroectodermal tumors. The neuroectodermal components are positive for one or more neural markers such as glial fibrillary acid protein (GFAP), neuron specific enolase (NSE), S-100 protein, myelin basic protein (MBP). In FNA specimens, the differential diagnosis includes squamous contamination due to transvaginal aspiration, normal colorectal mucosa, transitional epithelium, soft tissue and mesothelium that maybe sampled incidentally.

5.7. Mixed Malignant Germ Cell Tumors
5.7.1. General

These are tumors that contain a mixture of two or more types of germ cell neoplasia (dysgerminoma, yolk sac tumor, immature teratoma, embryonal carcinoma, choriocarcinoma, polyembryoma) and account for 8 - 10% of malignant germ cell tumors of the ovary.

5.7.2. Pathologic Findings

The microscopic findings reflect the components present within the tumor. Each component is listed in the diagnosis in decreasing order of quantity. Prognosis has been shown to correlate with the nature and quantity of the malignant components. Extensive sampling of grossly or radiologically different areas is essential to ensure representation of different components in biopsies and aspirate material respectively. A highly malignant component has to account for more than one third of the tumor to adversely affect prognosis(Kurman and Norris 1976).

REFERENCES

Austin, R.M. and H.J. Norris, Brenner tumor and transitional cell carcinoma of the ovary: a comparson. Int. J. Gynecol Pathol, 1987; 6: 29-39.

Arey, L.B., The origin and form of the Brenner tumor. Am J Obstet Gynecol, 1961; 81: 743-51.

Beckstead, J.H., Alkaline phosphatase histochemistry in human germ cell neoplasia. Am J Surg Pathol, 1983; 7:341-349.

Bell, D.A. and R.E. Scully, Atypical and borderline endometrioid adenofibromas of the ovary. A report of 27 cases. Am J Surg Pathol, 1985; 9: 205-14.

Berchuck, A., et al., Managing hereditary ovarian cancer risk. [Review]. Cancer 1999; 86(11): 2517-24.

Castilla, L.H., F.J. Couch, and M.R.e.a. Erdos, Mutations in the BRCA1 gene in families with early-onset breast and ovarian cancer. Nature Genet. 1994; 2:128-131.

Clement, P.B., Blaustein's pathology of the female genital tract. 4th edition ed. NY: Springer-Verlag, 1996.

Commerci, J.T., et al., mature cystic teratoma: a clinocpathologic evaluation of 517 cases and review of the literature. Obstet Gynecol, 1994; 84: 22-28

DePriest, P.D., E.R. Banks, and D.E.e.a. Powell, Endometrioid carcinoma of the ovary and endometriosis: the association in postmenopausal women. Gynecol Oncol, 1992; 47: 71-5.

Easton, D.F., D. Ford, and D.T. Bishop, Breast cancer linkage consortium. Breast and ovarian cancer incidence in BRCA-1 mutation carriers. Am J Hum Genet., 1995; 56: 265-271.

Erlich, C.E. and L. Roth, The Brenner tumor. A clinicopathologic study of 57 cases. Cancer, 1971; 27: 332-42.

Ford, D., et al., Breast cancer linkage consortium. Risk of cancer in BRCA1-mutation carriers. Lancet 1994; 343: 692-695.

Frank, T.S. and A.M. Braverman, The pros and cons of genetic testing for breast and ovarian cancer risk (review). International Journal of Fertility and Reproductive Medicine 1999; 44(3):139-45.

Fukunnaga, M., et al., Ovarian atypical endometriosis: its close association with malignant epithelial tumors. Histopathology, 1997; 30:249-55.

Futreal, P.A., Q.Y. Liu, and D.E.A. Shattuck-Eldens, BRCA1 mutations in primary breast and ovarian carcinomas. Science 1994; 266:120-122.

Gompel, E. and S.G. Silverberg, Chapter 6, in Pathology in Gyneclogy and Obstetrics. J.B. Lippincott Company, 1994.

Hall, J.M., M.K. Lee, and B.e.a. Newman, Linkage of early-onset familial breast cancer to chromosome 17q21. Science 1992:1684-1689.

Hart, W.R. and H.J. Norris, Borderline and malignant mucinous tumors of the ovary. Histologic riteria and clinical behavior. Cancer, 1973; 31(5): 1031-45.

Hendrickson, M.R., Surface epithelial neoplasms of the ovary, in State of the Art Reviews. Pathology. Hanley and Belfus: Philadelphia, 1992.

Katsube, Y., J.W. Berg, and S.G. Silverberg, Epidemiologic pathology of ovarian tumors: a histopathologic review of primary ovarian neoplasms diagnosed in the Denver standard metropolital statistical area, 1 July - 31 December 1969 and 1 July 31 December 1979. Int J Gynecol Pathol, 1982; 1: 3-16.

Kline RC et al., Endometrioid carcinoma of the ovary: retrospective review of 145 cases. Gynecol Oncol, 1990; 39: 337-46.

Koonings, P.P., et al., Relative frequency of primary ovarian neoplasms: a 10 year review. Obstet Gynecol, 1989; 74: 921-926.

Kurman, R.J. and H.J. Norris, Malignant mixed germ cell tumors of the ovary. A clinical and pathologic analysis of 30 cases. Obstet Gynecol, 1976; 48: 579-589.

Kurman, R.J. and H.J. Norris, Embryonal carcinoma of the ovary: a clinicopathologic entity distinct from endodermal sinus tumor resembling embryonal carcinoma of the adult testis. Cancer, 1976; 38: 2420-2433.

Lee, W.Y., et al., Immuno-localization of BRCA1 protein in normal breast tissue and sporadic breast invasive ductal carcinomas: a correlation with other biological parameters. Histopathology, 1999; 34:106-112.

Mostoufizadeh, M. and R.E. Sculley, Malignant tumors arising in endometriosis. Clin Obstet Gynecol, 1980; 23: 951-63.

McKay D.G., et al., The adult human ovary, a histochemical study. Obstet & Gynecol, 1961; 18: 13-39.

Nogales, F.F., et al., Immature teratoma of the ovary with neural component (solid teratoma): A clinicopathologic study of 20 cases. Hum Pathol, 1976; 7: 625-642.

O'Connor, D.M. and H.J. Norris, The influence of grade on the outcome of stage 1 ovarian immature (malignant) teratomas and the reproducibility of grading. Int J Gynecol Pathol, 1994;

Oliva, E., et al., Ovarian carcinomas with choriocarcinomatous differentiation. Cancer, 1993; 72:2441-2446.

Peterson, F. Annual report of treatment in gynecological cancer. in International Federation of Gynecology and Obstetrics.Stockholm, 1999.

Scully, E.R., R.H. Young, and P.B. Clement, Tumors of the ovary, maldeveloped gonads, fallopian tubes and broad ligament. third series ed. Atlas of tumor pathology. Vol. 23. 1998: AFIP.

Shih, I. and R. Kurman, Immunohistochemical localization of inhibin alpha in the placenta and gestational trophoblastic lesions. Intl J of Gyecol path, 1999; 18(2):144-150.

Simard, L., Polyembryonic embryoma of the ovary of pathogenic origin. Cancer, 1957; 10: 215-223.

Reagan, JW., Ceroid pigment in the human ovary. Am. J Obstet Gynecol, 1950; 59: 433-436.

Ruffner, H. and I.M. Verma, BRCA1 is a cell cycle-regulated nuclear phosphoprotein. Natl Acad Sci. 1997; 94:7138-7143.

Russell, P. and A. Farnsworth, Surgical pathology of the ovaries. second edition ed. United kingdom: Churchhill Livingstone, 1997.

Russell, P., Blaustein's pathology of the female genital tract. 4th edition ed. NY: Springer-Verlag, 1996.

Russell, P., The pathological assessment of ovarian neoplasms: I: Introduction to the common 'epithelial' tumors and analysis of benign 'epithelial' tumors. Pathology, 1979. 11: 493-532.

Sasaki, H., M. Furusato, and S.e.a. Teshima, Prognostic significance of histopathologic subtypes in stage I pure yolk sac tumor of the ovary. British J Cancer, 1994; 69:529-536.

Shen, D. and J.V. Vadgama, BRCA1 amd BRCA2 gene mutation analysis: visit to the breast cancer information core (BIC). Oncology Research, 1997; 11(2): 63-9.

Smith, T.E., Meeting to sort out BRCA1 confusion. Science 1996. 272: p. 799.

Snyder, R.R., H.J. Norris, and F. Tavassoli, Endometrioid proliferative and low malignant potential tumors of the ovary. A clinicopathologic study of 46 cases. Am J Surg Pathol, 1988; 12: 661-71.

Telium, G., Endodermal sinus tumors of the ovary and testis. comparative morphogenesis of the so-called mesonephroma ovarii (Schiller) and extraembryonic (yolk sac-allantoic) structures of rat placenta. Cancer, 1959; 12:1092-1105.

Wang, H., et al., BRCA1 proteins are transported to the nucleus in the absence of serum and splice variants BRCA1a, BRCA1b are tyrosine phosphoproteins that associate with E2F, cyclins and cyclin dependent kinases. Oncogene 1997; 15:143-157.

Wojcik, E.M. and B. Naylor, "Collagen balls" in peritoneal washings. Acta cytologica, 1992; 46:466-470.

Zaloudek, C.J., F.A. Tavassoli, and H.J. Norris, Dysgerminoma with syncytiotrophoblastic cells. A histologically and clinically distinctive subtype of dysgerminoma. Am J Surg Pathol, 1981; 5: 361-367.

Zhang, H.T., X. Zhang, and H.Z.e.a. Zhao, Relationship of p215BRCA1 to tyrosine kinase signaling pathways and the and the cell cycle in normal and transfomed cells. Oncogene 1997; 14:2863-2869.

FIGURE LEGENDS

Fig. 1. Scrape from the surface of normal ovary, depicting numerous small groups and isolated cells with rounded symmetrical nuclei. (Papanicolaou)

Fig. 2. Scrape from the ovarian surface of a patient with BRAC I and II chromosomal abnormalities, showing large cluster of hyperplastic cells and papillary fronds. (Papanicolaou)

Fig. 3. High power of cells from the case shown in Fig. 2. The cells are larger compare to Fig 1 depicting some irregular nuclear outlines. (Papanicolaou)

Fig. 4. Histological section of the ovarian surface from a patient with BRAC I and II chromosomal abnormalities. Deep invaginations and papillary structures lined by columnar epithelium are demonstrated. (H and E)

Fig. 5. Follicle cells, some surrounding a space occupied by homogeneous material characteristic of Call-Exner body. (Papanicolaou)

Fig. 6. Cluster of luteinized cells with abundant cytoplasm intermixed with small follicle cells. (Giemsa)

Fig. 7. Histological section of ovary, showing several germinal cystic structures lined by columnar epithelium. (H and E)

Fig. 8. Histological section of the ovarian surface and a collagen structure lined by columnar cells. (H and E)

Fig. 9. Collagen ball in fluid surrounded by epithelial cells detached from ovarian surface. (Papanicolaou) Same case as Fig 8.

Fig. 10. Cells from a follicle cyst showing limited cytoplasm granular chromatin and multiple small nucleoli. (Papanicolaou)

Fig. 11. Histological section of a papillary serous cystadenoma.(H and E)

Fig. 12. Histological section of borderline serous tumor, depicting papillary fronds lined by multilayered columnar epithelium. (H and E)

Fig. 13. Histological section of a poorly differentiated solid serous adenocarcinoma.(H and E)

Fig. 14. Monolayer of cells from a serous cystadenoma. The cells are uniform and the cytoplasm limited and the polarity maintained. (Papanicolaou)

Fig. 15. Cells from well-differentiated serous adenocarcinoma surrounding Psammoma bodies. (Papanicolaou)

Fig. 16. Histological section of a borderline serous tumor. Observe an area of greater cellular atypicality attached to the stroma. (H and E)

Fig. 17. Papillary fronds of small cells characteristic of borderline serous tumor. (Papanicolaou)

Fig. 18. Large monolayer of cells from a borderline serous tumor. The cells are larger than their benign counterpart (Fig 14) with less cytoplasm giving a crowded pattern. (Papanicolaou)

Fig. 19. Cluster of adenocarcinoma by cytology standards from a tumor histologically diagnosed as serous borderline tumor (same as shown in Fig. 16) showing marked cellular atypical features. (Papanicolaou)

Fig. 20. Cytology sample of a poorly differentiated serous carcinoma. The cellular morphology has deviated from recognizable classical serous neoplasm. (Papanicolaou)

Fig. 21. Clusters of cells with delicate cytoplasm depicting exaggerated distention of cytoplasm due to mucin content. (H and E)

Fig. 22. Histological section of mucinous cystadenoma. (H and E)

Fig. 23. Microscopic features of a borderline mucinous cystadenocarcinoma composed of tall columnar cells. (H and E)

208

Fig. 24. *Borderline mucinous adenocarcinoma, showing tall columnar cells with the cytoplasm distended by mucinous secretion. (Papanicolaou)*

Fig. 25. *Histological section of a clear cell adenocarcinoma with clear and hobnail cell component. (H and E)*

Fig. 26. *Cytology sample depicting malignant cells with clear abundant cytoplasm. (Papanicolaou)*

Fig. 27. *Histological section of granulosa cell tumor. (H and E)*

Fig. 28. *Isolated cells from a granulosa cell tumor depicting nuclear infolds. (Papanicolaou)*

Fig. 29. *Call – Exner body aspirated from a metastatic granulosa cell tumor. (Papanicolaou)*

Fig. 30. *Histological section of disgerminoma. (H and E)*

Fig. 31. *Malignant cells associated with lymphocytes from an ovarian disgerminoma. (Papanicolaou)*

Fig. 32. *Histological section of mature teratoma is depicting a variety of benign tissues. (H and E)*

Fig. 33. *Aspirate showing bronchial ciliated cells from a teratoma (Giemsa)*

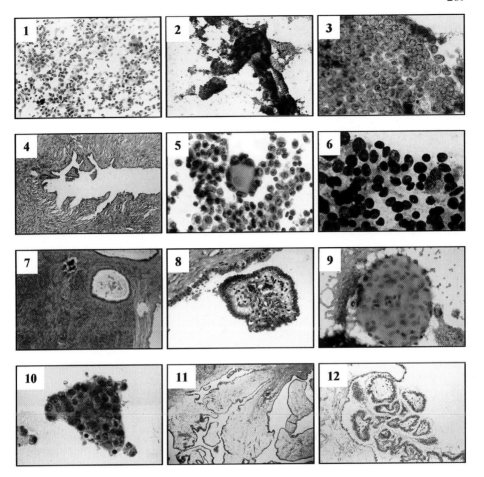

210

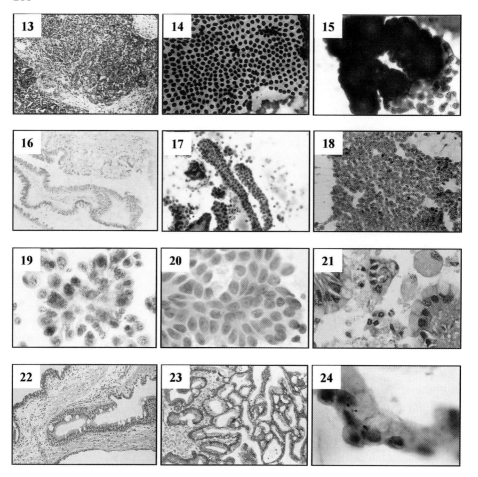

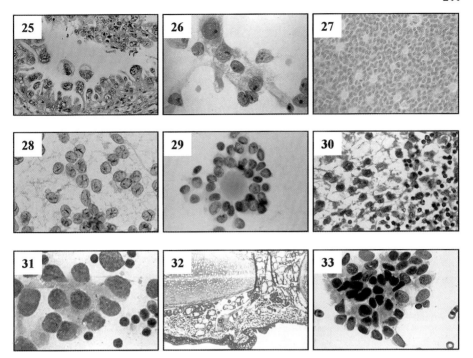

Chapter 9

TELOMERASE AND MALIGNANT TRANSFORMATION

Jiamei Yu and Louis Dubeau
Department of Pathology, Keck School of Medicine of the University of Southern California, USC/Norris Comprehensive Cancer Center, Los Angeles, California 90033

Recent progress in our understanding of the role of telomeres and telomerase in cell proliferation, malignant transformation, and genomic stability has opened new possibilities for cancer diagnosis, detection, and treatment. Novel approaches based on this knowledge are being investigated in different laboratories and are likely to have a significant impact on cancer management protocols in the future. This chapter gives an overview of our current knowledge of the function of telomeres and of the mechanisms responsible for their maintenance, followed by comments on potential applications of this knowledge in clinical medicine.

1. HISTORICAL PERSPECTIVES
1.1. Structure and Function of Telomeres

The term telomere was coined by early cytogeneticists to designate the tip of chromosomes. The first indications that telomeres are important for maintaining chromosomal integrity came in the 1930s and 1940s, when Muller and McClintock demonstrated that telomeric regions were essential for protecting chromosomes from degradation and recombination. In the 1950s and 1960s, the elucidation of the anti-parallel nature of the DNA double helix and the realization that DNA polymerase enzymes cannot initiate DNA replication from the very end of linear DNA molecules led to the speculation that telomeres must have unique structural features to allow overcoming of this 'end replication problem'. Although these observations underscored the importance of telomeres on chromosomal integrity and replication, it is only in 1978 that the first telomeric DNA sequence was reported Blackburn and Gall in *Tetrahymena*. Their finding that telomeres in this organism consisted of tandem repeats of short GC-rich DNA sequences was subsequently confirmed in several other species including humans (*1*). This basic structure of telomeres is now thought to be present in nearly all eukaryotes, although some organisms like drosophila contain telomeric DNA sequences that are significantly different (2).

The above work therefore led to the conclusion that in most eukaryotes, telomeres are made up of tandem repeats of a 5-8 nucleotide-long DNA sequence that is species-specific. In human telomeres, the sequence TTAGGG is repeated up to 2500 times. At least some structural features of telomeric DNA are conserved among species because Shampay *et al.* (3) showed that replacement of the telomeres of Saccharomyces by those of Tetrahymena was compatible with survival. When these authors characterized the telomeres of the Saccharomyces organisms several generations after the telomeric substitutions had been made, they found that Saccharomyces-specific telomeric sequences had been added onto the end of the *Tetrahymena*-specific sequence. Thus, *Saccharomyces* can use telomeric DNA from *Tetrahymena*, a distant relative, as substrate for the addition of its own telomeric sequence.

1.2. Discovery of Telomerase

This experiment led to the hypothesis that cells from a given organism must have an enzyme capable adding telomeric DNA sequences specific for that organism onto their chromosomal ends. Such enzymatic activity was first demonstrated by Greider and Blackburn (4) in extracts from *Tetrahymena*. The enzyme responsible for this activity is now being referred to as telomerase. These authors subsequently showed that the telomerase activity could be abolished by treatment of the *Tetrahymena* extracts with RNase (4). They isolated a 159 nucleotide RNA fragment that co-purified with telomerase activity and made the observation that a sequence complementary to the repeated telomeric unit of *Tetrahymena* was enclosed within the RNA fragment (4). These studies, as well as additional groundbreaking experiments performed by the same authors (5), provided strong support for the idea that telomerase is a riboprotein whose RNA component anchors onto chromosomal ends by hybridizing to complementary DNA sequence and serves as template for telomere sequence elongation. Elegant experiments subsequently showed that addition of the telomeric sequence to chromosomal fragments or any linear DNA was sufficient to generate functional telomeres (see Greider (6) for review).

1.3. Importance of Telomeres and Telomerase in Cancer

Telomeres are thought to act as a mitotic clock ensuring that most somatic cells are only able to undergo a limited number of division cycles during their lifespan. This is based on the notion that some telomeric sequences are lost during each cell division because of the 'end replication problem' mentioned above. Thus, each time a cell divides, its telomeres become shorter. Eventually, the telomeres will become too short to support further cell divisions. This hypothesis was first proposed by Olovnikov (7), who suggested that the gradual shortening of telomeres could be responsible for the finite lifespan on normal cells cultured *in vitro*. This insightful idea was later revisited by Harley *et al.* (8) and was strongly supported by Allsopp *et al.* (9), who determined that the *in vitro* longevity of normal diploid fibroblasts was directly proportional to telomere length.

Telomerase can maintain the length of telomeres in rapidly dividing cells and should therefore allow unlimited numbers of cell division. However, Kim *et al.* (10) showed that this enzyme was only expressed during embryological development in normal somatic cells. The only normal adult cells in which telomerase activity was observed by these authors using their novel Telomerase Repeat Amplification Protocol (TRAP) assay (10) were testicular germ cells. In contrast, cancer cells of various origins expressed high levels of the enzyme (10). This readily explained why cancer cells are able to sustain continuous growth. This also implied that activation of telomerase is a necessary step for malignant transformation (11). This led to the attractive hypothesis that interfering with telomerase expression either with drugs or by gene therapy could represent an effective mean of treating all cancers with little or no consequences on the patient's normal tissues.

2. COMPONENTS OF THE TELOMERE ELONGATION MACHINERY IN VERTEBRATES
2.1. Telomerase Enzyme

Three components of the human telomerase appear to be necessary for enzymatic activity. They are: (1) the RNA component (hTERC), which acts as an intrinsic template for telomeric repeat synthesis, (2) the telomerase catalytic subunit, hTERT, which shares several motifs with other known reverse transcriptases (12), and (3) a telomerase-associated protein called TEP1 that shares similarities with the Tetrahymena telomerase protein P^{80} (13,14).

2.1.1. The Telomerase RNA Component

The human telomerase RNA component is 560 nucleotides long and shares very little homology with that of lower eukaryotes. As is true in *Tetrahymena*, the human RNA component contains a region complementary to 1.5 repeat of the TTAGGG telomeric unit sequence. This RNA is thought to act as template during the telomere elongation reaction according to the mechanism illustrated in Fig. 1.

216

Telomeric end of genomic DNA

Newly synthesized telomeric sequence

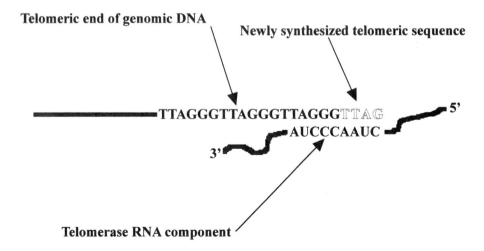

Figure 1. Role of the telomerase RNA component in telomere elongation. The 3' end of the telomerase RNA component hybridizes to complementary sequences at the 5' end of a telomere. The RNA component is then used as template for telomere chain elongation while the telomeric end acts as primer. In a subsequent step, the telomerase RNA component translocates to the 5' end of the newly synthesized telomeric end and the process is repeated.

The secondary structure of the telomerase RNA is important for telomerase assembly. In protozoa, disruption of a conserved pseudoknot structure prevents assembly (15). In vertebrates, four highly conserved structural domains are also probably important for assembly (16). Several proteins that bind to specific regions of the telomerase RNA molecule have been described that probably facilitate assembly into an active telomerase enzyme (17-19).

2.1.2. Telomerase Catalytic Subunit

The catalytic protein component of human telomerase was identified on the basis of its homology with yeast telomerases (13,14). The gene coding for this subunit has 16 exons, which encompass over 37 kb (20). Control of hTERT expression at the mRNA level appears to be the main regulatory determinant of telomerase enzymatic activity (21). At least 4 different splice forms of hTERT are expressed in various cells (22). In addition to the full-length hTERT transcript, which is 457 base pairs, there is a 421-base-pair transcript that lacks exon alpha, a 275-base-pair transcript that lacks exon beta, and a 239-base pair transcript that lacks both of these exons. Only the full length, 457-base pair transcript codes for an active telomerase. Exon alpha encompasses a conserved sequence motif critical for reverse transcriptase function. The product of the 275-base pair transcript that lacks exon beta is a protein that is truncated precisely at the end of the reverse transcriptase domain. Interestingly, exon beta contains a P-loop motif also found in a large number of protein families including a number of kinases, bacterial dnaA, recA, recF, mutS and ATP-binding helicases. The functional importance of this motif in the telomerase catalytic subunit is not clear. The splice variants are expressed in telomerase-negative cells lacking the full-length transcript. They show great variability in their relative expression levels in various normal and cancerous tissues or cell lines (22). Although this distribution suggests that these variants may have important cellular functions, their exact role(s) is/are not known.

2.1.3. Telomerase Associated Protein (TEP1)

The function of this protein is still unclear in humans. It was isolated based on its sequence similarity with telomerase P80 subunit of *Tetrahymena*. It has a potential ATP/GTP motif and WD repeats. The N-terminus of TEP1 is sufficient for binding of human telomerase RNA (13).

2.2. Structure of Telomeres

The first indication that telomeres may have a unique secondary structure came from Tommerup et al. (23), who reported that the chromatin structure of short human telomeres was unusual because it showed diffuse micrococcal nuclease patterns. This was not seen with longer mouse or human telomeres. The authors concluded that mammalian telomeres have a bipartite structure characterized by an unusual chromatin near their terminus (23). Subsequently, Griffith et al. (24) showed that the abnormal micrococcal nuclease pattern was due to a peculiar secondary structure involving telomerase termini. These authors showed that rather than ending as linear DNA as was previously thought, mammalian telomeres form large terminal loops where the potentially vulnerable single-stranded terminus forms hydrogen bonds with sequences several kilobases internal to the terminus. The resulting loop, called T-loop, protects the terminus. This also results in a small D-loop at the point of insertion of the G strand (24). The secondary structure of the terminal portion of telomeric DNA in vertebrates is illustrated diagrammatically in Fig. 2.

The presence of T-loops distinguishes a telomeric terminus from a DNA break and thus provides an explanation for the fact that telomeric ends are protected against degradation by nucleases. It is likely that a minimal telomeric length is required for T-loop formation, providing a potential explanation for the fact that chromosomes lose their ability to divide and become at risk of undergoing fusion well before all telomeric sequence is lost. It is not clear how the D-loop is unwound in order to provide access of the 3' terminus to the telomerase. Whether or not specific helicases are involved is not clear. The T-loop structure must be

218

dynamic and reform after each round of DNA synthesis. The unique structure of the T-loop might allow easy recognition by telomerase as the appropriate substrate for elongation.

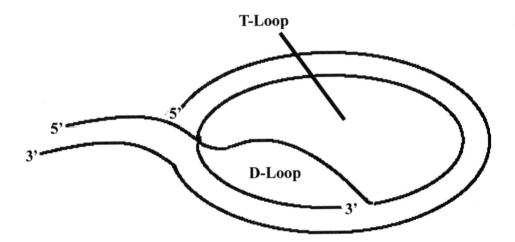

Fig. 2. *Telomeric secondary structure.*

2.3. Telomere-Associated Proteins

Telomeres are part of a nucleoprotein complex associated with the nuclear matrix. Four genes coding for telomere-associated proteins are currently known. The TERF1 gene encodes TRF1 and PIN2 (*25,26*). TRF1 is a negative regulator of telomere elongation. It has homology to the DNA-binding domain of the Myb family of transcription factors and may be a functional homologue of a yeast protein called Rap1 (*27,28*). It binds to telomeric DNA as a dimer. It has been suggested that TRF1-dependent changes in the conformation of telomeres are involved in the regulation of telomere length (*29*). TRF1 also promotes parallel pairing of telomeric DNA (*30*). A second gene, TIN2, binds to TRF1, localizes to telomeres, and is essential for the proper mediation of TRF1-dependent regulation of telomeric length (*31*). A third gene, TERF2, encodes a gene that is structurally similar to TRF1 called TRF2. This gene is important for the formation of the T-loops and binds to the D-loop region (*24*). Inhibition of TRF2 results in deprotection of chromosome ends, manifested by loss of the telomeric 3' overhang, activation of P63, and covalent fusion of chromosome ends (*32*). A fourth gene encodes tankyrase, a human poly - ADP ribosylase that interacts with TRF1 (*33,34*).

3. TELOMERASE AND CANCER DEVELOPMENT

The development of a sensitive assay for the telomerase enzyme by Kim *et al.* (*10*) allowed these authors to examine the spectrum of expression of this enzyme in various normal and cancerous tissues or cell lines. This work provided strong support for the notion that telomerase is widely expressed among cancers of practically all sources while it is not expressed in most normal somatic cells. As explained earlier, this apparent specificity of telomerase expression for the cancer phenotype gave rise to the attractive hypothesis that therapeutic protocols aimed at interfering with telomerase function may provide an effective strategy for the treatment of nearly all cancers. It also suggested that treatments based on this approach may have minimal or no consequences on the patients' normal tissues.

3.1. Anti-Telomerase Strategies in Cancer Therapy: Silver Bullet or Fool's Gold?

The specificity of telomerase expression for the cancer phenotype is not absolute. For example, this enzyme activity is detectable in activated lymphocytes (*35,36*), in normal ovaries (*37*), fallopian tubes (*37*), and endometrium (*38,39*), as well as in the gastro-intestinal tract (*40*). In addition, low levels of activity may be maintained in various stem cells (*41*). Conversely, although this enzyme is expressed in nearly all cancers, some cancers do not express it and it is now clear that alternate methods of telomere length maintenance are available in the absence of telomerase activity in yeast (*42*) as well as in humans (*43*). Finally, the merit of therapeutic approaches based on telomerase inhibition in cancer management can be seriously questioned in light of the results of Rudolph *et al.* (*44*), who used gene knock out technologies to create mice that are totally deficient for telomerase. These mice were able to develop and reproduce normally, at least for a few generations, and even developed malignancies (*44*). This raises the possibility that although inhibition of telomerase activity may indeed lead to the death of cancer cells eventually, these cells may be able to survive long enough to cause patient's death before any consequence of telomerase inhibition becomes manifested.

Should anticancer strategies based on interference with telomerase activity be discouraged in light of these observations? Such strategies should be ineffective against tumors relying on alternate mechanisms of telomere elongation or against tumors with long telomeres. However, most human cancer cells do express telomerase and have relatively short telomeres. Anti-telomerase strategies may prove very effective against such lesions. Inhibition of telomerase in cultured human cancer cell lines leads to cell death (*45,46*). The findings by Rudolph *et al.* (*44*) that total absence of telomerase activity has no immediate deleterious effect in mice can be used as an argument in favor anti-telomerase therapy, as they support the notion that therapeutic protocols based on this approach may have little or no toxicity effect in cancer patients. Given the small therapeutic window of most current anti-cancer agents, the prospects of a therapeutic approach with minimal side effects is appealing. Drugs with known anti-telomerase activity include reverse transcriptase inhibitors and deoxyguanosine analogs *(47,48)*.

3.2. Determinants of Telomerase Expression in Cancer Cells

Knowledge of the molecular genetic determinants of telomerase activation in cancer cells and of the signaling pathways involved in regulation of telomerase should facilitate our ability to modulate telomerase activity in therapeutic protocols. In addition, this knowledge is important for the development of cancer detection protocols based on the presence or absence of telomerase activity (see next section).

The current evidence suggests that the telomerase catalytic subunit is the main target for regulation of telomerase activity *(49)*. Studies of the promoter region of the gene for this subunit revealed that it contains binding sites for c-*myc* as well as for several transcription factors *(50-53)*. Several authors have also reported that c-*myc* expression can activate telomerase *(54-56)*, perhaps via cooperation with the Sp1 transcription factor *(57)*. The transcription factor Mad, in contrast, may act as a negative regulator of hTERT expression *(58)*. Other structural features of the promoter region of the hTERT gene include several potential DNA methylation sites, raising the possibility that this represents an important mechanism of regulation of this gene *(52,59)*. This is further supported by the fact that treatment with the methylation inhibitor 5-azacytidine led to induction of hTERT expression in 2 cell lines *(59,60)*.

Details of the signaling pathways important for regulation of telomerase expression are still unknown. Steroid hormone receptors may play a role *(61,62)*. In addition, there is evidence that the mitogen-activated protein kinase pathway is involved *(63)*. Negative cell cycle regulators such as p16INK4A and p53 can down-regulate hTERT expression *(64-66)*. This effect of p53 appears to be independent of its effect on cell growth *(65)*. Introduction of an intact chromosome 3 into a human breast carcinoma cell line led to down-regulation of telomerase activity while introduction of chromosomes 8, 12, or 20 had no measurable effect on expression of such activity *(67)*. Further mapping studies indicated that this effect was dependent on 2 separate regions of chromosome 3p *(67)*. Interestingly, this chromosomal region is often affected by losses of heterozygosity in human ovarian carcinomas *(68,69)*.

The hTERT protein is a phosphoprotein, raising the possibility of another level of regulation of this gene involving protein phosphorylation. In that regard, Li *et al.* *(70)* reported that protein kinaseC alpha mediates phosphorylation of hTERT as well as of TEP1. More recently, Kang *et al.* *(71)* reported that the Akt kinase enhances telomerase activity through phosphorylation of the hTERT protein. It is clear, based on this brief review, that telomerase expression is regulated at multiple levels using a variety of different mechanisms. Our arsenal for interfering with telomerase function using pharmacological agents is therefore likely to increase considerably in the future.

4. TELOMERASE AND CANCER DIAGNOSIS, PROGNOSTICATION, AND DETECTION

The strong association between telomerase expression and the malignant phenotype, together with the availability of a sensitive assay for the detection of telomerase activity, opens the possibility of using this enzyme as a cancer-specific marker in clinical tests. The fact that telomerase is remarkably stable at room temperature adds to the attractiveness of this approach in clinical settings, as it implies that clinical tests based on measurements of telomerase activity are not dependent on rapid sample processing or immediate refrigeration. Several investigators have examined the merit of applying this strategy to cancer diagnosis, prognostication, and detection.

4.1. Cancer Diagnosis

Biopsies or cytological aspirates or smears obtained from certain sites are notoriously difficult to evaluate for the presence or absence of malignancies using conventional pathological methods. Different authors have examined whether the presence of telomerase activity in such specimens could be used as a reliable indication of the presence of cancer cells. A good example in is the evaluation of patients with lesions of the pancreas. Distinction between pancreatic cancer and either benign tumors or inflammatory lesions of this organ is often very difficult. Recent studies have strongly suggested that testing for telomerase activity in such specimens can accurately determine whether a lesion is cancerous or not (72,73). Another example is in the evaluation of fine needle aspirates of thyroid lesions. A definitive diagnosis of malignancy can be made in only 60% of patients undergoing this procedure for suspicious thyroid nodules. Zeiger *et al.* (74) compared the outcome of cytopathological evaluations of such specimens to that of examining for hTERT RNA expression by RT-PCR. They concluded that the RT-PCR approach holds promise as a diagnostic test to complement more conventional approaches. Several authors have also compared the accuracy of testing for telomerase activity to that of cytological examination of body cavity effusions or washings (75-77). Distinction between cancer cells and reactive mesothelial cells in such specimens can be particularly difficult using conventional cytopathological methods. The telomerase assay was shown to outperform cytological examination in each of these studies (75-77).

The idea of measuring telomerase activity as an adjunct to cancer diagnostic methods is not applicable to all malignancies because detectable telomerase activity may be present in benign tumors or even normal tissues in some organs. For example, Pearson et al. (78) showed that benign breast tumors such as fibroadenomas could show telomerase activity. As mentioned earlier, telomerase is also expressed at high levels in normal endometrium during the follicular phase of the menstrual cycle (38,39), precluding the use of this enzyme as a marker for malignant transformation in endometrial specimens. Likewise, although telomerase activity is present in most high grade cervical intraepithelial neoplasias, the fact that this enzyme is also expressed in low grade intraepithelial neoplasias and reactive atypia and is also expressed, at least at the RNA level, in normal cervical mucosa precludes that use of this approach for the evaluation of cervical biopsies (79-81).

4.2. Cancer Prognostication

A number of authors have examined whether or not the mere presence of telomerase activity or levels of activity could provide independent prognostic information for specific tumor types. Dome et al. (82) reported that expression of hTERT mRNA above certain levels was a strong predictor of recurrence of Wilms tumor. In another study, the presence of telomerase activity was shown to be an independent prognostic indicator in neuroblastoma (83). Such studies suggest that the potential association between levels of telomerase expression and degree of biological aggressiveness in specific tumor types merits further investigation.

4.3. Cancer Detection

The high sensitivity of the TRAP assay suggests that it may provide a sensitive method of cancer detection, either for screening of populations at risk or for documenting residual disease or early recurrences in patients treated for cancer. Ramakumar et al. (84) concluded that urinary telomerase activity had the highest combination of sensitivity and specificity for bladder cancer screening when compared to various other tests including cytological examination. The telomerase test had superior accuracy in patients with grade 1/3 transitional cell carcinomas or with noninvasive papillary tumors and was extremely useful in patients with carcinoma in situ (84). This approach seems particularly attractive for the detection of residual disease in patients treated for ovarian carcinomas because of the mode of spread of these tumors. These cancers usually remain confined to the pelvis and abdomen after they spread outside the ovary, even at advanced disease stages. This implies that unlike most other cancers, it may be sufficient to focus our detection efforts on a single enclosed cavity. There is a need for a more sensitive method of detecting residual disease in patients treated for ovarian carcinoma. Up to 54% of patients in whom no evidence of disease is found at second-look laparotomy eventually undergo recurrences in spite of such negative findings (*85*). Thus, the sensitivity of second-look laparotomy, which is currently the most sensitive method of residual disease detection in ovarian carcinoma patients, is clearly suboptimal.

The merit of testing for telomerase activity in peritoneal washings or ascites of ovarian carcinoma patients as a mean of documenting the presence of residual disease was recently tested in the author's laboratory (*75*). Peritoneal washings were obtained from 42 patients undergoing either primary surgery or second-look laparotomies. Each patient had biopsy-proven ovarian cancer at the time of surgery. The sensitivity of the TRAP assay as a mean of detecting cancer cells in the washing specimens was compared to that of cytologic examination, which we used as gold standard (*75*). The results clearly showed that the telomerase assay was more sensitive than cytologic examination, even when performed under stringent conditions. The sensitivity of 88% that was observed for the telomerase assay when all common histological subtypes of ovarian carcinomas were considered could be raised to 95% when tumors with mucinous differentiation, which appeared to show frequent false-negativity, were eliminated. The only non-mucinous tumors with false-negative results were microscopic. These negative results may have been the consequence of inadequate sampling because there was little control over the thoroughness of the washing procedures in this preliminary study. In contrast, only 2 of 43 control patients showed telomerase activity, indicating a high degree of specificity. One of these 2 patients had a germ cell tumor, which could have accounted for the telomerase positivity. The other apparently false-positivite sample was from ascites of a patient with end-stage liver disease. The possibility of an occult malignancy in this patient could not be ruled out.

These results strongly support the idea that there is the merit in using the TRAP assay as a mean of ovarian cancer detection in the peritoneal cavity. It is still not clear whether or not the presence of telomerase activity in peritoneal washings from patients with otherwise negative second-look laparotomies can be used as an independent predictor of risk of recurrence. This question is currently being addressed in an ongoing multi-institutional study and should be answered in the near future. Since this approach involves measurement of an enzymatic activity, it may allow distinction between viable and dead cancer cells. Such distinction is important in this clinical setting because by definition, ovarian cancer patients who recently completed an adjuvant chemotherapy protocol undoubtedly harbor large quantities of dead cancer cell debris in their abdominal cavity.

224

5. CONCLUDING REMARKS

Still an obscure subject less than a decade ago, telomerase has become one of the most hotly debated topics in cancer research. Activation of this enzyme, although not sufficient to induce the malignant phenotype by itself, is now regarded as one of the necessary steps for such transformation (*11*). The exact impact of these developments in the future clinical management of the cancer patient is still not clear. The information reviewed in this chapter strongly suggests that interference with the activity of telomerase as a mean of anticancer therapy, or use of this enzyme as a cancer-specific marker in cancer detection strategies, are likely to become important components of clinical protocols.

REFERENCES

(*1*)   Blackburn EH: Structure and function of telomeres. Nature 1991; 350:569-573.
(*2*)   Levis RW, Ganesan R, Houtchens K, et al: Transposons in place of telomeric repeats at a Drosophila telomere. Cell 1993; 75:1083-1093.
(*3*)   Shampay J, Szostak JW, Blackburn EH: Cloning yeast telomeres on linear plasmid vectors. Cell 1982; 29:245-255.
(*4*)   Greider CW, Blackburn EH: The telomere terminal transferase of Tetrahymena is a ribonucleoprotein enzyme with two kinds of primer specificity. Cell 1987; 51:887-898.
(*5*)   Greider CW, Blackburn EH: A telomeric sequence in the RNA of Tetrahymena telomerase required for telomerase repeat synthesis. Nature 1989; 337:331-337.
(*6*)   Greider CW: Mammalian telomere dynamics: healing, fragmentation shortening and stabilization. Curr. Opinion Genet. Dev. 1994; 4:203-211.
(*7*)   Olovnikov AM: A theory of marginotomy. The incomplete copying of template margin in enzymic synthesis of polynucleotides and biological significance of the phenomenon. J. Theor. Biol. 1973; 41:181-190.
(*8*)   Harley CB, Futcher AB, Greider CW: Telomeres shorten during ageing of human fibroblasts. Nature 1990; 345:458-460.
(*9*)   Allsopp RC, Vaziri H, Patterson C, et al: Telomere length predicts replicative capacity of human fibroblasts. Proc. Natl. Acad. Sci. 1992; 89:10114-10118.
(*10*)   Kim NW, Piatyszek MA, Prowse KR, et al: Specific association of human telomerase activity with immortal cells and cancer. Science 1994; 266:2011-2015.
(*11*)   Hanahan D, Weinberg RA, 2000: The hallmarks of cancer. Cell 2000; 100:57-70.
(*12*)   Meyerson M, Counter CM, Eaton EN, et al: hEST2, the putative human telomerase catalytic subunit gene, is up-regulated in tumor cells and during immortalization. Cell 1997; 90:785-795.
(*13*)   Harrington L, McPhail T, Mar V, et al: A mammalian telomerase-associated protein. Science 1997; 275:973-977.
(*14*)   Nakayama J, Saito M, Nakamura H, et al: TLP1: a gene encoding a protein component of mammalian telomerase-associated protein. Science 1997; 275:973-977.
(*15*)   Gilley D, Blackburn EH: The telomerase RNA pseudoknot is critical for the stable assembly of a catalytically active ribonucleoprotein. Proc. Natl. Acad. Sci. 1999; 96:6621-6625.
(*16*)   Chen JL, Blasco MA, Greider CW: Secondary structure of vertebrate telomerase RNA. Cell 2000; 5:503-514.

(17)   Tesmer VM, Ford LP, Holt SE, et al: Two inactive fragments of the integral RNA cooperate to assemble active telomerase with the human protein catalytic subunit (hTERT) in vitro. Molec. Cell. Biol. 1999; 19:6207-6216.

(18)   Le S, Sternglanz R, Greider CW: Identification of two RNA-binding proteins associated with human telomerase RNA. Molec. Biol. Cell 2000; 11:999-1010.

(19)   Holt SE, Aisner DL, Baur J, et al: Functional requirement of p23 and Hsp90 in telomerase complexes. Genes Dev. 1999; 13:817-826.

(20)   Nakayama J, Tahara H, Tahara E, et al: Telomerase activation by hTRT in human normal fibroblasts and hepatocellular carcinomas. Nature Genet. 1998; 18:65-68.

(21)   Ramakrishnan S, Eppenberger U, Mueller H, et al: Expression profile of the putative catalytic subunit of the telomerase gene. Cancer Res. 1998; 58:622-625.

(22)   Kilian A, Bowtell DD, Abud HE, et al: Isolation of a candidate human telomerase catalytic subunit gene, which reveals complex splicing patterns in different cell types. Hum. Molec. Genet. 1997; 6:2011-2019,.

(23)   Tommerup H, Dousmanis A, de Lange T: Unusual chromatin in human telomeres. Mol. Cell. Biol. 1994; 14:5777-5785.

(24)   Griffith JD, Comeau L, Rosenfield S, et al: Mammalian telomeres end in a large duplex loop. Cell 1999; 97:503-514.

(25)   Chong L, van Steensel B, Broccoli D, et al: A human telomeric protein. Science 1995; 270:1663-1667.

(26)   Shen M, Haggblom C, Vogt M, et al: Characterization and cell cycle regulation of the related human telomeric proteins Pin2 and TRF1 suggest a role in mitosis. Proc. Natl. Acad. Sci. 1997; 94:13618-13623.

(27)   Conrad MN, Wright JH, Wolf AJ, et al: RAP1 protein interacts with yeast telomeres in vivo: overproduction alters telomere structure and decreases chromosome stability. Cell 1990; 63:739-750.

(28)   Kyrion G, Boakye KA, Lustig AJ: C-terminal truncation of RAP1 results in the deregulation of telomere size, stability, and function in Saccharomyces cerevisiae. Molec. Cell. Biol. 1992; 12:5159-5173.

(29)   van Steensel B, de Lange T: Control of telomere length by the human telomeric protein TRF1. Nature 1997; 385:740-743.

(30)   Griffith J, Bianchi A, de Lange T: TRF1 promotes parallel pairing of telomeric tracts in vitro. J. Molec. Biol. 1998; 278:79-88.

(31)   Kim SH, Kaminker P, Campisi J: TIN2, a new regulator of telomere length in human cells. Nature Genet. 1999; 23:405-412.

(32)   van Steensel B, Smogorzewska A, de Lange T: TRF2 protects human telomeres from end-to-end fusions. Cell 1998; 92:401-413.

(33)   Smith S, de Lange T: Cell cycle dependent localization of the telomeric PARP, tankyrase, to nuclear pore complexes and centrosomes. J. Cell Sci. 1999; 112:3649-3656.

(34)   Smith S, Giriat I, Schmitt A, et al: Tankyrase, a poly(ADP-ribose) polymerase at human telomeres. Science 1998; 282:1484-1487.

(35)   Broccoli D, Young JW, de Lange T: Telomerase activity in normal and malignant hematopoietic cells. Proc. Natl. Acad. Sci. 1995; 92:9082-9086.

(36)   Hiyama K, Hirai Y, Kyoizumi S, et al: Activation of telomerase in human lymphocytes and hematopoietic progenitor cells. J. Immunol. 1995; 155:3711-3715.

(37)   Yokoyama Y, Takahashi Y, Shinohara A, et al: Telomerase activity in the female reproductive tract and neoplasms. Gynecol. Oncol. 1998; 68:145-149.

(38)   Yokoyama Y, Takahashi Y, Morishita S, et al: Telomerase activity in the human endometrium throughout the menstrual cycle. Molec. Hum. Reprod. 1998; 4:173-177.

(39)   Tanaka M, Kyo S, Takakura M, et al: Expression of telomerase activity in human endometrium is localized to epithelial glandular cells and regulated in a menstrual phase-dependent manner correlated with cell proliferation. Am. J. Pathol. 1998; 153:1985-1991.

226

(40)   Nakamura Y, Tahara E, Tahara H, et al: Quantitative reevaluation oftelomerase activity in cancerous and noncancerous gastrointestinal tissues. Molec. Carcinog. 1999; 26:312-320.

(41)   Kolquist KA, Ellisen LW, Counter CM, et al: Expression of TERT in early premalignant lesions and a subset of cells in normal tissues. Nature Genet. 1998; 19:182-186.

(42)   Le S, Moore JK, Haber JE, et al: RAD50 and RAD51 define two pathways that collaborate to maintain telomeres in the absence of telomerase. Genetics 1999; 152:143-152.

(43)   Bryan T, Marusic L, Bacchetti S, et al: The telomere lengthening mechanism in telomerase-negative immortal human cells does not involve the telomerase RNA subunit. Hum. Molec. Genet.1997; 6:921-926.

(44)   Rudolph KL, Chang S, Lee HW, et al: Longevity, stress response, and cancer in aging telomerase-deficient mice. Cell 1999; 96:701-712.

(45)   Herbert B, Pitts AE, Baker SI, et al: Inhibition of human telomerase in immortal human cells leads to progressive telomere shortening and cell death. Proc. Natl. Acad. Sci. 1999; 96:14276-14281.

(46)   Hahn WC, Stewart SA, Brooks MW, et al: Inhibition of telomerase limits the growth of human cancer cells. Nature Med. 1999; 5:1164-1170.

(47)   Murakami J, Nagai N, Shigemasa K, et al: Inhibition of telomerase activity and cell proliferation by a reverse transcriptase inhibitor in gynaecological cancer cell lines. Eur. J. Cancer 1999; 35:1027-1034.

(48)   Tendian SW, Parker WB: Interaction of deoxyguanosine nucleotide analogs with human telomerase. Mol. Pharmacol. 2000; 57:695-699.

(49)   Xu D, Gruber A, Bjorkholm M, et al: Suppression of telomerase reverse transcriptase (hTERT) expression in differentiated HL-60 cells: regulatory mechanisms. Br. J. Cancer 1999; 80:1156-1161.

(50)   Horikawa I, Cable PL, Afshari C, et al: Cloning and characterization of the promoter region of human telomerase reverse transcriptase gene. Cancer Res. 1999; 59:826-830.

(51)   Takakura M, Kyo S, Kanaya T, et al: Cloning of human telomerase catalytic subunit (hTERT) gene promoter and identification of proximal core promoter sequences essential for transcriptional activation in immortalized and cancer cells. Cancer Res. 1999; 59:551-557.

(52)   Wick M, Zubov D, Hagen G: Genomic organization and promoter characterization of the gene encoding the human telomerase reverse transcriptase (hTERT). Gene 1999; 232:97-106.

(53)   Cong YS, Wen J, Bacchetti S: The human telomerase catalytic subunit hTERT: organization of the gene and characterization of the promoter. Hum. Mo.l Genet. 1999; 8:137-142.

(54)   Greenberg RA, O'Hagan RC, Deng H, et al: Telomerase reverse transcriptase gene is a direct target of c-Myc but is not functionally equivalent in cellular transformation. Oncogene 1999; 18:1219-1226.

(55)   Wu KJ, Grandori C, Amacker M, et al: Direct activation of TERT transcription by c-MYC. Nature Genet. 1999; 21:220-224.

(56)   Wang J, Xie LY, Allan S, et al: Myc activates telomerase. Genes Dev. 1998; 12:1769-1774.

(57)   Kyo S, Takakura M, Taira T, et al: Sp1 cooperates with c-Myc to activate transcription of the human telomerase reverse transcriptase gene (hTERT). Nucleic Acids Res. 2000; 28:669-677.

(58)   Oh S, Song YH, Yim J, et al: Identification of Mad as a repressor of the human telomerase (hTERT) gene. Oncogene 2000; 19:1485-1490.

(59)   Dessain SK, Yu H, Reddel RR, et al: Methylation of the human telomerase gene CpG island. Cancer Res. 2000; 60:537-541.

(60)   Devereux TR, Horikawa I, Anna CH, et al: DNA methylation analysis of the promoter region of the human telomerase reverse transcriptase (hTERT) gene. Cancer Res. 1999; 59:6087-6090.

(61)   Aldous WK, Marean AJ, DeHart MJ, et al: Effects of tamoxifen on telomerase activity in breast carcinoma cell lines. Cancer 1999; 85:1523-1529.

(62)   Kyo S, Takakura M, Kanaya T, et al: Estrogen activates telomerase. Cancer Res. 1999; 59:5917-5921.

(63)   Seimiya H, Tanji M, Oh-hara T, et al: Hypoxia up-regulates telomerase activity via mitogen-activated protein kinase signaling in human solid tumor cells. Biochem. Biophy.s Res. Commun. 1999; 260:365-370.

(64)   Sawa H, Kamada H, Ohshima TA, et al: Exogenous expression of p16INK4a is associated with decrease in telomerase activity. J. Neurooncol. 1999; 42:45-57.

(65)   Kusumoto M, Ogawa T, Mizumoto K, et al: Adenovirus-mediated p53 gene transduction inhibits telomerase activity independent of its effects on cell cycle arrest and apoptosis in human pancreatic cancer cells. Clin. Cancer Res. 1999; 5:2140-2147.

(66)   Li H, Cao Y, Berndt MC, et al: Molecular interactions between telomerase and the tumor suppressor protein p53 in vitro. Oncogene 1999; 18:6785-6794.

(67)   Cuthbert AP, Bond J, Trott DA, et al: Telomerase repressor sequences on chromosome 3 and induction of permanent growth arrest in human breast cancer cells. J. Natl. Cancer Inst. 1999; 91:37-45.

(68)   Cheng PC, Gosewehr JA, Kim TM, et al: Potential role of the inactivated X chromosome in ovarian epithelial tumor development. J..Natl..Cancer Inst. 1996; 88:510-518.

(69)   Cliby W, Ritland S, Hartmann L, et al: Human epithelial ovarian cancer allelotype. Cancer Res. 1996; 53:2393-2398.

(70)   Li H, Zhao L, Yang Z, et al: Telomerase is controlled by protein kinase Calpha in human breast cancer cells. J. Biol. Chem. 1998; 273:33436-33442.

(71)   Kang SS, Kwon T, Kwon DY, et al: Akt protein kinase enhances human telomerase activity through phosphorylation of telomerase reverse transcriptase subunit. J. Biol. Chem. 1999; 274:13085-13090.

(72)   Uehara H, Nakaizumi A, Tatsuta M, et al: Diagnosis of pancreatic cancer by detecting telomerase activity in pancreatic juice: comparison with K-ras mutations. Am. J. Gastroenterol. 1999; 94:2513-2518.

(73)   Yeh TS, Cheng AJ, Chen TC, et al: Telomerase activity is a useful marker to distinguish malignant pancreatic cystic tumors from benign neoplasms and pseudocysts. J. Surg. Res. 1999; 87:171-177.

(74)   Zeiger MA, Smallridge RC, Clark DP, et al: Human telomerase reverse transcriptase (hTERT) gene expression in FNA samples from thyroid neoplasms. Surgery 1999; 126:1195-1199.

(75)   Duggan B, Wan M, Yu M, et al: Detection of ovarian cancer cells: Comparison of a telomerase assay and cytologic examination. J. Natl. Cancer Inst. 1998; 90:238-242.

(76)   Toshima S, Arai T, Yasuda Y, et al: Cytological diagnosis and telomerase activity of cells in effusions of body cavities. Oncol. Res. 1999; 6:199-203.

(77)   Tangkijvanich P, Tresukosol D, Sampatanukul P, et al: Telomerase assay for differentiating between malignancy-related and nonmalignant ascites. Clin. Cancer Res. 1999; 5:2470-2475.

(78)   Pearson AS, Gollahon LS, O'Neal NC, et al: Detection of telomerase activity in breast masses by fine-needle aspiration. Ann. Surg. Oncol. 1998; 5:186-193.

(79)   Shroyer KR, Thompson LC, Enomoto T, et al: Telomerase expression in normal epithelium, reactive atypia, squamous dysplasia, and squamous cell carcinoma of the uterine cervix. Am. J. Clin. Pathol. 1998; 109:153-162.

(80)   Snijders PJ, van Duin M, Walboomers JM, et al: Telomerase activity exclusively in cervical carcinomas and a subset of cervical intraepithelial neoplasia grade III lesions: strong association with elevated messenger RNA levels of its catalytic subunit and high-risk human papillomavirus DNA. Cancer Res. 1998; 58:3812-3818.

(*81*)   Nakano K, Watney E, McDougall JK: Telomerase activity and expression of telomerase RNA component and telomerase catalytic subunit gene in cervical cancer. Am. J. Pathol. 1998; 153:857-864.

(*82*)   Dome JS, Chung S, Bergemann T, et al: High telomerase reverse transcriptase (hTERT) messenger RNA level correlates with tumor recurrence in patients with favorable histology Wilms' tumor. Cancer Res. 1999; 59:4301-4307.

(*83*)   Poremba C, Willenbring H, Hero B, et al: Telomerase activity distinguishes between neuroblastomas with good and poor prognosis. Ann. Oncol. 1999; 10:715-721.

(*84*)   Ramakumar S, Bhuiyan J, Besse JA, et al: Comparison of screening methods in the detection of bladder cancer. J. Urol. 1999; 161:388-394.

(*85*)   Muderspach L, Muggia FM, Conti PS: Second-look laparotomy for stage III epithelial ovarian cancer: rationale and current issues. Cancer Treatment Rev. 1996; 21:499-511.

II.   RESEARCH

B. Growth Control

Chapter 10

HOMEOBOX GENE EXPRESSION IN OVARIAN CANCER

Susan M. Pando and Hugh S. Taylor
Department of Obstetrics and Gynecology
Yale University School of Medicine, New Haven, CT

1. INTRODUCTION

Homeobox genes control embryogenesis in both vertebrates and invertebrates. They are named after the highly conserved 180 bp sequence, the homeobox. There are two families of vertebrate homeobox genes. The first is the Hox genes and members of this family are clustered on the chromosome. These genes are classified according to sequence similarities as well as their position within the cluster[1]. The second group is divergent and members of this group are found throughout the genome. In invertebrates, the cluster is known as the homeotic complex, or HOM-C. The vertebrate family of homeobox genes is large; greater than 0.2% of the estimated 100,000 genes per genome may contain a homeobox with only a small number residing in the Hox cluster[2]. The HOM-C and Hox complexes contain homologous genes that are similar in both sequence and function in different organisms. These genes dictate body design in all embryos. The effects of vertebrate HOX genes can be ascertained from their expression pattern during mouse development and from the phenotype of mice with a targeted deletion, disruption or overexpression of a specific Hox gene [1].

The development of the female Müllerian system, which consists of the upper vagina, cervix, uterus and oviducts, is controlled in part by Hox genes [3]. The female reproductive system originates from the embryonic paramesonephric duct. Differential gene expression within this duct with maturation aids in giving a separate identity to the different components. Hox genes encode the proteins which direct the expression of downstream target genes which in turn direct the development of the female reproductive system along the anterior-posterior axis [3]. HOXA9 is expressed in the area that will become the fallopian tube. HOXA10 is expressed in the developing uterus. HOXA11 is expressed in the primordia of the uterus and cervix. There is no evidence of a HOXA12 gene. Finally, HOXA13 is expressed in the developing vagina.

HOX genes encode proteins that direct the growth, proliferation and differentiation of all organ systems. Aberrant regulation of growth and differentiation are characteristic of cancer; knowledge of the genes that control this process in the reproductive tract will undoubtedly lead to a better understanding of factors that regulate gynecologic tumors. In this paper we present background on HOX gene expression in normal and malignant tissues. We also present preliminary data on the role of these genes in the detection, regulation and/or formation of gynecological malignancies such as ovarian cancer.

2. BACKGROUND

The fruit fly, *Drosophila melanogaster*, serves as a model for Hox gene function. In the fly, these genes are referred to as the HOM genes that are part of the HOM complex. It is estimated that these gene sequences evolved between 600 million and one billion years ago[1]. The highly conserved nature of these genes indicates their essential role in development. Distantly related organisms rely on the same or similar genes for their structure and function. The homeobox sequences of many mammalian genes are strikingly similar to those found in *Drosophila*.

The role of Hox genes in development is best exemplified in *Drosophila* in which embryonic design was studied extensively. Originally, flies with homeotic mutations were described [4]. These mutations produced a characteristic phenotype; one body part or segment is replaced by another. Examples include flies with two second thoracic segments and therefore two pair of wings or flies with legs protruding from the head in place of antennae. Each phenotype was mapped to a single locus, therefore the development of an entire body segment is controlled by one gene. All of these genes also mapped to a single cluster. The first described set of fly homeotic genes was named the *Bithorax* complex. Defects in the posterior half of the body were mapped to genes in this complex. Homeotic genes relay positional information. They assign spatial identities to cells in different regions of the anterior-posterior axis [1].

Genetic crosses and gene mapping revealed that the linear order on the chromosome parallels the order of body regions on the anterior-posterior axis where each gene is expressed. Phenotypic alterations resulting from a mutation in a single gene occur in an expected region as predicted by the expression pattern. The organization of these genes relays positional information [1]. Further, if three genes in the *Bithorax* complex [specifically, *Ultrabithorax* (*Ubx*), *abdominal-A* (*abd-A*) and *Abdominal-B* (*Abd-B*)] were removed, a lethal mutation would result. These mutant embryos survived long enough to develop identifiable structures in which all eight abdominal segments are changed into thoracic segments [5]. The posterior genes clustered in the *Bithorax* complex give rise to posterior identity; in their absence, only thoracic identity is possible. A second set of fly homeotic genes referred to as the *Antennapedia* complex was identified. Mutations in this complex altered body design in the anterior half of the fly. For example, a mutation in the *Antennapedia* gene results in a fly that has legs growing in place of antennae. The genes of the *Antennapedia* complex determine specific anterior identity.

3. HOX: ORGANIZATION, STRUCTURE & FUNCTION

In the 1980s, this set of developmental control genes was cloned and found to contain a conserved 180 base pair sequence element referred to as the homoebox [6]. This element encodes a 60 amino acid homeodomain that is the primary determinant of the regulatory specificity of these proteins. The homeodomain functions as a sequence-specific DNA binding domain; the HOX protein contains this domain and acts as a transcription factor which controls the expression of target genes [7].

The mammalian Hox genes are homologous to the HOM-C genetic complex of *Drosophila* [1]. There are a minimum of 39 Hox genes grouped into four clusters: Hoxa, Hoxb, Hoxc and Hoxd. Each of these clusters is compromised of 9-11 genes that are localized to four separate chromosomes. Specifically, HOX clusters A-D are located on human chromosomes 7, 17, 12 and 2 respectively. Homeodomains have a 25% conservation of amino acid identity. The recognized homeodomains have nearly identical backbone structures. X-ray crystallography and NMR analysis revealed that the protein structure of the homeodomain contains three alpha helical parts that make up a hydrophobic core [8-10]. One of these helices makes sequence-specific contacts by inserting into the major groove of the DNA. The homeodomain protein also makes contact with the minor groove via the N terminus which stabilizes the association with DNA. The homeodomain acts as a DNA-binding domain via a helix-turn-helix structure similar to those found in prokaryotic transcription factors [11].

It is believed that these gene sequences evolved approximately one billion years ago thereby creating an evolutionary pattern of different phyla that contain homeotic genes [12]. Hox genes are very similar in sequence and genomic organization to the HOM-C genes. As described above, homeodomains are organized into four Hox loci or clusters [1]. It is hypothesized that the vertebrate clusters evolved due to a quadruplication of an ancestral complex common to both the HOM-C and Hox clusters [13]. Homeodomains may be divided into subclasses based on their sequence [1].

These sequence similarities as well as their location within groups have been used to classify the genes into 13 paralagous groups [14]. Evolutionary conservation is evidenced by the similarities in paralog function, sequence and location. Genes that are homologous across species are referred to as orthologous. Homeobox genes in other species remain in the same relative order as in Drosophila [15, 16]. For example, the Hox/HOX genes that are orthologous to the *Antennapedia* gene in Drosophila are locate at the 3' end of the chromosome. This evidence supports the hypothesis that Hox genes arose from one cluster and are conserved throughout evolution. These clusters were expanded and partially replicated (due to an uneven distribution of genetic material during meiosis) during lateral gene duplication [13]. Although conserved, this complex is also a determining factor for creating morphological diversity among multicellular animals [12]. Subtle changes in their regulation underlie differences in many body structures between species.

Hox genes are detected at gastrulation and are expressed in all three germ layers. The organization on the chromosome paralleled with the expression pattern along the anterior-posterior axis of the embryo. Specifically, the genes located in the 5' region are expressed in the posterior while the anterior regions express the 3' genes. Specifically, the 3' Hox genes of the first four paralogs dictate the development of the embryonic region corresponding to the head and brain [17]. The thoracic portion of the body is controlled by central Hox genes of the middle four paralogs. Finally, the 5' Hox genes of the last five paralogs determine identity in the lumbosacral region. Hox genes are unique in that their organization is both spatial and temporal. The temporal expression pattern of Hox genes has been determined in the mouse. The relationship between gene order on the chromosome and time of appearance during embryogenesis is known as temporal colinearity. The most anteriorly expressed Hox genes which are located at the 3' end of the Hox cluster, are also sequentially activated earlier than those at the 5' end of the cluster between gestational days 8-10 in the mouse [18]. Alterations in Hox expression domains may lead to structural abnormalities[19], indicating that the expression pattern is essential to normal embryogenesis.

Mutations in *Drosophila* homeobox genes result in dramatic changes in segmental identity, typically anterior transformation. These variations are not as severe in mammals. This may be due to an overlap in genetic function between the Hox clusters. Gene targeting experiments using murine models have determined that Hox genes provide regional developmental identity along the vertebrate anterior-posterior axis. For example, mice with a homozygous Hoxa3 mutation expired after birth and post mortem examination revealed cranial, glandular and vascular deformities [20]. When the Hoxc-8 gene was inactivated, the first lumbar vertebra was converted into a more anterior thoracic vertebra that resulted in a 14th pair of ribs [20]. Ectopic expression of Hoxd-4 anteriorly under control of a Hoxa-1 promoter, led to the formation of neural arches on the basioccipital bone [21]; overexpression of Hoxd-4 caused anterior structures to transform into posterior structures [21]. Each of the aforementioned phenotypic changes was caused by changes in expression leading to structural transformations.

The molecular mechanism underlying typical anterior transformation has been revealed by the effect of Hox genes on downstream targets. The study of both gain and loss of function mutations in both *Drosophila* and mice revealed that the more posterior-acting Hox and homeotic proteins are dominant to the anterior-acting proteins [1]. This occurrence is referred to as "phenotypic suppression" in the fruit fly or "posterior prevalence" in mice [12]. This suppression or prevalence may function in maintaining homeotic gene expression via transcriptional downregulation [12]. Specifically, if the DNA-binding domains of homeotic proteins overlap, autoregulatory sites will be filled and be blocked by the suppressing product [12]. Second, this hierarchy suggests that there may be gradients in the binding efficiencies of gene products, specifically, posterior products may bind more effectively. Third, posterior gene products may compete more efficiently for interactions with cofactors necessary for homeotic function. In summary, of the many Hox genes expressed in any given segment, body segment development is thought to be dictated by the Hox gene that is most posterior (most 5'-located) in the cluster. However, it should also be noted that the overlapping functional domains of the homeotic genes suggest that these genes may have a combinational component and may not necessarily act in a strictly hierarchical manner. This functional hierarchy may be a method of silencing a gene's function without shutting off transcription. Finally, both gain and loss of function mutations can disrupt gene regulation that may lead to decreased function. In addition to loss of that gene function, cross regulation of Hox genes may result in changes in other Hox gene functions.

4. HUMAN HOX GENE MUTATIONS

Two human developmental defects have been described that result from mutations in HOX genes. Human synpolydactaly is an autosomal dominant inherited limb abnormality resulting from a mutation of the HOXD13 gene[22]. This mutation presents as webbing between fingers and a duplication of fingers. This mutation is caused by a short amplification of a polyalanine stretch in the N-terminal region of HOXD13 [22]. Surprisingly, this mutation is more severe than the Hoxd-13(-/-) mutation observed in mice [23]. It is possible that the mutated human protein is transcriptionally inactive although it retains its DNA binding properties and functions as a dominant negative. Digit alterations may be more severe than with Hoxd-13(-/-) because mutated HOXD13 may suppress the other homeoproteins involved in digit morphogenesis such as HOXA13 via binding site occupancy [22].

Human hand-foot-genital (HFG) syndrome is an autosomal dominant syndrome due to a HOXA13 mutation [24]. This anomaly affects appendages such as the thumb and large toe as well as the development of the urethra and Mullerian tract. In a murine model, Mullerian tract defects include a hypoplastic urogenital sinus and incomplete extension of the paramesonephric duct into the urogenital sinus by day 13.5 post coitum [25]. These mice usually expire between days 11.5-15.5 post coitum due to umbilical artery stenosis [25]. The HFG mutation involves a nucleotide substitution that changes a Trp to a stop codon [26]. This abnormality is similar to synpolydactaly in that the Hoxa-13(-/-) murine mutation is less severe, again, likely due to a dominant negative effect of the mutated HOXA13 in the hand-foot-genital syndrome[24].

5. REPRODUCTIVE TRACT DEVELOPMENT

As described above, HOX genes act as master regulators of developmental identity. We have recently shown that Hox genes are also involved in the partitioning of the paramesonephric duct into the mature female reproductive system [3]. Specifically, HOXA9 is expressed in the area that will become the fallopian tube. HOXA10 is expressed in the developing uterus. HOXA11 is expressed in the uterus and cervix. There is no evidence of a HOXA12 gene. Finally, HOXA13 is expressed in the primordia of the vagina. All of the Hox genes of the Müllerian axis are simultaneously expressed in the paramesonephric duct at embryonic day 15.5 [3]. Temporal colinearity or sequential activation, which is typically seen with Hox genes, is not observed in the female reproductive tract. Spatial colinearity was maintained in this system, however. This divergence from temporal colinearity may allow late expression of these genes and thereby allow the delayed development of the murine female reproductive tract. The murine Müllerian system is rudimentary at birth with the most differentiation occurring later in development [27]. These genes are also expressed in the adult and may function to maintain the developmental plasticity that characterizes the female reproductive tract.

The pattern of HOX/Hox gene expression is conserved between the human and murine female reproductive systems [3]. This data support the hypothesis that Hox genes play a role in defining functional and tissue identity rather than a structural identity. Structurally, the two uteri are different; the human uterus is unicornuate which results from the fusion of the two paramesonephric ducts. The murine uterus is bicornuate and allows for multiple gestations. However despite these differences, the uteri both express Hoxa-10/HOXA10 and Hoxa-11/HOXA11 genes.

6. ADULT EXPRESSION

The female reproductive system retains Hox/HOX expression in the adult to maintain functions such as the continued differentiation of the endometrium. The endometrium undergoes growth and differentiation in the adult on par with many embryonic developmental processes. Further, Hox/HOX expression is menstrual cycle dependent and is regulated by estrogen and progesterone [28]. This developmental plasticity may help to establish and maintain pregnancy by allowing the system to respond to various hormonal changes. We have shown that estrogen and progesterone are direct regulators of HOX gene expression [29]. Northern Blot analysis and *In Situ* Hybridization established the levels and location of HOXA10 expression during the menstrual cycle. HOXA10 is expressed in the endometrium in a menstrual cycle stage-dependent manner [28, 29]. During the proliferative phase of the menstrual cycle, when estrogen is the predominant hormone, northern analysis has shown significant HOXA10 expression. During the proliferative phase, the endometrium thickens two to three-fold; due to proliferation and differentiation of surface epithelium, glands, stroma and blood vessels. Progesterone (P4) levels increase prior to the midsecretory phase of the menstrual cycle driving further differentiation. Northern analysis has shown a dramatic increase in HOXA10 mRNA levels at midsecretory phase [28]. It is at this point that the uterus becomes receptive to implantation. This expression pattern also suggests that adult HOXA10 expression is necessary for successful uterine implantation. Expression persists into the late luteal phase and the decidua of pregnancy.

A targeted disruption of the Hoxa-10 gene results in mice with female infertility [30]. These mice will ovulate normally and produce zygotes that develop in pseudopregnant surrogates, however, these mice have a reproductive tract that cannot support the preimplantation embryo or implantation. These murine data support the findings described above which suggest that adult HOXA10 expression is essential to human endometrial receptivity and implantation.

Mice with a targeted mutation of Hoxa11 display limb deformities, axial skeletal defects and a sexually dimorphic reproductive phenotype in which the female has uterine factor infertility [31, 32]. Like HOXA10, HOXA11 expression in women is increased under the influence of estrogen and progesterone and is expressed in a cyclic manner [29]. HOXA11 directs the embryonic development of the uterus and cervix and may later continue this developmental regulation during the menstrual cycle. Northern blot analysis of human endometrium has shown that HOXA11 is expressed in moderate levels throughout the menstrual cycle [29]. However, during the mid-secretory phase a significant increase in HOXA11 expression was noted - also corresponding to the time of implantation. Northern analysis was also used to determine whether HOXA11 functioned in the decidualization and maintenance of pregnancy. The examination of first trimester uterine decidua revealed that HOXA11 expression persists into pregnancy at similar levels as seen in the secretory endometrium. In situ hybridization was used to localize cellular distribution of HOXA11 in the endometrium [29]. HOXA11 was expressed in both glandular and stromal cells with higher levels in the latter. This data suggests that HOXA11 directs endometrial differentiation which aids in receptivity to implantation. Decidual expression also suggests that HOXA11 may play a role in the maintenance of pregnancy.

Hox genes and their mutations have been linked to pathologies other than those of the female reproductive tract. These genes have been studied in regard to the role they play in skin and hair follicles. It has been established that a gene's position within each homeotic complex determines the anterior limits of its expression. As previously stated, the anterior regions express the 3' genes while the expression of the 5' genes are more posterior. In addition to spatial colinearity, temporal colinearity also plays a role in gene expression. Specifically, the genes located in the 3' region are expressed before the more posterior genes in the 5' region. Therefore, when studying a gene such as Hoxc13, (the 5' most gene of the C cluster) using targeted mutation in mice, one would expect to find defects in the caudal region of the axial skeleton and the nails which are the most distal regions of the limb [33]. Hoxc13 gene expression in normal mice and genetic defects in mice with a Hoxc13 mutation were noted in other areas as well. Hoxc13 was expressed in facial vibrissae and the filiform papillae of the tongue, which suggests that using spatial colinearity as a predictor of development may not always be accurate at later embryological stages [33]. It has also been observed that Hoxc13 is not restricted to a specific area, but is expressed in hair follicles throughout the body. The Hoxc13 mutant mice are hairless; the mouse is able to produce hair, however, the follicle breaks at the skin surface resulting in alopecia. Hoxc13 may code for the development of hair and filiform papilla. HOX genes may have a significant unexpected role outside of their predicted spatially restricted expression domain.

7. HOX GENES AND SOLID TUMORS

As described above, homeoproteins are transcription factors that give spatial and temporal developmental signals to various organ systems. Specifically, these genes control cell growth, proliferation and differentiation as well as communication and apoptosis. Variations in the aforementioned cellular processes are characteristic of cancer. The molecular mechanisms of oncogenesis and the physiology of homeoproteins may be related; both processes deal with the acquisition, regulation and maintenance of cell identity. Indeed abnormal HOX gene expression has been identified in several tumors.

Homeobox genes have been associated with colon cancer. Northern analysis of primary tumors and metastatic liver lesions originating from colorectal tumors demonstrated misexpression of HOXA9, HOXB7 and HOXD11 [34]. Other studies have shown misexpression of HOXB6, HOXB8 and HOXC9 at various stages of colon cancer [35]. HOXB6, HOXB8, HOXC8 and HOXC9 were overexpressed in both premalignant polyps and colorectal cancer [35]. HOX gene expression is increased in early colorectal cancer. Early malignancy is characterized by changes in cell identity and gene expression. As HOX genes impart developmental identity, changes in cell identity and in developmental programs may well involve changes in HOX expression. HOX gene expression is decreased in more advanced cancer; there is a loss of HOX expression as cells dedifferentiate. HOX genes control differentiation during development and it is not surprising to find a loss of such expression in undifferentiated cells. Increased HOX gene expression may serve as an early indicator of malignancy aiding in patient diagnosis and treatment whereas loss of HOX expression may be predictive of loss of differentiation and poor prognosis.

As described above, Northern analysis has shown that HOXA9 is strongly expressed in primary colonic tumors [36]. A primary breast malignancy that metastasized to the colon did not express HOX genes typically associated with the colon [36]. HOX expression is retained in these tumors and they do not vary in their HOX expression with metastasis to take on the pattern of HOX gene expression normally observed at the metastatic site [36]. Nor did either primary or secondary gastric carcinomas express any of the HOX genes that typify colon cancer. Gastrointestinal adenocarcinomas express HOX genes according to their rostral-caudal tumor location. For example, HOXA9 was not expressed in gastric carcinomas but was consistently expressed in colon malignancies. Variations in HOX gene expression associated with gastrointestinal cancers may be used as a molecular marker to determine origin and state of differentiation of the disease.

Homeobox genes that are orthologous of the *Drosophila Abdominal-B* (*Abd-B*) genes are found in gastrointestinal carcinomas. These genes may potentially aid in the diagnosis and treatment of malignancies. First, the genes retain the rostral-caudal boundaries of their organ of origin. HOX expression patterns are maintained in tumor metastasis and aid in the diagnosis of secondary tumors from unknown origins. Second, different types of tumors found within one organ may be distinguished on the basis of their HOX gene expression patterns. Third, several organ systems express various HOX genes and tumors of these tissues demonstrate abnormal HOX gene expression patterns, thus serving as tumor markers.

HOX gene expression has also been found in the kidney. There is marked variation in gene expression in renal carcinomas and compared to normal human kidneys [37]. HOX genes can be upregulated (HOXC11) or downregulated (HOXB5, HOXB9) in primary kidney tumors [37]. These tumors may also exhibit different-sized transcripts compared to normal kidneys [37]. These differences in gene expression between benign and malignant tissues suggest an association between renal cancer and HOX genes. These genetic differences may be used as a marker for malignancy.

The kidney forms from the metanephric intermediate mesoderm following induction by the mesonephric bud [36]. Transitional epithelial tumors originate at this bud and display decreased and differential HOX expression. It is hypothesized that congenital mesoblastic nephroma is derived from the metanephric mesoderm before induction and expresses HOXA9, HOXC9 and HOXD10 [36]. HOXD10 expression was the highest in Wilm's tumors but is rare in renal adenocarcinomas which expressed only HOXA9 [36]. Specifically, HOXA9, HOXC9 and HOXD10 act as indicators of the histological subtypes. Northern analysis has shown that these three genes are expressed in the normal kidney [36]. However, tumors of different histologic subtypes showed different expression patterns which suggests that these genes are cell specific.

HOX genes are involved in tissue differentiation during embryogenesis and, as shown, maintenance of a differentiated state in the adult. Abnormal HOX gene expression is known to cause congenital anomalies and possibly pediatric cancers. There is an increased incidence of pediatric cancers in individuals affected with a cervical rib. Patients with this congenital defect display skeletal abnormalities resembling those of transgenic mice with mutant homeobox genes [38]. The possible misexpression of HOX genes may underlie both conditions. Frequent correlation exists between developmental regulation, embryogenesis and oncology.

8. HOX GENES AND LEUKEMIA

Hematopoietic stem cells have self-renewal and proliferative capabilities and can give rise to several types of mature blood cells [39]. Although the molecular pathology leading to the proliferation and differentiation of the stem cells is not fully understood, it has been suggested that homeobox genes may regulate hematopoiesis [39]. Homeobox genes are expressed in blood cells and their differentiation correlates with the activation and/or inactivation of several HOX genes. Further, hematopoietic cells express several HOX genes in a temporal fashion, therefore, modulation of this gene expression may alter the proliferative, differentiative or phenotypic characteristics of hematopoietic cells.

Alterations in HOX genes have been described in leukemic cells leading to oncogenesis. Lymphoid cells express several HOX genes. HOXB7 has been detected in normal peripheral blood lymphocytes [40]. Experimental overexpression of HOXA10 and HOXB8 may be a precursor to leukemia [39]. Changes in HOX genes that are normally expressed in the peripheral blood may lead to malignancy. The mixed lineage leukemia, MLL, is a gene encoding a zinc finger protein [41]. A murine model with a *Mll* deficiency resulted in an embryonic lethal mutation [42]. This deficiency was also associated with altered Hox gene expression along the anterior-posterior axis [42]. The MLL gene was discovered at translocation breakpoints in human acute leukemias and may function to maintain the initiation of HOX gene expression in normal hematopoiesis as well as in the embryo.

A form of human acute myeloid leukemia involves the translocation t(7;11)(p15;p15) [43, 44]. This translocation involves the fusion of HOXA9 to NUP98, a gene coding for nucleoporin [43, 44]. This results in a chimeric NUP98-HOXA9 protein, in which the amino terminal half of NUP98 is fused in the frame to HOXA9 This protein may inhibit the normal function of NUP98 or HOXA9 in a dominant negative fashion and may be leukemogenic [45, 46].

HOX genes are clearly useful molecular markers of malignancy. Specific overall patterns of HOX expression characterize different types of human leukemias [47] as well as renal and gastrointestinal malignancies. HOX gene expression may be used to characterize cell type and degree of differentiation [47]. They may also play a role in the early detection of these tumors.

9. OVARIAN CANCER

This year in the United States approximately 24,000 women will be diagnosed with ovarian cancer and 14,200 will die from the disease [48]. Ovarian cancer is the leading cause of death from gynecological malignancies. Advanced epithelial ovarian cancer (EOC) is a clinical challenge with a poor outcome, therefore, the ability to detect this disease at an early stage would have a significant impact on morbidity and mortality.

CA-125 is a glycoprotein antigen located on the surface of several EOCs and is released into the bloodstream by tumors [49]. CA-125 levels aid in predicting ovarian tumor biology; an increased CA-125 level correlates with poorly differentiated tumors as well as metastasis. In 90% of advanced stage EOC, the serum CA-125 level was elevated (>35 U/mL) while less than 50% of Stage I patients display abnormal levels [50]. Although this is the only widely used test in current use, it has little value in detecting malignancy at an early stage. There is clearly a need for more and better early markers of ovarian cancer.

Ovarian cancer may eventually be characterized at the molecular level although currently the exact nature of the mutations and number of mutations that cause ovarian cancer are still unknown [51]. Many interesting candidate genes including HOX genes have been described. HOX genes play an essential role in the female reproductive system. As described above, previous work has shown a relation of HOX genes to multiple malignancies. Therefore, it is of interest to determine if these genes might play a role in the detection and/or formation of gynecological malignancies such as ovarian cancer. HOX genes may act as novel molecular markers of this malignancy.

Preliminary data from our laboratory using Northern Blot analysis has shown that there is decreased HOXA10 expression in ovarian cancer as compared to normal ovary. This data was obtained using normal and malignant ovarian tissue and confirmed using several established ovarian cancer cell lineages. Trizol was used to extract RNA from both primary tissue samples and established cell lines. Total RNA was run on an agarose gel, transferred to a nylon membrane and hybridized with a ^{32}P-labeled riboprobe. pGEM plasmids containing sequences from the 3' untranslated region of HOXA10 were linearized with EcoR1, ethanol precipitated, and used as a riboprobe template. The riboprobe was generated using the RNA polymerase SP6, and ^{32}P-UTP. Hybridization was performed for three hours at 68°C and the membrane washed twice at 60°C for 20 minutes in 0.1x SSC and SDS. The film was exposed overnight at −70°C. G3PDH, a housekeeping gene, was used for normalization. The autoradiographs were normalized and HOXA10 expression was compared.

HOXA10 is expressed in the normal ovary at significant levels and this expression is decreased in tumor samples. Forty percent of the ovarian cancer samples demonstrate HOXA10 expression whereas 60% lack HOXA10 expression. This preliminary data indicates that HOXA10 may be a useful marker in the detection of ovarian cancer. Studies are underway to determine if the loss of expression is dependent on tumor grade, stage or other clinically relevant parameters.

Homeobox genes such as HOXA10 dictate cell differentiation. A decrease in HOX gene expression may be a necessary part of the dedifferentiation process seen in carcinogenesis. HOXA10 may be useful as a tumor marker. HOXA10 gene expression may be a beneficial marker of changing physiology of the ovary and perhaps part of the process of oncogenesis.

10. CONCLUSION

Homeobox genes may be useful in the diagnosis and treatment of cancers. First, these genes have unique expression patterns in several tissues and have demonstrated spatial colinearity. This characterization may help to determine the specific cell lineage of primary tumors [52-54]. Second, the expression patterns of these genes remains constant and may be used to identify the origin of metastatic tumors [55]. Third, HOX genes determine and maintain differentiation in all cells. Therefore, decreased HOX gene expression could lead to loss of differentiation which is characteristic of malignancies. Finally, HOX genes may play a role in disease treatment as well as detection. Gene therapy using HOX genes may replace the mutated genes or alter misexpressed genes that lead to malignancy [56].

We are in the process of exploring which other HOX genes are expressed in the ovary and at what level. Preliminary data indicated at least one, HOXA10, is misexpressed in ovarian cancer. Other HOX genes normally expressed in the ovary may likely be misexpressed in ovarian cancer. This data could add to a molecular definition of ovarian cancer and to the treatment and detection of this disease. Increased expression of developmental genes, such as HOX genes, may induce differentiation of these tumors.

REFERENCES

1. McGinnis, W. and R. Krumlauf, Homeobox genes and axial patterning. Cell 1992; 68(2):283-302.
2. Stein, S., et al., Checklist: vertebrate homeobox genes. Mech Dev 1996; 55(1): 91-108.
3. Taylor, H.S., G.B. Vanden Heuvel, and P. Igarashi, A conserved Hox axis in the mouse and human female reproductive system: late establishment and persistent adult expression of the Hoxa cluster genes. Biol Reprod 1997; 57(6): 1338-45.
4. Lewis, E.B., A gene complex controlling segmentation in Drosophila. Nature, 1978; 276(5688):565-70.
5. Sanchez-Herrero, E., et al., Genetic organization of Drosophila bithorax complex. Nature 1985; 313(5998):108-13.
6. McGinnis, W., et al., A homologous protein-coding sequence in Drosophila homeotic genes and its conservation in other metazoans. Cell 1984; 37(2):403-8.
7. Scott, M.P. and A.J. Weiner, Structural relationships among genes that control development: sequence homology between the Antennapedia, Ultrabithorax, and fushi tarazu loci of Drosophila. Proc Natl Acad Sci U S A 1984; 81(13):4115-9.
8. Kissinger, C.R., et al., Crystal structure of an engrailed homeodomain-DNA complex at 2.8 A resolution: a framework for understanding homeodomain-DNA interactions. Cell 1990; 63(3):579-90.
9. Qian, Y.Q., et al., The structure of the Antennapedia homeodomain determined by NMR spectroscopy in solution: comparison with prokaryotic repressors [published erratum appears in Cell 1990 May 4;61(3):548]. Cell 1989; 59(3):573-80.
10. Wolberger, C., et al., Crystal structure of a MAT alpha 2 homeodomain-operator complex suggests a general model for homeodomain-DNA interactions. Cell 1991; 67(3):517-28.
11. Manak, J.R. and M.P. Scott, A class act: conservation of homeodomain protein functions. Dev Suppl 1994: 61-77.
12. Duboule, D. and G. Morata, Colinearity and functional hierarchy among genes of the homeotic complexes. Trends Genet 1994; 10(10):358-64.
13. Ruddle, F.H., et al., Evolution of chordate hox gene clusters. Ann N Y Acad Sci 1999; 870: 238-48.

14. Scott, M.P., Vertebrate homeobox gene nomenclature [letter]. Cell 1992; 71(4):551-3.

15. Duboule, D. and P. Dolle, The structural and functional organization of the murine HOX gene family resembles that of Drosophila homeotic genes. EMBO J 1989; 8(5): 1497-505.

16. Graham, A., N. Papalopulu, and R. Krumlauf, The murine and Drosophila homeobox gene complexes have common features of organization and expression. Cell 1989; 57(3): 367-78.

17. Lumsden, A. and R. Krumlauf, Patterning the vertebrate neuraxis. Science 1996; 274(5290):1109-15.

18. Izpisua-Belmonte, J.C., et al., Murine genes related to the Drosophila AbdB homeotic genes are sequentially expressed during development of the posterior part of the body. EMBO J 1991; 10(8): 2279-89.

19. Davis, A.P. and M.R. Capecchi, A mutational analysis of the 5' HoxD genes: dissection of genetic interactions during limb development in the mouse. Development 1996; 122(4):1175-85.

20. Le Mouellic, H., Y. Lallemand, and P. Brulet, Homeosis in the mouse induced by a null mutation in the Hox-3.1 gene. Cell 1992; 69(2):251-64.

21. Lufkin, T., et al., Homeotic transformation of the occipital bones of the skull by ectopic expression of a homeobox gene. Nature 1992; 359(6398): 835-41.

22. Muragaki, Y., et al., Altered growth and branching patterns in synpolydactyly caused by mutations in HOXD13 [see comments]. Science 1996; 272(5261):548-51.

23. Dolle, P., et al., Disruption of the Hoxd-13 gene induces localized heterochrony leading to mice with neotenic limbs. Cell 1993; 75(3):431-41.

24. Mortlock, D.P. and J.W. Innis, Mutation of HOXA13 in hand-foot-genital syndrome [see comments]. Nat Genet 1997; 15(2):179-80.

25. Warot, X., et al., Gene dosage-dependent effects of the Hoxa-13 and Hoxd-13 mutations on morphogenesis of the terminal parts of the digestive and urogenital tracts. Development 1997; 124(23):4781-91.

26. Devriendt, K., et al., Haploinsufficiency of the HOXA gene cluster, in a patient with hand- foot-genital syndrome, velopharyngeal insufficiency, and persistent patent Ductus botalli [letter]. Am J Hum Genet 1999; 65(1):249-51.

27. Cunha, G.R., Stromal induction and specification of morphogenesis and cytodifferentiation of the epithelia of the Mullerian ducts and urogenital sinus during development of the uterus and vagina in mice. J Exp Zool 1976; 196(3):361-70.

28. Taylor, H.S., et al., HOXA10 is expressed in response to sex steroids at the time of implantation in the human endometrium. J Clin Invest 1998; 101(7):1379-84.

29. Taylor, H.S., et al., Sex steroids mediate HOXA11 expression in the human peri-implantation endometrium. J Clin Endocrinol Metab 1999; 84(3):1129-35.

30. Satokata, I., G. Benson, and R. Maas, Sexually dimorphic sterility phenotypes in Hoxa10-deficient mice. Nature 1995; 374(6521):460-3.

31. Small, K.M. and S.S. Potter, Homeotic transformations and limb defects in Hox A11 mutant mice. Genes Dev 1993; 7(12A):2318-28.

32. Hsieh-Li, H.M., et al., Hoxa 11 structure, extensive antisense transcription, and function in male and female fertility. Development 1995; 121(5): 1373-85.

33. Godwin, A.R. and M.R. Capecchi, Hoxc13 mutant mice lack external hair. Genes Dev 1998; 12(1):11-20.

34. De Vita, G., et al., Expression of homeobox-containing genes in primary and metastatic colorectal cancer. Eur J Cancer 1993; 6: 887-93.

35. Vider, B.Z., et al., Human colorectal carcinogenesis is associated with deregulation of homeobox gene expression. Biochem Biophys Res Commun 1997; 232(3):742-8.

36. Redline, R.W., et al., Expression of AbdB-type homeobox genes in human tumors. Lab Invest 1994; 71(5): 663-70.

37.   Cillo, C., et al., HOX gene expression in normal and neoplastic human kidney. Int J Cancer 1992; 51(6): 892-7.

38.   Anbazhagan, R. and V. Raman, Homeobox genes: molecular link between congenital anomalies and cancer. Eur J Cancer 1997; 33(4):635-7.

39.   Magli, M.C., C. Largman, and H.J. Lawrence, Effects of HOX homeobox genes in blood cell differentiation. J Cell Physiol 1997; 173(2):168-77.

40.   Deguchi, Y., J.F. Moroney, and J.H. Kehrl, Expression of the HOX-2.3 homeobox gene in human lymphocytes and lymphoid tissues. Blood 1991; 78(2):445-50.

41.   Ziemin-van der Poel, S., et al., Identification of a gene, MLL, that spans the breakpoint in 11q23 translocations associated with human leukemias. Proc Natl Acad Sci U S A 1991; 88(23):10735-9.

42.   Yu, B.D., et al., Altered Hox expression and segmental identity in Mll-mutant mice. Nature, 1995 378(6556):505-8.

43.   Borrow, J., et al., The t(7;11)(p15;p15) translocation in acute myeloid leukaemia fuses the genes for nucleoporin NUP98 and class I homeoprotein HOXA9. Nat Genet 1996; 12(2):159-67.

44.   Nakamura, T., et al., Fusion of the nucleoporin gene NUP98 to HOXA9 by the chromosome translocation t(7;11)(p15;p15) in human myeloid leukaemia. Nat Genet 1996; 12(2) :154-8.

45.   Weis, K., et al., Retinoic acid regulates aberrant nuclear localization of PML-RAR alpha in acute promyelocytic leukemia cells. Cell 1994; 76(2):345-56.

46.   Yergeau, D.A., et al., Embryonic lethality and impairment of haematopoiesis in mice heterozygous for an AML1-ETO fusion gene. Nat Genet 1997; 15(3):303-6.

47.   Celetti, A., et al., Characteristic patterns of HOX gene expression in different types of human leukemia. Int J Cancer 1993; 53(2):237-44.

48.   Greenlee, R.T., et al., Cancer statistics, 2000. CA Cancer J Clin; 2000; 50(1):7-33.

49.   Bast, R.C., Jr., et al., A radioimmunoassay using a monoclonal antibody to monitor the course of epithelial ovarian cancer. N Engl J Med 1983; 309(15):883-7.

50.   Jacobs, I. and R.C. Bast, Jr., The CA 125 tumour-associated antigen: a review of the literature. Hum Reprod 1989; 4(1):1-12.

51.   Mutch, D.G., Molecular characteristics of cancers: the way of the future?. Gynecol Oncol 2000; 77(1):8-10.

52.   Scott, M.P., J.W. Tamkun, and G.W.d. Hartzell, The structure and function of the homeodomain. Biochim Biophys Acta 1989; 989(1):25-48.

53.   Holland, P.W. and B.L. Hogan, Expression of homeo box genes during mouse development: a review. Genes Dev 1988; 2(7):773-82.

54.   Redline, R.W., et al., Homeobox genes and congenital malformations. Lab Invest 1992; 66(6):659-70.

55.   Beddington, R.S., A.W. Puschel, and P. Rashbass, Use of chimeras to study gene function in mesodermal tissues during gastrulation and early organogenesis. Ciba Found Symp 1992; 165: 61-74.

56.   Bagot, C.N., P.J. Troy, and H.S. Taylor, Alteration of maternal Hoxa10 expression by in vivo gene transfection affects implantation. Gene Ther 2000; 7(16):1378-84.

Chapter 11

EGF/ErbB RECEPTOR FAMILY IN OVARIAN CANCER

Maihle, N. J., Baron, A. T., *Barrette, B. A., *Boardman, C. H., Christensen, T. A., **Cora, E. M., Faupel-Badger, J. M., Greenwood, T., Juneja, S. C., Lafky, J. M., Lee, H., Reiter, J. L., and *Podratz, K. C.
*Tumor Biology Program, *Department of Obstetrics/Gynecology, Mayo Clinic, Rochester, MN 55905 and **Department of Biochemistry & Nutrition, University of Puerto Rico, Medical Sciences Campus, School of Medicine, P.O. Box 365067, San Juan PR 00936-5067*

1. THE EGF/ErbB RECEPTOR FAMILY

The EGF/ErbB receptor family is comprised of four members: ErbB1, ErbB2, ErbB3 and ErbB4 (Fig. 1). The human EGF receptor (i.e., EGFR/ErbB1) is the prototype in this family, and is distinguished by its ability to interact with a large number of polypeptide growth factors with high affinity (Fig. 2). The two most widely studied members of this ligand family are epidermal growth factor (EGF) and transforming growth factor-alpha (TGF-α). Overexpression of ErbB1 results in ligand-dependent, anchorage independent growth of primary cells in culture (1-4). Although a causative link between perturbation of expression of human EGFR and human cancers has not yet been established, *EGFR* gene amplification and rearrangements have been reported in a variety of human carcinomas, including breast and ovarian cancer. The molecular biology and biochemistry of human EGFR have been studied extensively. The gene encoding this receptor has been isolated and characterized, the promoter region has been mapped, and several transcripts have been identified in normal human tissues (5-10). Furthermore, the biochemical characterization of EGFR has been pioneering in the field of polypeptide hormone receptor research. In 1980, Stanley Cohen and his colleagues demonstrated, for the first time, that the human EGFR expressed intrinsic tyrosine kinase activity (11). Numerous studies have since contributed to our current understanding of the biosynthesis, post-translational processing, and cellular trafficking of this receptor, and these studies have been reviewed (12-14).

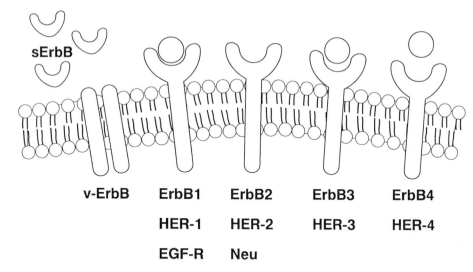

sErbB

v-ErbB	ErbB1	ErbB2	ErbB3	ErbB4
	HER-1	HER-2	HER-3	HER-4
	EGF-R	Neu		

Figure 1. The EGF/ErbB receptor family is comprised of four members. The human EGFR/ErbB1 is prototypic in the family and is structurally homologous to the retroviral oncogene vErbB. ErbB2 is also referred to as HER-2 or Neu. ErbB3 and ErbB4 are the most recently described members of this family. All four members share sequence homology that is highest in the conserved tyrosine kinase region; however, ErbB3, while capable of binding to ATP, is catalytically defective. ErbB2 is distinguished as the only orphan receptor in the family, and recently has been proposed to function solely as a coreceptor for the other ErbB receptors (15). Soluble truncated receptor isoforms also have recently been described (9,10,16-19).

Biochemical studies indicate that the mature form of the EGF receptor is a 170,000 Da protein. This protein is divided by the transmembrane region into two major domains: a cysteine-rich extracellular ligand-binding domain (containing multiple asparagine-linked carbohydrate residues), and an intracellular cytoplasmic domain, which can be further subdivided into a tyrosine kinase domain and a carboxy-terminal regulatory domain (Fig. 2). Several models have been proposed to explain the mechanism of information relay (signal transduction) during/following ligand-binding by this receptor, and most of these propose a conformational change in the receptor followed by receptor dimerization, receptor autophosphorylation, and phosphorylation of exogenous substrates (Fig. 3). Although a conformational change in EGFR structure occurs upon ligand binding, the precise nature of this allosteric change has not been well established. Similarly, although the propensity of this receptor to form dimers (and higher order complexes) has been correlated with ligand binding, it is unclear if the kinase active form of the receptor is monomeric or dimeric (20-27). At this time, no single molecular model for ligand-dependent signal transduction has been established for EGFR. Nonetheless, ligand-dependent signalling by human EGFR is one of the best characterized pathways of signal transduction for any receptor tyrosine kinase. More recently, ligand-independent signalling pathways have been established for oncogenic mutant forms of EGFR and ErbB2 (28-30).

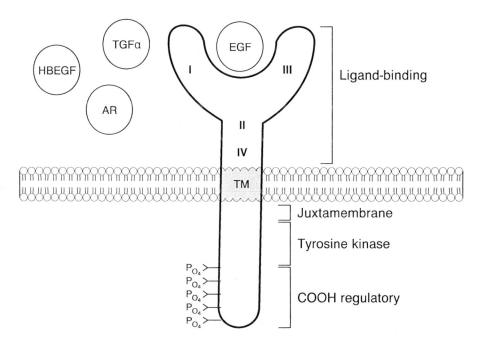

Figure 2. *All four EGFR/ErbB family members share structural similarities, as exemplified in this diagram of the EGFR. Ligands for these receptors typically bind to either the EGFR or to ErbB3 or 4 (heregulins); recently, however, certain ligands have been shown to bind to both EGFR and ErbB4 (e.g., epiregulin, betacellulin) (31,32). Ligand binding to the EGFR involves subdomains I and III of the ligand binding domain. Receptor contact sites for the heregulins have not yet been mapped. The transmembrane domain has been implicated in receptor:receptor interactions (i.e., dimerization). In addition to the kinase domain, the cytoplasmic aspect of these receptors includes key regulatory sequences in both the juxtamembrane and carboxy-terminal regions.*

250

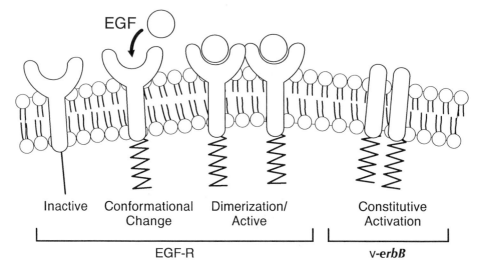

Figure 3. *A model of ligand-dependent EGFR/ErbB receptor activation.*

2. DISCOVERY AND STRUCTURE OF SOLUBLE EGF/ErbB RECEPTORS

Our laboratory was one of the first to report the natural occurrence of truncated/secreted forms of receptor tyrosine kinases (33-35) (Fig. 4). Over the past decade numerous growth factor/cytokine receptors have been reported to have soluble, ligand-binding receptor forms detectable in the conditioned medium of cells in culture and in biological fluids, such as serum and urine. Soluble receptors, i.e., receptors lacking their transmembrane and cytoplasmic domains, have now been reported for ligands as diverse as acidic and basic fibroblast growth factor (FGF), (36) colony stimulating factor (CSF) (37), growth hormone (38), nerve growth factor (39), tumor necrosis factor (40), lutropin/choriogonadotropin (LH/CG) (41), and several of the interleukins (e.g., IL-2, IL-4, IL-6, and IL-7) (42-45). Two mechanisms appear to be responsible for the generation of soluble receptors. One involves the proteolytic processing of full-length receptors. For example, formation of a soluble CSF-1 receptor occurs by proteolytic cleavage and is a down-modulatory response to ligand-binding and protein kinase C activation (37). The other mechanism of generating soluble receptors involves alternative splicing or processing of primary RNA transcripts. Soluble receptors generated by this mechanism include the avian, rat, and human *EGFR* products, human ErbB2 and ErbB3, and the receptors for FGF, LH/CG, and the interleukins (9,10,16-19,33,35,36,41-45).

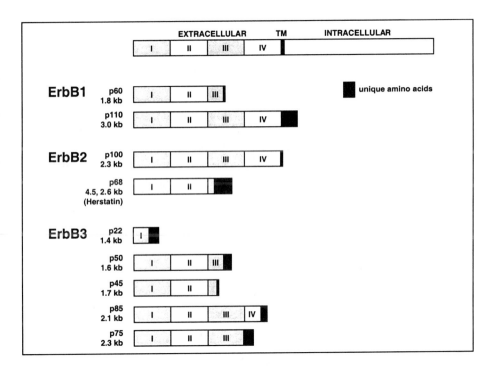

Figure 4. Summary of the structure of the known human soluble EGFR/ErbB receptors (sErbB) that arise via alternative messenger RNA processing/transcription.

In addition, soluble receptors occasionally arise from aberrant transcription products in carcinoma derived cell lines, as exemplified by the truncated *EGFR* product in the human vulvar carcinoma line, A431 (5). In this cell line, the *EGFR* gene is amplified and rearranged, and synthesis of a 2.8 kb transcript is due to a genomic rearrangement resulting in the fusion of DNA sequence encoding the ligand-binding domain (LBD) of the EGF receptor to an unidentified region of genomic DNA (5,46).

3. GROWTH REGULATORY FUNCTIONS OF sErbB RECEPTORS

The widespread distribution of soluble receptors suggests that these molecules may play important physiological roles. Proposed functions include: (*i*) interaction with membrane-bound growth factor precursor molecules; (*ii*) soluble ligand-binding serum proteins (soluble receptors could potentially function as transport molecules and/or as competitive inhibitors of ligand stimulation of the native receptor); (*iii*) receptor down-modulation through proteolytic removal of the LBD (37); (*iv*) modulation of ligand degradation by specific degrading enzymes (47); (*v*) interaction with the extracellular matrix affecting availability/release of growth factors; and (*vi*) regulation of tyrosine kinase activity, perhaps by modulation of receptor dimerization (48). In this regard, Basu and colleagues (48) have demonstrated that the mutant p115 sErbB1 receptor isolated from A431 cells could inhibit the tyrosine kinase activity of the full-length p170 EGFR by forming heterodimers. In these studies inhibition did not appear to be the result of competition for ligand binding or for binding to the active site of the kinase. In addition, Ilekis and colleagues have identified an 80 kDa truncated EGFR in ovarian tumors that was capable of inhibiting EGF receptor autophosphorylation *in vitro* (49). Although it is currently unclear which of these proposed functions for soluble receptors are physiologically relevant to the ErbB family, our laboratory has demonstrated previously that the avian sErbB1 product can block ligand-dependent transformation *in vitro* (35). In addition, sErbB3 can inhibit heregulin-dependent tyrosine kinase activity and cell proliferation in breast carcinoma cells (Lee *et al.*, submitted).

Soluble cytokine receptors recently have been used as potent immunomodulators. For example, systemic administration of soluble IL-1 receptor in mouse allograft recipients (heart) blocks *in vivo* alloreactivity (50); hence, the survival of allograft recipients can be significantly prolonged in mice systemically treated with soluble IL-1 receptor. Similarly, soluble human complement receptor has been used in rats as an inhibitor of complement and as an anti-inflammatory agent (51). In addition, soluble receptors have been used to block systemic infection by HIV-1 (52,53), Epstein-Barr virus (54), and rhinovirus (55). These studies on the neutralizing effects of soluble viral receptors have led to the development of recombinant soluble receptor-immunoglobulin chimeras which have enhanced potency in preventing viral infection, and can function as anti-inflammatory reagents (51). Given the relatively recent discovery of this novel class of truncated receptor molecules, and the rapid establishment of the utility of these soluble receptors as modulators of native receptor function, it is reasonable to predict a significant role for this novel class of growth factor receptors in the development of targeted therapies for selected human malignancies.

4. EGFR/ErbB AND sErbB EXPRESSION IN OVARIAN CANCER

Epithelial ovarian cancer (EOC) is a major women's health problem, as reviewed in this text. Approximately 1 woman in 70 will be diagnosed with EOC in her lifetime, and an estimated 14,500 women will die from this disease in the United States this year. The high mortality rate of EOC is primarily because early clinical symptoms are vague and nonspecific; hence, this disease often goes undetected and untreated until in its advanced stages. Sensitive and reliable methods for detecting earlier stages of EOC are, therefore, urgently needed. EGF/ErbB receptor family members have been shown to play a key role in normal ovarian follicle development, and cell growth regulation of the ovarian surface epithelium (56). It is, therefore, not surprising that overexpression of EGFR, ErbB2, and ErbB3 is common in human ovarian carcinoma-derived cell lines and tumors, and this growth factor receptor family is thought to play a critical role in both ovarian tumor etiology and progression (57-59). Furthermore, EGFR overexpression is associated with disease recurrence and decreased survival in ovarian cancer patients (57). Several studies demonstrate that normal and malignant cells synthesize soluble forms of EGFR in addition to the transmembrane form of this molecule. One 80 kDa truncated EGFR has been reported by Ilekis and colleagues (49). As mentioned above, this protein is capable of inhibiting the autophosphorylation of EGFR *in vitro* (49). Interestingly, the levels of this truncated isoform of EGFR appear to be significantly reduced in metastatic *vs.* primary ovarian carcinomas (49). Together, these observations led us to hypothesize that soluble EGFR (also referred to as sErbB1) levels in human body fluids might be altered during ovarian carcinogenesis and/or tumor progression. We, therefore, developed an acridinium-linked immunosorbent assay (ALISA) to detect sErbB1 in human body fluids (60). In recent studies, we have shown that our ALISA detects a ~110-kDa sErbB1 protein in serum samples from healthy men and women (60). We also have demonstrated that serum p110 sErbB1 levels are significantly lower in EOC patients with stage III or IV disease prior to and shortly after cytoreductive staging laparotomy, in comparison to healthy women of similar ages (61). For those EOC patients who received cytoreductive surgery followed by combination chemotherapy, we have shown that sErbB1 levels increased over time for many patients (61). Our most recent results show that serum p110 sErbB1 levels are significantly reduced in Stage I/II EOC patients, but not in women with different benign pelvic diseases (Baron *et al.,* in preparation). These studies demonstrate that serum p110 sErbB1 levels are significantly different in patients with EOC, and suggest that altered and/or changing serum p110 sErbB1 levels may provide important information useful for the management of patients with epithelial ovarian cancer.

In contrast, elevated serum levels of soluble ErbB2 have been reported in EOC patients with an incidence that ranges from 10-54% (62-67). In addition, McKenzie *et al.* have demonstrated that serum-protein levels of soluble ErbB2 in EOC patients correlate with ErbB2 overexpression in tumors (65). Soluble ErbB2 levels also have been reported to correlate with poor clinical outcomes in patients with EOC (67). Recently, our laboratory has isolated four alternative ErbB3 transcripts from a human carcinoma derived cell line (19). Three of these four alternate ErbB3 products are secreted (19). Moreover, one of the secreted products, i.e., p85 sErbB3, is a potent inhibitor of heregulin-stimulated breast carcinoma cell growth, and may, therefore, be an excellent candidate for the development of novel therapeutics in both breast cancer and EOC patients (Lee et al., submitted). Together, these studies suggest that soluble forms of ErbB receptors may be key regulators of EGF and heregulin stimulated EOC cell growth, and that their expression levels may serve as useful serum biomarkers which have both diagnostic and prognostic utility. In addition, this naturally occurring class of cell growth inhibitors may provide a basis for well tolerated therapeutics targeting receptor tyrosine kinases of the EGF/ErbB receptor family.

5. SUMMARY AND CONCLUSIONS

In summary, the EGF/ErbB family of receptor tyrosine kinases has been shown to play a key role in normal ovarian follicle development, and cell growth regulation of the ovarian surface epithelium. Disregulation of these normal growth regulatory pathways, including overexpression and/or mutation of EGFR/ErbB receptor family members, as well as elements of their downstream signalling pathways, have been shown to contribute to the etiology and progression of epithelial ovarian cancer. It is, therefore, not surprising that these gene products, and their related soluble receptor isoforms may have clinical utility as tumor and/or serum biomarkers of disease activity. Moreover, since several of these soluble receptor isoforms have potent growth inhibitory activity, and are naturally occurring in the circulation, they are ideal candidates for the development of novel therapeutics for the treatment of ovarian cancer patients.

REFERENCES

1. Di Fiore, P.P., Pierce J.H., Fleming T.P., Hazan R., Ullrich A., King C.R., Schlessinger J. and Aaronson S.A. Overexpression of the human EGF receptor confers an EGF-dependent transformed phenotype to NIH 3T3 cells. Cell 1987; 51: 1063-1070.
2. Lax, I., Johnson A., Howk R., Sap J., Bellot F., Winkler M., Ullrich A., Vennstrom B., Schlessinger J. and Givol D. Chicken epidermal growth factor (EGF) receptor: cDNA cloning, expression in mouse cells, and differential binding of EGF and transforming growth factor alpha. Mol. Cell. Biol. 1988; 8: 1970-1978.

3. Riedel, H., Massoglia S., Schlessinger J. and Ullrich A. Ligand activation of overexpressed epidermal growth factor receptors transforms NIH 3T3 mouse fibroblasts. Proc. Natl. Acad. Sci. 1988; 85: 1477-1481.

4. Velu, T.J., Beguinot L., Vass W.C., Willingham M.C., Merlino G.T., Pastan I. and Lowy D.R. Epidermal growth factor-dependent transformation by a human EGF receptor proto-oncogene. Science 1987; 238: 1408-1410.

5. Ullrich, A., Coussens L., Hayflick J.S., Dull T.J., Gray A., Tam A.W., Lee J., Yarden Y., Libermann T.A., Schlessinger J., Downward J., Mayes E.L.V., Whittle N., Waterfield M.D. and Seeburg P.H. Human epidermal growth factor receptor cDNA sequence and aberrant expression of the amplified gene in A431 epidermoid carcinoma cells. Nature 1984; 309: 418-425.

6. Lin, C.R., Chen W.S., Kruiger W., Stolarsky L.S., Weber W., Evans R.M., Verma I.M., Gill G.N. and Rosenfeld M.G. Expression cloning of human EGF receptor complementary DNA: gene amplification and three related messenger RNA products in A431 cells. Science 1984; 224: 843-848.

7. Ishii, S., Xu Y.-h., Stratton R.H., Roe B.A., Merlino G.T. and Pastan I. Characterization and sequence of the promoter region of the human epidermal growth factor receptor gene. Proc. Natl. Acad. Sci. 1985; 82: 4920-4924.

8. Haley, J., Whittle N., Bennett P., Kinchington D., Ullrich A. and Waterfield M. The human EGF receptor gene: structure of the 110 kb locus and identification of sequences regulating its transcription. Oncogene Res. 1987; 1: 375-396.

9. Reiter, J.L. and Maihle N.J. A 1.8 kb alternative transcript from the human epidermal growth factor receptor gene encodes a truncated form of the receptor. Nucl. Acids Res.1996; 24: 4050-4056.

10. Reiter, J.L., Threadgill D.W., Eley G.D., Strunk K.E., Danielsen A.J., Schehl Sinclair C., Pearsall R.S., Green P.J., Yee D., Lampland A.L., Balasubramaniam S., Crossley T.D., Magnuson T.R., James C.D. and Maihle N.J. Comparative genomic sequence analysis and isolation of human and mouse alternative EGFR transcripts encoding truncated receptor isoforms. Genomics 2001; In Press.

11. Cohen, S., Carpenter G. and King L., Jr. Epidermal growth factor-receptor-protein kinase interactions. Co-purification of receptor and epidermal growth factor-enhanced phosphorylation activity. J. Biol. Chem. 1980; 255: 4834-4842.

12. Carpenter, G. and Cohen S. Epidermal growth factor. J. Biol. Chem.1990; 265: 7709-7712.

13. Carpenter, G. and Wahl M.I. The epidermal growth factor family. In Sporn, M.B. and Roberts, A.B. (eds), Peptide Growth Factors and Their Receptors. Springer-Verlag, New York, pp. 69-171, 1990.

14. Prigent, S.A. and Lemoine N.R. The type I (EGFR-related) family of growth factor receptors and their ligands. Prog. Growth Factor Res. 1992; 4: 1-24.

15. Klapper, L.N., Glathie S., Vaisman N., Hynes N.E., Andrews G.C., Sela M. and Yarden Y. The ErbB-2/HER2 oncoprotein of human carcinomas may function solely as a shared coreceptor for multiple stroma-derived growth factors. Proc. Natl. Acad. Sci. USA 1999; 96: 4995-5000.

16. Scott, G.K., Robles R., Park J.W., Montgomery P.A., Daniel J., Holmes W.E., Lee J., Keller G.A., Li W.-L., Fendly B.M., Wood W.I., Shepard H.M. and Benz C.C. A truncated intracellular HER2/neu receptor produced by alternative RNA processing affects growth of human carcinoma cells. Mol. Cell. Biol. 1993; 13: 2247-2257.

17. Doherty, J.K., Bond C., Jardim A., Adelman J.P. and Clinton G.M. The HER-2/neu receptor tyrosine kinase gene encodes a secreted autoinhibitor. Proc. Natl. Acad. Sci. USA 1999; 96: 10869-10874.

18. Katoh, M., Yazaki Y., Sugimura T. and Terada M. c-erbB3 gene encodes secreted as well as transmembrane receptor tyrosine kinase. Biochem. Biophys. Res. Commun. 1993; 192: 1189-1197.

19. Lee, H. and Maihle N.J. Isolation and characterization of four alternate c-erbB3 transcripts expressed in ovarian carcinoma-derived cell lines and normal human tissues. Oncogene 1998; 16: 3243-3252.

20. Yarden, Y. and Schlessinger J. Epidermal growth factor induces rapid, reversible aggregation of the purified epidermal growth factor receptor. Biochem. 1997; 26: 1443-1551.

21. Spaargaren, M., Defize L.H.K., Boonstra J. and de Laat S.W. Antibody-induced dimerization activates the epidermal growth factor receptor tyrosine kinase. J. Biol. Chem.1991; 266: 1733-1739.

22. Spivak-Kroizman, T., Rotin D., Pinchasi D., Ullrich A., Schlessinger J. and Lax I. Heterodimerization of c-erbB2 with different epidermal growth factor receptor mutants elicits stimulatory or inhibitory responses. J. Biol. Chem.1992; 267: 8056-8063.

23. Zhou, M., Felder S., Rubinstein M., Hurwitz D.R., Ullrich A., Lax I. and Schlessinger J. Real-time measurements of kinetics of EGF binding to soluble EGF receptor monomers and dimers support the dimerization model for receptor activation. Biochem.1993; 32: 8193-8198.

24. Biswas, R., Basu M., Sen-Majumdar A. and Das M. Intrapeptide autophosphorylation of the epidermal growth factor receptor: regulation of kinase catalytic function by receptor dimerization. Biochem.1985; 24: 3795-3802.

25. Koland, J.G. and Cerione R.A. Growth factor control of epidermal growth factor receptor kinase activity via an intramolecular mechanism. J. Biol. Chem.1988; 263: 2230-2237.

26. Northwood, I.C. and Davis R.J. Activation of the epidermal growth factor receptor tyrosine protein kinase in the absence of receptor oligomerization. J. Biol. Chem.1988; 263: 7450-7453.

27. Carraway, K.L., III and Cerione R.A. Inhibition of epidermal growth factor receptor aggregation by an antibody directed against the epidermal growth factor receptor extracellular domain. J. Biol. Chem.1993; 268: 23860-23867.

28. Boerner, J.L., Danielsen A.J., McManus M.J. and Maihle N.J. Activation of Rho is required for ligand-independent oncogenic signaling by a mutant EGF receptor. J. Biol. Chem.2000; In Press.

29. McManus, M.J., Boerner J.L., Danielsen A.J., Wang Z., Matsumura F. and Maihle N.J. An oncogenic epidermal growth factor receptor signals via a p21-activated kinase-caldesmon-myosin phosphotyrosine complex. J. Biol. Chem. 2000; 275: 35328-35334.

30. Hung, M.-C. and Lau Y.-K. Basic science of HER-2/neu: A review. Semin. Oncol. 1999; 26 (Suppl 12): 51-59.

31. Riese, D.J., II and Stern D.F. Specificity within the EGF family/ErbB receptor family signaling network. BioEssays 1998; 20: 41-48.

32. Olayioye, M.A., Neve R.M., Lane H.A. and Hynes N.E. The ErbB signaling network: receptor heterodimerization in development and cancer. EMBO J. 2000; 19: 3159-3167.

33. Petch, L.A., Harris J., Raymond V.W., Blasband A., Lee D.C. and Earp H.S. A truncated, secreted form of the epidermal growth factor receptor is encoded by an alternatively spliced transcript in normal rat tissue. Mol. Cell. Biol.1990; 10: 2973-2982.

34. Maihle, N.J., Flickinger T.W., Raines M.A., Sanders M.L. and Kung H.-J. Native avian c-erbB gene expresses a secreted protein product corresponding to the ligand-binding domain of the receptor. Proc. Natl. Acad. Sci.1991; 88: 1825-1829.

35. Flickinger, T.W., Maihle N.J. and Kung H.-J. An alternatively processed mRNA from the avian c-erbB gene encodes a soluble, truncated form of the receptor that can block ligand-dependent transformation. Mol. Cell. Biol. 1992; 12: 883-893.

36. Johnson, D.E., Lee P.L., Lu J. and Williams L.T. Diverse forms of a receptor for acidic and basic fibroblast growth factors. Mol. Cell. Biol. 1990; 10: 4728-4736.

37. Downing, J.R., Roussel M.F. and Sherr C.J. Ligand and protein kinase C downmodulate the colony-stimulating factor 1 receptor by independent mechanisms. Mol. Cell. Biol. 1989; 9: 2890-2896.

38. Baumbach, W.R., Horner D.L. and Logan J.S. The growth hormone-binding protein in rat serum is an alternatively spliced form of the rat growth hormone receptor. Genes Dev 1989; 3: 1199-1205.

39. DiStefano, P.S. and Johnson E.M., Jr. Identification of a truncated form of the nerve growth factor receptor. Proc. Natl. Acad. Sci. 1988; 85: 270-274.

40. Schall, T.J., Lewis M., Koller K.J., Lee A., Rice G.C., Wong G.H.W., Gatanaga T., Granger G.A., Lentz R., Raab H., Kohr W.J. and Goeddel D.V. Molecular cloning and expression of a receptor for human tumor necrosis factor. Cell 1990; 61: 361-370.

41. Loosfelt, H., Misrahi M., Atger M., Salesse R., Vu Hai-Luu Thi M.T., Jolivet A., Guiochon-Mantel A., Sar S., Jallal B., Garnier J. and Milgrom E. Cloning and sequencing of porcine LH-hCG receptor cDNA: variants lacking transmembrane domain. Science 1989; 245: 525-528.

42. Rubin, L.A., Kurman C.C., Fritz M.E., Biddison W.E., Boutin B., Yarchoan R. and Nelson D.L. Soluble interleukin 2 receptors are released from activated human lymphoid cells in vitro. J. Immunol. 1985; 135: 3172-3177.

43. Mosley, B., Beckmann M.P., March C.J., Idzerda R.L., Gimpel S.D., VandenBos T., Friend D., Alpert A., Anderson D., Jackson J., Wignall J.M., Smith C., Gallis B., Sims J.E., Urdal D., Widmar M.B., Cosman D. and Park L.S. The murine interleukin-4 receptor: molecular cloning and characterization of secreted and membrane bound forms. Cell 1989; 59: 335-348.

44. Lust, J.A., Donovan K.A., Kline M.P., Greipp P.R., Kyle R.A. and Maihle N.J. Isolation of an mRNA encoding a soluble form of the human interleukin-6 receptor. Cytokine 1992; 4: 96-100.

45. Goodwin, R.G., Friend D., Ziegler S.F., Jerzy R., Falk B.A., Gimpel S., Cosman D., Dower S.K., March C.J., Namen A.E. and Park L.S. Cloning of the human and murine interleukin-7 receptors: demonstration of a soluble form and homology to a new receptor superfamily. Cell 1990; 60: 941-951.

46. Merlino, G.T., Ishii S., Whang-Peng J., Knutsen T., Xu Y.-H., Clark A.J.L., Stratton R.H., Wilson R.K., Ma D.P., Roe B.A., Hunts J.H., Shimizu N. and Pastan I. Structure and localization of genes encoding aberrant and normal epidermal growth factor receptor RNAs from A431 human carcinoma cells. Mol. Cell. Biol. 1985; 5: 1722-1734.

47. Garcia, J.V., Gehm B.D. and Rosner M.R. An evolutionarily conserved enzyme degrades transforming growth factor-alpha as well as insulin. J. Cell. Biol. 1989; 109: 1301-1307.

48. Basu, A., Raghunath M., Bishayee S. and Das M. Inhibition of tyrosine kinase activity of the epidermal growth factor (EGF) receptor by a truncated receptor form that binds to EGF: role for interreceptor interaction in kinase regulation. Mol. Cell. Biol. 1989; 9: 671-677.

49. Ilekis, J.V., Gariti J., Niederberger C. and Scoccia B. Expression of a truncated epidermal growth factor receptor-like protein (TEGFR) in ovarian cancer. Gynecologic Oncol. 1997; 65: 36-41.

50. Fanslow, W.C., Sims J.E., Sassenfeld H., Morrissey P.J., Gillis S., Dower S.K. and Widmer M.B. Regulation of alloreactivity in vivo by a soluble form of the interleukin-1 receptor. Science 1990; 248: 739-742.

51. Weisman, H.F., Bartow T., Leppo M.K., Marsh H.C., Jr., Carson G.R., Concino M.F., Boyle M.P., Roux K.H., Weisfeldt M.L. and Fearon D.T. Soluble human complement receptor type 1: in vivo inhibitor of complement suppressing post-ischemic myo. 'ial inflammation and necrosis. Science 1990; 249: 146-151.

52. Berger, E.A., Fuerst T.R. and Moss B. A soluble recombinant polypeptide comprising the amino-terminal half of the extracellular region of the CD4 molecule contains an active binding site for human immunodeficiency virus. Proc. Natl. Acad. Sci.1998; 85: 2357-2361.

53. Fisher, R.A., Bertonis J.M., Meier W., Johnson V.A., Costopoulos D.S., Liu T., Tizard R., Walker B.D., Hirsch M.S. and Schooley R.T. HIV infection is blocked in vitro by recombinant soluble CD4. Nature 1988; 331: 76-8.

54. Nemerow, G.R., Mullen J.J., III, Dickson P.W. and Cooper N.R. Soluble recombinant CR2 (CD21) inhibits Epstein-Barr virus infection. J. Virol.1990; 64: 1348-1352.

55. Marlin, S.D., Staunton D.E., Springer T.A., Stratowa C., Sommergruber W. and Merluzzi V.J. A soluble form of intercellular adhesion molecular-1 inhibits rhinovirus infection. Nature 1990; 344: 70-72.

56. Doraiswamy, V., Parrott J.A. and Skinner M.K. Expression and action of transforming growth factor alpha in normal ovarian surface epithelium and ovarian cancer. Biol. Reprod.2000; 63: 789-796.

57. Berchuck, A., Rodriguez G.C., Kamel A., Dodge R.K., Soper J.T., Clarke-Pearson D.L. and Bast Jr. R.C. Epidermal growth factor receptor expression in normal ovarian epithelium and ovarian cancer. I. Correlation of receptor expression with prognostic factors in patients with ovarian cancer. Am. J Obstet. Gynecol. 1991; 164: 669-674.

58. Gullick, W.J. Prevalence of aberrant expression of the epidermal growth factor receptor in human cancers. Br. Med. Bull.1991; 47: 87-98.

59. Salomon, D.S., Brandt R., Ciardiello F. and Normanno N. Epidermal growth factor-related peptides and their receptors in human malignancies. Crit. Rev. Oncol./Hematol.1995; 19: 183-232.

60. Baron, A.T., Lafky J.M., Connolly D.C., Peoples J.J., O'Kane D.J., Suman V.J., Boardman C.H., Podratz K.C. and Maihle N.J. A sandwich type acridinium-linked immunosorbent assay (ALISA) detects soluble ErbB1 (sErbB1) in normal human sera. J. Immunol. Methods 1998; 219: 23-43.

61. Baron, A.T., Lafky J.M., Boardman C.H., Balasubramaniam S., Suman V.J., Podratz K.C. and Maihle N.J. Serum sErbB1 and epidermal growth factor levels as tumor biomarkers in women with stage III or IV epithelial ovarian cancer. Cancer Epidemiol. Biomarkers Prev., 1999; 8: 129-137.

62. Yazici, H., Dolapcioglu K., Buyru F. and Dalay N. Utility of c-erbB-2 expression in tissue and sera of ovarian cancer patients. Cancer Invest.2000; 18: 110-114.

63. Slamon, D.J., Godolphin W., Jones L.A., Holt J.A., Wong S.G., Keith D.E., Levin W.J., Stuart S.G., Udove J., Ullrich A. and Press M.F. Studies of the HER-2/neu proto-oncogene in human breast and ovarian cancer. Science 1989; 244: 707-712.

64. Wu, J.T., Astill M.E. and Zhang P. Detection of the extracellular domain of c-erbB-2 oncoprotein in sera from patients with various carcinomas: correlation with tumor markers. J. Clin. Lab. Anal. 1993; 7: 31-40.

65. McKenzie, S.J., DeSombre K.A., Bast B.S., Hollis D.R., Whitaker R.S., Berchuck A., Boyer C.M. and Bast R.C., Jr. Serum levels of HER-2 neu (c-erbB-2) correlate with overexpression of p185neu in human ovarian cancer. Cancer 1993; 71: 3942-3946.

66. Molina, R., Jo J., Filella X., Bruix J., Castells A., Hague M. and Ballesta A.M. Serum levels of c-erbB-2 (HER-2/neu) in patients with malignant and non-malignant diseases. Tumor Biol. 1997; 18: 188-196.

67. Cheung, T.H., Wong Y.F., Chung T.K., Maimonis P. and Chang A.M. Clinical use of serum c-erbB-2 in patients with ovarian masses. Gynecol. Obstet. Invest.1999; 48: 133-137.

Chapter 12

CRITICAL ROLE OF LYSOPHOSPHOLIPIDS IN THE PATHOPHYSIOLOGY, DIAGNOSIS, AND MANAGEMENT OF OVARIAN CANCER

Gordon B. Mills[1], Astrid Eder[1], Xianjun Fang[1], Yutaka Hasegawa[1], Muling Mao[1], Yiling Lu[1], Janos Tanyi[1], Fazal Haq Tabassam[1], Jon Wiener[1], Ruth Lapushin[1], Shiangxing Yu[1], Jeff A. Parrott[2], Tim Compton[2], Walter Tribley[2], David Fishman[3], M. Sharon Stack[3], Douglas Gaudette[4], Robert Jaffe[5], Tatsuro Furui[6], Junken Aoki[7], and James R. Erickson[8]

1   Department of Molecular Therapeutics, MD Anderson Cancer Center, 1515 Holcombe Boulevard, Houston Texas 77030

2   Atairgin Technologies, 101 Theory, Irvine, California 92612

3   Department of Obstetrics and Gynecology, Northwestern University, 333 East Superior Street, Chicago, Illinois 60611

4   Department Human Biology & Nutrition Science, University of Guelph, ANNU Building, Room 341A, Guelph, Ontario, Canada N1G 2W1

5   Department of Obstetrics, Gynecology and Reproductive Sciences, University of California San Francisco, 513 Parnassus Avenue, San Francisco, California 94122

6   Department of Obstetrics and Gynecology, Gifu University, School of Medicine, 40 Tsukasa-machi, Gifu, Gifu 500-8705, Japan.

7   Graduate School of Pharmaceutical Sciences, The University of Tokyo, 7-3-1 Hongo, Bunkyo-Ku, Tokyo 113-0033, Japan

8   AGY Therapeutics, 290 Utah Avenue, S. San Francisco, California 94080

Abstract: Lysophosphatidic acid (LPA), the simplest of all phospholipids, exhibits pleiomorphic functions in multiple cell lineages. The effects of LPA appear to be mediated by binding of LPA to specific members of the endothelial differentiation gene (Edg) family of G protein-coupled receptors (GPCR). Edg 2, Edg4, and Edg7 are high affinity receptors for LPA, and Edg1 may be a low affinity receptor for LPA. PSP24 has been shown to be responsive to LPA in Xenopus oocytes, however, its role in mammalian cells is unclear. The specific biochemical events initiated by the different Edg receptors, as well as the biological outcomes of activation of the individual receptors, are only beginning to be determined. LPA levels are consistently elevated in the plasma and ascites of ovarian cancer patients, but not in most other epithelial tumors, with the exception of cervix and endometrium, suggesting that LPA may be of particular importance in the pathophysiology of ovarian cancer. In support of this concept, ovarian cancer cells constitutively and inducibly produce high levels of LPA and demonstrate markedly different responses to LPA than normal ovarian surface epithelium. Edg4 and Edg7 levels are consistently increased in malignant ovarian epithelial cells contributing to the aberrant response of ovarian cancer cells to LPA. Edg2 may represent a negative regulatory LPA receptor inducing apoptosis in ovarian cancer cells. Thus, increased levels of LPA, altered receptor expression and altered responses to LPA may contribute to the initiation, progression or outcome of ovarian cancer. Over 40% of known drugs target GPCR, making LPA receptors attractive targets for molecular therapeutics. Indeed, using the structure-function relationship of LPA in model systems, we have identified selective Edg2 antagonists, as well as Edg4 and Edg7 agonists. These lead compounds are being assessed in preclinical model systems. Understanding the mechanisms regulating LPA production, metabolism and function could lead to improved methods for early detection and to new targets for therapy in ovarian cancer.

1. BACKGROUND
1.1. LPA is a Potent Cell Activator

Several different lysophospholipids have been demonstrated to exhibit potent growth-regulatory activity suggesting that this family of molecules may be of equal importance as peptide growth factors in the pathophysiology of cancer (1-26). The bioactive lysophospholipid family includes LPA, sphingosine-1-phosphate (S1P), lysophosphatidylcholine (LPC), sphingosyl-phosphorylcholine (SPC), and platelet-activating factor (PAF) (Figure 1). LPA and the related lysophospholipid sphingosine-1-phosphate (S1P) appear to constitute the major growth-promoting activity present in serum and may contribute, along with insulin-like growth factor 1 (IGF-1), to the ability of serum to promote cell viability (1-4,27). LPA and S1P consist of a hydrophobic fatty acyl chain attached to a glycerol or sphingosine backbone, which has an underivatized phosphate at the *sn*-3 position. LPA has a relatively high solubility in aqueous solutions and is likely to exist in plasma and serum as monomers, carried on proteins such as serum albumin and potentially higher affinity carriers such as gelsolin (28). The hydrophilic nature of LPA suggests that it exerts most of its activity extracellularly. Indeed, microinjection of LPA fails to recapitulate many of the activities of exogenous LPA (1). The fatty acyl chain in LPA can be of variable length and saturation and can be located at the *sn*-1 or *sn*-2 site of the glycerol backbone (1,16). Although *sn*-2 fatty acyl chains can transmigrate to the *sn*-1 site at physiological pH, this is a relatively inefficient process. The generic term LPA thus represents a family of molecules, which, dependent on the fatty acyl chain present and the location of the chain, may exhibit markedly different functions.

261

The ability of LPA to alter cellular functions is highly conserved through ontogeny affecting diverse organisms including dictyostelium, plants, and Xenopus (1-4,16). It however, has no detectable effects in yeast (Saccharomyces) and insect cells (14,16,25,29-31). LPA is a potent regulator of cell growth increasing proliferation and survival in multiple lineages with the exception of neurons where it can apparently induce both necrosis and apoptosis (1-4,16,32). LPA is a critical mediator of ion homeostasis inducing increases in cytosolic calcium which in turn opens chloride channels leading to smooth muscle contraction and neurotransmitter release (1-4,16). LPA also induces Rho-dependent stress fiber and focal adhesion formation through changes in expression of adhesion molecules, and alterations in cell shape and motility (1-4). This cytoskeletal reorganization contributes to retraction of neurites, platelet aggregation and adhesion as well as stimulation of chemotaxis, migration and invasion thus likely contributing to metastases. LPA also regulates the secretion or activation of multiple peptide growth factors including TGFα, TGFβ, heparin-binding EGF (HB-EGF), insulin-like growth factor-II (IGF-II), and endothelin 1 (ET-1) and proteases (13,16,33-40). Thus LPA may alter cellular function both by direct signaling and by the induction or activation of other ligands. The increased production and activity of other ligands likely contributes to the ability of LPA to transactivate tyrosine kinases including Src, the epidermal growth factor receptor (EGFR), the human EGFR family member erbB2/HER2/neu, the platelet-derived growth factor receptor (PDGFR) and insulin-like growth factor receptor I (IGFR I, 33-40).

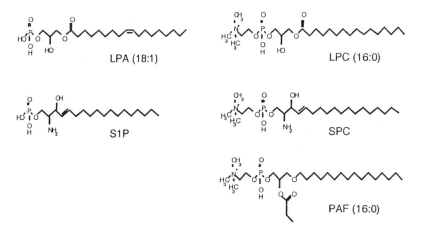

Figure 1. Schematic representation of the structure of LPA, S1P, LPC, SPC and PAF. Note that the structures of these bioactive lysophospholipids are quite similar.

1.2. Signaling by LPA Receptors

LPA binds to specific G protein-coupled receptors (GPCR) of the Edg family and potentially PSP24, leading to activation of pertussis toxin-sensitive and -insensitive $G\alpha/\beta/\gamma$ heterotrimers (1,16,29-31,43-49). As assessed by homology searching, the eight identified Edg receptors likely constitute the complete complement of family members (7). Whether additional non-Edg LPA receptors remain to be identified is unknown. The outcomes of LPA signaling are determined by the spectrum of LPA receptors on the cell surface, the specific G proteins expressed by the cell and the integration of signals from other ligands in the environment.

Edg receptors exhibit high affinity binding for LPA and S1P. Edg1,Edg3,Edg5,Edg6 and Edg8 exhibit a high affinity for S1P, whereas Edg2,Edg4 and Edg7 have a high affinity for LPA (31,35,41-50). Edg 1,Edg3 and Edg5 have been reported to respond to SPC and LPA has been reported to bind to Edg1 (3,44,51-55), however, the low affinity of the interactions questions whether SPC or LPA are functional ligands for these receptors in mammalian cells.

Edg2, Edg4 and Edg7 are broadly expressed with the exception of liver commensurate with the effects of LPA in multiple cell lineages (3-7, 30,42,47). Edg2 and Edg4 are expressed in the brain, indeed, Edg2 was independently identified as ventricular zone gene 1 (VZG1) (3-6,56,57). Edg2 and Edg4 have both been reported to signal through the intracellular small G protein Rho. Edg2, which may be the only Edg capable of activating Rho, initiates Rho-dependent changes in cytoskeletal function including cell rounding, stress fiber formation, and neurite retraction (3-7,43,47). Rho also contributes to increases in cytosolic calcium and inositol trisphosphate, fibronectin production, decreases in cAMP, and activation of PLC and the serum response element (3-7,43,47,58).

The signaling pathways and responses induced by Edg receptors may be determined, at least in part, by the spectrum of G proteins expressed by responding cells. For example, although Edg2 has been reported to mediate increases in cytosolic calcium and activation of extracellular response kinase (ERK), in some cell types Edg2 does not mediate changes in cytosolic calcium or activation of ERK. Similarly, depending on the cell assayed, specific responses to Edg2 or Edg4 can be more or less sensitive to the effects of pertussis toxin (1-9).

The ability to activate ERK correlates with LPA-induced cell proliferation (1). Edg2 and Edg4, but not Edg7, have been reported to couple to ERK (1,30,49). However, in some cell systems, Edg2 does not couple to ERK. Further, our studies suggest that Edg2 may induce apoptosis, questioning its role in inducing cell proliferation (23), making Edg4 and Edg7 the most likely candidates for signaling leading to cell proliferation. We have demonstrated that the ability to activate both the phosphatidylinositol 3-kinase (PI3K) pathway and Ras/ERK pathway contributes to LPA-induced cell proliferation

(19). The ability to activate ERK appears to be the major contributor to LPA-induced maintenance of cell viability (19). Compatible with this model, the p110β isoform of PI3K appears to be required for LPA-induced mitogenesis (59) and is selectively activated by LPA in ovarian cancer cells (not presented). The ability of LPA to activate the PI3K pathway is modulated by the atypical protein kinase C isoforms including PKCζ and PKCι (15). Depending on the cell line analyzed, LPA-induced activation of the EGFR or the PDGR is required for LPA-induced PI3K activation and cell proliferation (33,35,37). Although LPA clearly couples to PI3K in multiple cell systems (19,20,33,59), the Edg receptor(s) involved is not known. Thus the identity of the LPA receptor(s) that mediates cell proliferation remains controversial.

PSP24, originally cloned from Xenopus oocytes (41), is expressed in most cell lineages. Although PSP24 appears to mediate LPA-induced opening of chloride channels in Xenopus oocytes, its functions and signaling pathways and, indeed, whether it is responsive to LPA in mammalian cells, have not been determined.

1.3. LPA Metabolism

Little is known about the mechanisms regulating LPA levels in vivo; however, the low LPA levels in plasma (60) indicate that production, metabolism and/or clearance of LPA are tightly controlled. LPA can be produced by activated platelets, adipocytes, leukocytes, fibroblasts, endothelial cells and, of particular importance, ovarian cancer cells (1,3-7,16,18,61-64). Membrane phospholipids with the exception of phosphatidylethanolamine (PE), which has significant amounts of unsaturated and non-acyl-linked fatty acids at the *sn*-1 position, have mainly saturated fatty acyl chains at the *sn*-1 position and unsaturated fatty acyl chains at the *sn*-2 position. The most likely pathway for LPA production in response to cellular activation is sequential activity of PLD on phosphatidylcholine (PC) producing phosphatidic acid (PA), followed by PLA2-mediated deacylation of PA (1,3-7,16,18,61-64). This would produce LPA with saturated fatty acyl chains at the *sn*-1 position. In contrast to PLA2, PLA1 would produce LPA with unsaturated fatty acyl chains at the *sn*-2 position, which could migrate to the *sn*-1 position. PLA1 may thus contribute to the production of LPA with unsaturated fatty acyl chains and in particular the *sn*-2 fatty acyl chains that selectively activate Edg7 (30,31). PA-specific PLA1 has recently been cloned and is related to phosphatidylserine-specific PLA1 (65, not presented). PLD may play a dual role in LPA production, contributing to the production of PA, the major precursor of LPA, and also contributing to the formation of microvesicles which are targets for secretory PLA2 (sPLA2) (63,64). LPA can induce LPA production (16,18) which may be explained by its ability to activate PLD and PLA2 (1-4,18). An alternative pathway for LPA production would be sequential activity of PLA1 or PLA2 on membrane lipids followed by removal of the head group by lysophospholipase D (lysoPLD). PLD1 and

PLD2 have little or no activity against lysophospholipids with their activity restricted to phospholipids (63,64,66). Although lysoPLD has not yet been cloned, lysoPLD activity has been detected in multiple tissues as well as in rat serum (63,67). The lysoPLD activity in rat serum selectively targets LPC with unsaturated fatty acyl chains (67) potentially contributing to the production of LPA with unsaturated fatty acyl chains.

LPA can be metabolized by being acylated by lysophospholipid acyl transferase (LPAT) or endophilin (63,68,69) to produce phosphatidic acid, which is also bioactive (1,2,69), deacylated by lysophospholipases (LYPL) to produce glycerol phosphate (63-70), or dephosphorylated by lysophosphatidic acid phosphatases (PAP2a,b,c) producing monoacylglycerol (21,63). The cloned LYPL I and II do not have activity against LPA, and indeed are inhibited by LPA (63,70); thus, reacylation and dephosphorylation are the most likely pathways for LPA metabolism. Indeed, overexpression of PAP2 both decreases the amount of LPA associated with the cell membrane and also decreases the effects of LPA on cellular functions (71). In ovarian cancer cells, a gonadotropin-releasing hormone (GNRH)-regulated phosphatidic acid phosphatase is the major mediator of LPA degradation (21). Intracellular and plasma LPA levels are low, and the half-life of LPA is very short (seconds) suggesting that these degradative or resynthetic enzymes are highly active (3,4,60,63, not presented).

1.4. Signaling Requirements for LPA Functions

Table 1 Signaling requirements for LPA functions

Pathways	PI3K AKT	RAS ERK	p38	JNK	PLC PKC
Activation	++	++++	++	+	+++
Proliferation	++++	++++	?	?	?
Survival	+	+++	?	?	?
uPA secretion	+	+	+++	?	?
LPA release	?	?	?	?	?

Pathways	Tyrosine Kinases	PLD	sPLA2	G Proteins
Activation	++	?	?	++++
Proliferation	++++	?	?	++++
Survival	+++	++	?	++++
uPA	+++	-	?	?
LPA release	++++	++	++++	?

Inhibitors used: PI3K: LY294002 and wortmannin, MEK: PD098059, p38: SB203580/SB202190, heterotrimeric G proteins: pertussis toxin, tyrosine kinases: herbimycin, PLD: 1-butanol, sPLA2: OOEPC. uPA = urokinase plasminogen activator, ? = not assessed.

LPA is an efficient activator of the PLC pathway, increasing cytosolic calcium and activation of PKC, the Ras/ERK cascade and p38. LPA is a relatively inefficient activator of tyrosine phosphorylation, the PI3K pathway and JNK (15,16,19). Pertussis toxin-sensitive activation of both the PI3K and Ras/ERK pathways is critical to LPA-induced cellular proliferation (19), whereas the Ras/ERK pathway appears to be sufficient to regulate cell viability, at least in model systems (19). LPA increases phosphorylation of Bax, a critical regulator of cell viability, likely through activation of the Ras/ERK cascade and RSK2. LPA also regulates expression of Bax (72), a critical mediator of apoptosis. LPA-induced survival may be due to activation of the Ras/ERK pathway, potentially through activation of the PDGFR, EGFR and Src (33-35,39). Indeed, decreasing the levels of Src in ovarian cancer cells inhibits LPA-induced proliferation and urokinase plasminogen activator (uPA) production (20). The identity of the specific Edg receptors and G proteins mediating these effects remains controversial.

1.5. Structural Requirements for LPA Signaling

Over 40% of all current drugs target GPCR, with most of the drugs being structural analogs of the cognate ligand. GPCR-specific agonists and antagonists, based on ligand analogs, are also powerful tools in dissecting the functions of individual members of a GPCR subfamily. We have thus begun to explore the structural requirements for the activation of specific Edg receptors to facilitate generation of receptor-selective agonists and antagonists to study the outcome of activation of specific LPA receptors and as potential lead compounds for molecular therapeutics aimed at treatment of ovarian cancer. LPA is the simplest phospholipid with 5 potential key points for structural activity (Figure 1): **1)** the backbone structure, **2)** the *sn*-3 phosphate **3)** the length, saturation and location of the fatty acid chain, **4)** the *sn*-2 hydroxyl, and **5)** the linkage of the fatty acid chain to the glycerol backbone.

As described above, the LPA-responsive Edg receptors are broadly expressed resulting in most mammalian cell lines expressing multiple LPA receptors (1-7). When mammalian cells are studied, it is thus difficult to attribute responses to LPA or LPA analogs to activation of a specific LPA receptor. To define the structural requirements for activation of specific Edg receptors, we have utilized two non-mammalian model systems. The first system consists of transformation of specific Edg receptors into yeast with stably integrated *FUS1::lacZ* or *FUS1::His3* reporters (16,22,29). To complement this system, we have used Sf9 insect cells that do not respond to LPA with increases in cytosolic calcium likely due to the absence of functional LPA receptors (30,31,73). Using the baculovirus system, we have transiently introduced Edg receptors into Sf9 cells and assessed the ability to induce increases in cytosolic calcium. To confirm the results, we have transiently transfected specific LPA receptors into human cell lines lacking specific Edg receptors as assessed by reverse transcriptase polymerase chain reaction (RT-PCR) assays.

Optimal activation of Edg2 by LPA is dependent on the presence of an acyl-linked fatty acid chain of 16-18 carbons, optimally 18:1 or 18:2, however, saturated 16:0 and 18:0 are highly effective whereas shorter carbon chains are inactive or inhibit the function of Edg2 (16,22,29-31,73). Similar activity occurs with the fatty acyl chain being located at either the *sn*-1 or *sn*-2 position. Efficient activation of Edg2 requires a *sn*-3 free phosphate. In contrast, the structure of the *sn*-2 position is not particularly important, with deoxy, methyl and Br derivatives being highly active (16,22,29). This lack of requirement for a free *sn*-2 hydroxyl potentially allows development of relatively selective Edg2 analogs. Activation of Edg2 requires fairly high concentrations of LPA, with IC_{50}s in the high nanomolar to micromolar range in both yeast and insect cells (16,22,29-31,73).

Similar to Edg2, the optimal fatty acyl chain length on LPA for activation of Edg4 is 16-20 carbons. The fatty acyl chain can be located at either the *sn*-1 or *sn*-2 position on the glycerol backbone. In contrast to Edg2, Edg4 is activated by LPA with 14:0 and 12:0 fatty acyl chains making these analogs relatively selective for Edg4 (31). Indeed, short chain LPA functions as a competitive inhibitor of Edg2, potentially increasing the utility of this analog. Edg4 has a much higher affinity for LPA than Edg2, with IC_{50}s in the low nanomolar range in insect cells. As with Edg2, a free *sn*-3 phosphate is critical for activation of Edg4. In contrast to Edg2, a free *sn*-2 hydroxyl is required for optimal activation of Edg4, and the type of linkage of the fatty acid to the glycerol backbone is less important than for Edg2 (16,31). Once again this structural specificity potentially allows the development of Edg4-selective analogs.

Although there is some controversy potentially arising from studies of mammalian cells that express multiple LPA receptors (49), Edg7 is remarkable in its specificity responding only to LPA with unsaturated fatty acyl chains of 16-20 carbons (30,31,73). Further, the location of the double bond is critical suggesting that the length and structure of the fatty acyl chain contributes to the selectivity of binding (31). In contrast to both Edg2 and Edg4, a free *sn*-3 phosphate is not critical for activation. Strikingly, *sn*-2 LPA is much more effective than *sn*-1 LPA in activating Edg7 (31). The IC_{50} for unsaturated *sn*-2 LPA is in the low nanomolar range with unsaturated *sn*-1 LPA being in the high nM range, and saturated LPA in the high micromolar range or not effective (31). LPA with acyl linkages are much more active on Edg7 than those with alkyl or alkenyl linkages (31).

These preliminary structure-function studies potentially point the way to methods to develop receptor-selective analogs. For example, LPA with saturated fatty acids linked to the glycerol backbone will activate Edg2 or Edg4 but not Edg7. 14:0 or 12:0 LPA appears to selectively activate Edg4. Derivatization of the phosphate may allow the development of Edg7-selective analogs. Manipulation of the *sn*-2 site could result in development of Edg2-selective analogs, and altering the fatty acid linkage could contribute to the development of Edg4-selective analogs. It is important in studies of each of these alterations to ensure that the analogs are not so structurally diverse as to activate receptors for other lysophospholipids such as PAF, S1P or SPC.

We have used the structure-function relationship of LPA with specific receptors to develop highly potent, stable Edg7 selective analogs. These analogs efficiently increase cytosolic calcium, viability and proliferation. Indicative of specificity, the analogs do not induce shape changes or alteration in stress fibers (not presented) which has been linked to RhoA, which is activated by Edg2 and Edg4 (3-7,48). As the analogs effectively activate Edg7, Edg7 may not activate RhoA. The analogs are highly active in vivo. This suggests that molecular therapeutics targeting specific LPA receptors may soon be a reality.

Earlier studies noted that lysophosphatidylglycerol (LPG) inhibits LPA-induced changes in calcium and ERK activation (9). Unfortunately, LPG functions as a partial agonist in cell proliferation and cell survival assays, likely through the conversion of LPG to LPA by the action of lysoPLD (not presented).

1.6. Structural Dependence of Activation of Specific Signaling Events and Functional Outcomes by LPA

In mammalian cells, the ability of LPA analogs to activate ERK is dependent on a free hydroxyl at the *sn*-2 position (16). LPA with either an ester or ether linkage retains the ability to activate ERK (16). This structure-function relationship is more concordant with the ability to activate Edg4 than Edg2 (16,31). This is compatible with our observation that transfection of Edg2 into A2780 cells (23) does not alter the ability of LPA to activate the Ras/ERK cascade. Indeed, in several model systems, Edg4 but not Edg2 has been demonstrated to activate ERK. In support of a potential role of Edg4 in activating ERK, Edg7 has been reported to fail to activate ERK in model systems (30,49). The ability of LPA analogs to activate JNK is dependent on a *sn*-1 acyl linkage and not dependent on a free *sn*-2 hydroxyl, concordant with the ability to activate Edg2, but not Edg4 or potentially Edg7 (16,31). This suggests that the pathways leading to activation of JNK are different from those regulating activation of ERK and may involve different LPA receptors.

In contrast to ERK activation, LPA with either acyl or ether linked fatty acids, with or without a free hydroxyl, in the presence or absence of an underivatized phosphate can mediate the cell survival activity of LPA (16). This structural non-dependence does not correlate with the structure-function relationship of any of the LPA receptors. This is also compatible with our recent observation that the cell survival activity of LPA can be mediated by either the PI3K or Ras/ERK cascade (19). LPA analogs, which in model systems selectively target Edg4 and Edg7, can increase cell viability. This suggests that Edg4 and Edg7 may both mediate cell viability with activation of either of the receptors by a specific LPA analog being sufficient. This also underscores the difficulty of attempting to define receptor-specific responses in mammalian cells.

2. LPA IS A CRITICAL MEDIATOR IN OVARIAN CANCER PATHOPHYSIOLOGY
2.1. Ovarian Cancer Ascites Contains *in vitro* and *in vivo* Growth-Promoting Activity, Which is Mediated by LPA

Ascites from ovarian cancer patients contains potent growth factor activity (16,17,74,75). Co-injection of the HEY ovarian cancer cell line with partially purified ascites from ovarian cancer patients increases the ability of the HEY ovarian cancer cell line to grow in the peritoneal cavity of nude mice (75). A short (7 day) treatment with exogenous ascites was sufficient to allow the growth of HEY ovarian cancer cells in the peritoneal cavity (75). The HEY cells-carrying nude mice eventually develop intraperitoneal ascites indistinguishable from that in human patients. This "murine" ascites fluid was also sufficient to facilitate growth of the human HEY ovarian cancer cell line both in vitro and in vivo (75). Strikingly, treatment of mice with human ovarian cancer ascites also induced distant metastases of the HEY ovarian cancer cell line, from 0% to approximately 30%. Thus ascites from ovarian cancer patients not only includes growth-promoting activity but also increases metastatic potential. The growth-promoting activity in ovarian cancer ascites is considerably more potent than that contained in fetal calf serum (16,17,74).

Growth-promoting activity can be detected in all ovarian cancer ascites samples when the samples are assayed at dilute concentrations. However, approximately 1/4 of all ascites samples contains growth inhibitory activity when assayed at high concentrations. This growth inhibitory activity is "dominant" over the growth-stimulatory activity both in vitro and in vivo. The inhibitory activity does not appear to be mediated by TGFβ as the cell line used in the assays (HEY) is not growth- inhibited by exogenous TGFβ.

Ascites from more than 50 patients both increased the proliferation of ovarian cancer cell lines and induced activation of ovarian cancer cells as indicated by the ability to increase cytosolic calcium (74). Ascitic fluid from ovarian cancer patients increased cytosolic calcium in ovarian cancer cells freshly isolated from patients (16,74). The growth factor activity in ascites was designated ovarian cancer growth factor (OCGF) (74,75) whereas the activity that induced changes in cytosolic calcium was designated ovarian cancer activating factor (OCAF) (17). Subsequent purification and characterization, demonstrated that OCGF and OCAF activity are mediated by multiple forms of LPA present in ascites from ovarian cancer patients (16,17,74,75).

2.2. LPA Exhibits Pleiomorphic Activities on Ovarian Cancer Cells

LPA is present at concentrations between 1 and 80 μM in ascites from ovarian cancer patients (16-18,76). This suggests that ovarian cancer cells in the patient are "bathed" in an LPA-rich environment. Indeed, large numbers of ovarian cancer cells (up to 10^9/ml), either as single cells or small clumps, are present in ascites. At concentrations present in ascites from ovarian cancer patients, LPA has marked effects on proliferation of ovarian cancer cells, increasing thymidine incorporation, cell number, and colony formation under anchorage-dependent and -independent conditions (16,17). The increase in cell number is likely due to increased cell cycle entry and progression as well as decreased frequency of apoptosis (16) and anoikis (not presented). In ovarian cancer cells, LPA also contributes to multiple processes critical to the metastatic cascade. LPA induces cytoskeletal reorganization, change of shape, motility and invasiveness. The increased invasiveness is associated with increased production of urinary plasminogen activator (uPA, 13), and the uPA receptor (unpublished) as well as activation of uPA and the MMP2 matrix metalloproteinase. Bypassing anoikis, a form of apoptosis that occurs when cells are dissociated from their underlying matrix, is particularly important for ovarian cancer cells to survive and seed across the peritoneal cavity and to metastasize (77,78). LPA markedly decreases anoikis in ovarian cancer cell lines suggesting that LPA plays a role in preventing anoikis and increasing metastases in vivo. Similar to LPA, vascular endothelial growth factor (VEGF), also known as vascular permeability factor (VPF), is present at high concentrations in ascites (25). VEGF appears to be important both for the accumulation of ascites in the peritoneal cavity of ovarian cancer patients and for neovascularization. LPA is a potent inducer of VEGF production by ovarian cancer cells (14). LPA also increases the levels of mRNAs for multiple growth factors and other important mediators including LPA itself (18, not presented). In some ovarian cancer cell lines, incubation with LPA induces increases in tyrosine phosphorylation of the EGFR, and erbB2/HER2/neu tyrosine kinase-linked receptors (9). In other systems, LPA-induced tyrosine phosphorylation has been demonstrated to be due to LPA-induced processing and activation of HB-EGF by extracellular proteases (34). LPA, at least in the HEY ovarian cancer cell line, decreases sensitivity to cisplatin, the most effective drug in ovarian cancer (10).

LPA increases the secretion, activation and transcription of uPA by ovarian cancer cells, but not normal ovarian surface epithelium (OSE), Large T Antigen (Tag)-immortalized OSE (IOSE) or breast cancer cells (13,20). LPA-induced uPA production is absolutely dependent on functional p38 Hog, and appears to represent a convergence of signaling through the PI3K and the Ras/ERK cascades (20). Tyrosine kinases including Src are required for p38 activation and uPA secretion in ovarian cancer cells. Blocking p70S6 kinase or PLD (20) does not inhibit LPA-induced uPA production. LPA also induces increased expression of the uPA receptor, which focuses uPA activity at the cell surface and contributes to uPA- mediated cell activation and proliferation (not presented). The ability of LPA to increase production and activity of proteases correlates with LPA-induced invasiveness in in-vitro models.

Thus, the pathways by which LPA mediates its pleiomorphic activities in ovarian cancer bifurcate at multiple points. Further, specific LPA responses can be attributed to the relative activation of a particular branch of the LPA signaling cascade. This likely represents activation of specific LPA receptors, selective recruitment of particular G proteins and activation of specific downstream mediators. As ovarian cancer cells express multiple LPA receptors (16,26, Figure 2), it has been difficult to ascertain the role of each of the receptors in responses of ovarian cancer cells to LPA. However, preliminary data using potentially receptor-selective ligands implicates Edg2 in cell motility and cytoskeletal changes, and Edg4 and Edg7 in changes in cytosolic calcium, ERK and PI3K activation, cell proliferation and uPA production. Thus LPA plays a critical role in the regulation of proliferation, viability, drug sensitivity, invasion and metastasis of ovarian cancer cells. Therefore, LPA, its receptors and signaling pathways are potential targets for therapy of ovarian cancer.

2.3. Ovarian Cancer Cells Acquire Expression of Edg4 and Edg7 During Transformation

LPA has modest if any biological activity on normal ovarian surface epithelium (OSE) or TAg-immortalized OSE (IOSE) (13,14,16,18). However, transformation of IOSE by enforced expression of E-cadherin (IOSE-EC, 79) results in acquisition of responsiveness to LPA. OSE and IOSE express Edg1, Edg2, Edg3 and Edg5 mRNA, but have low levels of Edg4 and Edg7 mRNA (13,16,18,23,26, Figure 2). In contrast, most ovarian cancer cells express low levels of Edg1 and Edg5, modestly decreased levels of Edg3, elevated levels of Edg4 and markedly elevated levels of Edg7 mRNA (13,16,18,23,26, Figure 2). HEY, which is unusual in having an activating Ras mutation, has high Edg1 mRNA levels (16, Figure 2). Levels of Edg2 mRNA vary markedly among ovarian cancer cell lines and OSE or IOSE without a consistent pattern (16,23,26, Figure 2). In IOSE and the OV202 and OVCAR3 ovarian cancer cell lines, mRNA levels for Edg2, Edg3, Edg4 and Edg5 correlate with protein levels (26 and not presented). The genetic mechanisms underlying the altered Edg expression by ovarian cancer cells are not known. Expression of Edg1, Edg3 and Edg5 suggests that OSE are primarily S1P-dependent, whereas loss of Edg1 and Edg5 expression, combined with novel Edg4 and Edg7 expression, suggests that ovarian cancer cells have shifted to a LPA-dependent phenotype. However, ovarian cancer cells do retain modest responses to S1P potentially through Edg3 (26,80). Combined with increased secretion of LPA by ovarian cancer cells (16,18), this suggests that ovarian cancer cells, in contrast to OSE, have an autocrine LPA loop. Compatible with this model, IOSE cells are more responsive to S1P than to LPA with respect to proliferation, SRE activation and IGF-II production, and ovarian cancer cells are more responsive to LPA than to S1P (26) while retaining modest responses to S1P (9,80). Further, antibodies to Edg4, in the presence of phorbol esters, can induce cellular proliferation and SRE activation in ovarian cancer cells but not IOSE (26). Thus, the responsiveness of ovarian cancer cells, but not normal ovarian surface epithelium, to LPA is likely a consequence of the novel expression of Edg4 and Edg7.

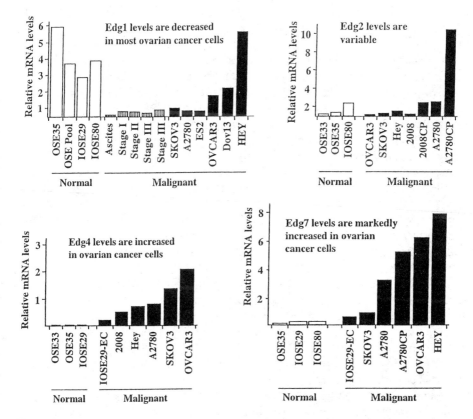

Figure 2. Northern blot analysis of Edg receptor expression in various cell lines and patient samples. Blots were hybridized with ^{32}P-labeled Edg1, Edg2, Edg4 and Edg7 probes using total RNA from the indicated cell lines or patient samples (ascites, stage I-III; Edg1 panel). Edg receptor mRNA was quantitated by PhosphorImager. OSE, normal ovarian surface epithelial cells; IOSE, immortalized ovarian surface epithelial cells; IOSE29-EC, IOSE transfected with E-cadherin. Note that the scales for the relative mRNA levels differ in each panel.

2.4. Structural Dependence of Activation of Ovarian Cancer Cells by LPA

As indicated by the ability to increase cytosolic calcium in ovarian cancer cells, the length and degree of saturation of the fatty acid chain (18:2>18:1>20:4>22:6>18:0>>16:0=14:0) of LPA is critically important (16). Further, LPA analogs with the fatty acyl chain at the *sn*-2 site (18:0, 18:1, 18:2) are consistently more active than their *sn*-1 counterparts (16). Compatible with this structural dependency, *sn*-2 18:2 LPG is the most effective inhibitor of LPA-induced changes in cytosolic calcium in ovarian cancer cells. Analogs with an ester-linked fatty acyl chain are more active than ether analogs (18:1 alkyl LPA). A free hydroxyl is also important for activity with *sn*-2 O-methyl or *sn*-2 deoxy LPA being much less active than LPA itself (16). The concentration-dependence of LPA-induced increases in cytosolic calcium in ovarian cancer cells forms a complex curve suggesting that multiple Edg receptors can induce increases in cytosolic calcium in ovarian cancer cells (not presented). Indeed, desensitization of Edg7 with Edg7-selective analogs only partially inhibits LPA-induced increases in cytosolic calcium in ovarian cancer cells (not presented). Nevertheless, the structure-function relationship of LPA-induced changes in cytosolic calcium, particularly the increased activity of *sn*-2 and unsaturated LPA argues that Edg7 plays a critical role in mediating the effects of LPA on cytosolic calcium in ovarian cancer cells (13,16,18,23,26).

The majority of LPA in ascites has saturated fatty acyl chains (17). However, LPA with unsaturated (18:1) and polyunsaturated fatty acyl chains (18:2, 20:4 and 22:6) are present at high concentrations (17). As treatment with lipoxygenase or PLA2 markedly decreases the ability of ascites to induce increases in cytosolic calcium in ovarian cancer cells (17), the polyunsaturated and *sn*-2 LPA present in ascites are highly active. As Edg2 and Edg4 are equally responsive to LPA with saturated or unsaturated fatty acyl chains at the *sn*-1 or *sn*-2 position, and Edg7 is selectively activated by LPA with unsaturated fatty acyl chains and, in particular, fatty acyl chains at the *sn*-2 position (16,30,31,73), the increased expression of Edg7 by ovarian cancer cells may contribute to the initiation, progression, metastases or pathophysiology of ovarian cancer (16,17).

Taken together, the data argues that targeting Edg7 may result in decreased proliferation and survival of the cancer cells as well as increased responsiveness to therapy thus likely ameliorating the dismal prognosis in ovarian cancer. Nevertheless, it is important to note that ovarian cancer cells express both Edg2 and Edg4, which may bypass the effects of a specific Edg7 inhibitor. While this is likely for Edg4, it is less likely for Edg2, as Edg2 may be a negative regulator (see below). Indeed, our preliminary data suggests that Edg4- and Edg7-selective LPA analogs can induce both increases in cytosolic calcium and proliferation in ovarian cancer cells. Further, Goetzl and colleagues have demonstrated that cross-linking Edg4 on the surface of ovarian cancer cells is sufficient to induce a number of different functional outcomes in ovarian cancer cells (26). Thus targeting Edg7 and potentially Edg4 may prove efficacious in improving the outcome for ovarian cancer patients.

2.5. Edg2 May be a Negative Growth Regulator in Ovarian Cancer Cells

Most normal ovarian epithelial cells express low levels of Edg2 (16,23,26, Figure 2). Some, but not all, ovarian cancer cells express elevated levels of Edg2 (16,23,26, Figure 2). The A2780 ovarian cancer cell line expresses low levels of Edg2 mRNA, whereas the cisplatin-resistant and more slowly growing 2780CP subclone expresses very high levels of Edg2 mRNA and elevated levels of Edg2 protein (16,23, Figure 2). This suggested the intriguing possibility that Edg2 may mediate resistance to cisplatin, compatible with our observation that LPA decreased cisplatin-induced apoptosis in the HEY ovarian cancer cell line (10). Unexpectedly, several stable Edg2-transfectants of A2780 cells did not exhibit altered responses to cisplatin. However, the second phenotype of 2780CP, decreased growth, was recapitulated by overexpression of Edg2. The decreased growth rates of 2780CP and the Edg2-transfectants were due to an increased rate of LPA-independent but fetal calf serum-dependent apoptosis and anoikis (16,23). This effect of Edg2 expression was also seen in the Jurkat T cell line (23). Overexpression of Edg2 by baculovirus-mediated expression in insect cells leads to LPA-independent coupling of Edg2 to Gα (81), potentially due to dimerization of the high number of Edg2 receptors on the cell surface. This is compatible with the observation that Edg2-mediated apoptosis is LPA-independent in 2780CP cells and in the Edg2-transfectants of A2780 (16,23). As the Edg2 LPA receptor may represent a negative growth regulator, the net effect of LPA on ovarian cancer cells is likely determined by the relative expression and activity of multiple receptors. As a corollary, Edg2-selective agonists may inhibit ovarian cancer cell growth and viability.

3. OVARIAN CANCER CELLS ARE RESPONSIVE TO MULTIPLE LYSOPHOSPHOLIPIDS

In addition to LPA, SPC, S1P, LPC, PAF and lysophosphatidylserine (LPS) are potent stimulators of ovarian cancer cells indicated by changes in cell activation or proliferation (9,16,26,80). Several of the bioactive lysophospholipids increase cytosolic free calcium as well as tyrosine phosphorylation of multiple proteins including focal adhesion kinase (FAK) (9,16,80). Whereas LPA induced a significant increase in cell proliferation, LPS did not substantially alter cell proliferation, and SPC inhibited cell proliferation (9). Phosphatidic acid (PA), while not increasing cytosolic free calcium in ovarian cancer cells, increased proliferation (9). Whether this represents conversion of PA to LPA during tissue culture is not known. LPC increases cytosolic calcium in all ovarian cancer cell lines assessed. LPC does not cross-desensitize with LPA suggesting that they utilize different receptors. In contrast to LPA, which is a potent activator of ERK and a weak activator of JNK kinases, LPC is a potent activator of JNK and weak activator of ERK kinases (9,12). While many of the effects of LPA on ovarian cancer cells are sensitive to pertussis toxin implicating Gi, the effects of LPC are generally insensitive to pertussis toxin (9, not presented), suggesting that different pathways are involved, and that the activity of LPC is not mediated by conversion to LPA. Further, the most effective LPC contains a 16:0 fatty acyl chain, whereas 16:0 LPA is relatively inactive providing further support for a lack of inter-conversion of LPA and LPC (12). S1P efficiently induces proliferation of normal ovarian epithelial cells, but is less efficient than LPA at inducing proliferation of ovarian cancer cells (9,26,80). The ability of normal ovarian epithelium to respond to S1P, and the switch to a LPA-responsive phenotype in ovarian cancer cells correlates with the relative expression of S1P-(Edg1,Edg3,Edg5) and LPA-responsive Edg receptors (Edg4,Edg7) on normal ovarian epithelial cells as compared to ovarian cancer cells (13,16,18,23,26). SPC binds to ovarian cancer G-protein coupled receptor 1 (OGR1, 82), which is expressed on some ovarian cancer cells (83,84). OGR1 appears to be a growth-inhibitory receptor despite the ability to induce increases in cytosolic calcium and activation of ERK kinase (82). As described above, LPA and S1P, which only differ in having a glycerol vs. sphingosine backbone (Figure 1) share the Edg receptor family. Likewise, LPC and SPC only differ in having a glycerol vs. sphingosine backbone and are similar in structure to PAF (Figure 1). Thus LPC and SPC and potentially PAF may share a family of GPCR. OGR1 and the related GPR4 (82,84) may be the defining members of a family of SPC and LPC receptors. Thus multiple different lysophospholipids have the ability to activate ovarian cancer cells through specific cell surface receptors.

In addition to elevated LPA levels, LPC (11), SPC (82), and lysophosphatidylinositol (LPI) (85) are increased in ascites or plasma of ovarian cancer patients. Thus not only are ovarian cancer cells responsive to multiple different lysophospholipids, but elevated levels of these lysophospholipids are present in ovarian cancer patients. The coordinate elevation of LPA, LPC and LPI in ovarian cancer patients is most compatible with the initial step in production of LPA being PLA1- or PLA2-mediated cleavage of membrane lipids followed by the action of lysophospholipase D on LPC or LPI producing LPA. As noted above, the primary mechanism of LPA degradation by ovarian cancer cells and potentially other cells is removal of the phosphate group by phosphatidic acid phosphatase producing monoacylglycerol rather than hydrolysis of the acyl linkage producing glycerol-3-phosphate (21) or reacylation producing phosphatidic acid.

4. LPA MAY BE A SCREENING MARKER FOR OVARIAN CANCER
4.1. LPA Levels are Elevated in the Plasma of Ovarian Cancer Patients

LPA is present at high levels in the ascites of ovarian cancer patients (17,18). If LPA migrates from the peritoneal cavity into the circulation, it could be an early diagnostic marker, a prognostic indicator, or a monitor of response to therapy. Our data indicates that LPA levels are higher in ascites than in matched plasma samples (18), indicating that LPA is likely produced in the peritoneal cavity and migrates to the peripheral circulation. As LPA can be produced by platelets during coagulation (62), LPA levels, as a reflection of in vivo concentrations, are preferably measured in plasma, precluding the use of serum banks. However, levels of LPA in carefully collected serum samples may be representative of LPA levels in vivo. Plasma is collected in EDTA tubes to prevent coagulation and activation of calcium-dependent lipases. LPA levels do not change significantly post-collection if samples are collected on ice, processed within 4h of collection and then frozen at $-80^{\circ}C$ allowing assessment of in vivo LPA levels.

In our initial report of purification of LPA from ascites, we noted that LPA levels were elevated in plasma from ovarian cancer patients (17). Dr. Yan Xu and colleagues, using the thin layer chromatography (TLC)-gas chromatograph (GC) assay developed to assess LPA levels in ascites (17), and a electrospray ionization mass spectrometry analysis of a limited number of patient samples (60,85), suggest that LPA levels are elevated in patients with advanced ovarian cancer and, with very small sample numbers, early, curable ovarian cancer (>90%). A smaller proportion of patients with benign intraperitoneal tumors, renal dialysis patients, endometrial cancer, cervical cancer, and multiple myeloma (60,76,85-87), all of which can be distinguished from ovarian cancer by medical management, may have elevated levels of LPA. LPA levels do not appear to be significantly elevated in several other major cancers including breast, bowel, lung and leukemia.

In collaboration with Atairgin Technologies, we have utilized an enzyme-based assay that gives highly sensitive, specific and reproducible LPA quantification. LPA in plasma is converted to glycerol-3-phosphate (G3P) by incubation with bacterial lysophospholipase. G3P is detected using a second enzymatic reaction, providing a second level of specificity. Endogenous G3P, which is present in plasma at low levels, can be removed by solid-phase extraction, enzymatic pre-treatment or subtracted as reaction background without addition of the lysophospholipase. Product is detected spectrophotometrically in an ELISA reader or standard clinical chemistry machines making the assay readily applicable to high throughput screening. Preliminary results demonstrate that the assay has a sensitivity of 0.1 µM, a linear range of 0.1-30 µM, an intra-assay variability of approximately 4% and an inter-assay variability of approximately 6%. The enzymatic assay shows greater than 1000-fold selectivity for LPA as compared to PA, with no detectable activity on other phospholipids or lysophospholipids. The enzymatic reaction generates a similar separation of patients from controls as does TLC-GC or ion spray mass spectrometry. An enzyme assay using PAP2a and detection of phosphate release shows similar operating characteristics (Andrew Morris, Stoneybrook, personal communication).

In stage I ovarian cancer, where the cure rate is greater than 90%, CA125 is elevated in only 50% of patients (88). In preliminary experiments using the enzymatic reaction, LPA levels are elevated in more than 80% of stage I ovarian cancer patients with a false positive rate of under 5%. Surprisingly, there is no obvious stage distribution for LPA levels (not presented, 60). Further, in contrast to CA125 levels, which are higher prior to menopause, there is no obvious age distribution for LPA levels in normal healthy women. LPA levels are elevated in ovarian cancer patients with normal CA125 levels, suggesting that the two assays may be complementary.

4.2. Mechanisms for Increased LPA Levels in Ovarian Cancer Patients

Ovarian cancer ascites contains LPA with both saturated (61%) and unsaturated (39%) fatty acyl chains located at the *sn*-1 or *sn*-2 position of the glycerol backbone (17). As noted above, most membrane phospholipids (with the exception of phosphatidylethanolamine, significant amounts of polyunsaturated fatty acyl chains at the *sn*-1 position) primarily have saturated fatty acyl chains at the *sn*-1 position and unsaturated fatty acyl chains at the *sn*-2 position. Thus, PLA2-mediated hydrolysis of membrane phospholipids followed by lysoPLD activity would produce a *sn*-1 LPA with primarily saturated fatty acyl chains. In contrast, PLA1 would produce a *sn*-2 LPA with primarily polyunsaturated fatty acyl chains. As *sn*-2 fatty acyl chains undergo a pH-dependent migration to the *sn*-1 position, PLA1-mediated cleavage could contribute to the production of *sn*-1 LPA with unsaturated fatty acyl chains. Therefore, both PLA1 and PLA2 likely contribute to the production of LA in ovarian cancer cells.

Ovarian cancer cell lines constitutively secrete almost 6 times more LPA than breast cancer cell lines cultured under the same conditions (18). The SKOV3 cancer cell line is particularly remarkable in that LPA is the major phospholipid in cell supernatants (18). Compatible with ovarian cancer cells contributing to the elevated LPA levels in ovarian cancer patients, LPA levels are on average 4-fold higher in ascites than in plasma, and higher in ascites than in matched plasma samples (18). LPA (OVCAR3) (18) or phorbol esters (HEY, OCC1) (61) increase the release of LPA from ovarian cancer cell lines, but not from breast cancer cell lines. In contrast, normal ovarian epithelial cells and TAg-immortalized normal ovarian epithelial cells produce much lower levels of LPA than do ovarian cancer cells, and exogenous LPA does not increase LPA production (18).

Constitutive and LPA-induced LPA production by ovarian cancer cells is dependent on functional PLD (18). Group IB (pancreatic) sPLA2 plays a critical role in both constitutive and LPA-induced LPA production, whereas Group IIA (synovial) sPLA2 contributes to LPA-induced LPA production only. Cytosolic PLA2s contribute to constitutive LPA synthesis but not LPA-induced LPA formation (18), in contrast to phorbol ester-induced LPA release, which is dependent on cytosolic PLA2 (61). Although the enzymes involved in LPA production are beginning to be characterized, the underlying genetic events remain elusive.

5. SUMMARY

During transformation, ovarian cancer cells acquire the ability to produce LPA and increase the expression of the Edg4 and Edg7 receptors for LPA. Novel receptor expression and LPA production result in the formation of an autocrine and potentially paracrine LPA loop resulting in increased proliferation, viability and metastatic capability. The ability to respond to and produce LPA, at least in in-vitro models of ovarian cancer, appears to be acquired at the step between immortalization and transformation (4,13,16). The presence of high levels of LPA in the ascites of ovarian cancer patients (17) also argues for a major role of LPA in the pathophysiology of ovarian cancer. This suggests that LPA production and metabolism are potential targets for therapy. Further, as over 40% of all drugs in current use target GPCR, LPA receptors are ready targets for development of molecular therapeutics. Indeed, studies from several different laboratories (16,29-31,47,56,57,89) have begun to define the structure-function relationships of specific LPA receptors. The efficacy and toxicity of potential therapeutic mediators will likely be determined by the necessity of the pathways in malignant cells, the distribution of the receptors on normal tissues (56), particularly in the brain, and the redundancy of the pathways activated. In addition to being a potential therapeutic target, LPA may play a role in early diagnosis and monitoring response to therapy. Additional studies of other lysophospholipids in ovarian and other cancers may demonstrate similar critical roles.

ACKNOWLEDGMENTS

These studies are supported by PO1 CA64602 to GBM and by Sponsored Research Grants to X.F. and D.G. from Atairgin Technologies, Irvine, California.

REFERENCES

1. Moolenaar W, Jalink K, and Van Corven E. Lysophosphatidic Acid: A bioactive phospholipid with growth factor-like properties Rev Physiol Biochem Pharmacol 1992; 119:47-65.
2. Tigyi G and Miledi R. Lysophosphatidinates bound to serum albumin activate membrane currents in *Xenopus Iaevis* oocytes and neurite retraction in PC12 pheochromocytoma cells. J Biol Chem 1992; 267:21360-21367.
3. Goetzl EJ, An S. Diversity of cellular receptors and functions for the lysophospholipid growth factor lysophosphatidic acid and shingosine 1-phosphate. FASEB J 1998.
4. Nietgen GW, Durieux ME. Intercellular Signaling By Lysophosphatidate recent developments. Cell Adhesions and Comm 1998; 5:221-235.
5. Moolenaar WH. Bioactive lysophospholipids and their G protein-coupled receptors. Exp Cell Res 1999; 253(1):230-38.
6. Chun J, Contos JJ, Munroe D. A growing family of receptor genes for lysophosphatidic acid (LPA) and other lysophospholipids (LPs). Cell Biochem Biophys 1999; 30(2):213-42.
7. Lynch KR, Im I. Life on the edg. Trends Pharmacol Sci 1999; 20(12):473-75.
8. Xu Y, Casey G, Mills GB. Effect of lysophospholipids on signaling in the human Jurkat T cell line. J Cell Physiol 1995; 163(3):441-450.
9. Xu Y, Fang XF, Casey G, and Mills GB. Lysophospholipids activate ovarian and breast cancer cells Biochem J 1995; 309:933-940.
10. Frankel A, and Mills G.B. Peptide and lipid growth factors decrease cisplatin-induced cell death in human ovarian cancer cells Clinical Cancer Res 1996; 2:1307-1313.
11. Okita M, Gaudette DC, Mills GB and Holub BJ. Elevated levels of plasma lysophosphatidylcholine (LysoPC) in ovarian cancer patients. Int J Cancer 1997; 71:31-34.
12. Fang XJ, Gibson S, Flowers M, Furui T, Bast RC and Mills GB. Lysophosphatidylcholine stimulates AP-1 and the c-Jun N-terminal kinase activity. J Biol Chem 1997; 272:13683-13689.
13. Pustilnik TB, Estrella V, Wiener J, Mao M, Eder A, Watt MAV, Bast RC, and Mills GB. Lysophosphatidic acid induces urokinase secretion in ovarian cancer cells. Clinical Cancer Research 1999; 5:3704-10.
14. Hu YL, Goetzl EJ, Mills GB, Ferrara N, and Jaffe RB. Induction of vascular endothelial growth factor expression by lysophosphatidic acid in normal and neoplastic human ovarian epithelial cells Submitted, 2000.
15. Mao M, Fang XJ, Lu Y, Lapushin R, Bast RC, and Mills GB. Inhibition of growth factor-induced phosphorylation and activation of PKB/AKT by atypical PKCζ in breast cancer cells Biochem J. In press, 2000.
16. Fang XJ, Gaudette D, Furui T, Mao M, Estrella V, Eder A, Putstilnik T, Sasagawa T, Lapushin R, Yu S, Jaffe R, Wiener J, Erickson J, and Mills GB. Lysophospholipid growth factors in the initiation, progression, metastases and management of ovarian cancer. Annals of the New York Academy of Science 2000; 95:188-208.
17. Xu Y, Gaudette D, Boynton JD, Frankel A, Fang XJ, Sharma A, Hurteau J, Casey G, Goodbody A, Mellors A, Holub B and Mills GB. Characterization of an ovarian cancer activating factor (OCAF) in ascites from ovarian cancer patients Clin Canc Res 1995; 1:1223-1232.

18. Eder A, Sasagawa T, Mao M, Aoiki J, Mills G. Constitutive and LPA induced LPA production: Role of PLD and PLA2 Clinical Cancer Research: In press, 2000.

19. Fang XJ, Yu S, Lapushin R, Lu Y, Furui T, Penn LZ, Stokoe DF, Erickson JR, Bast RC, and Mills GB. Lysophosphatidic acid prevents apoptosis in fibroblasts through Gi Protein-mediated activation of mitogen-activated protein kinase Biochem J 2000; 6:2482-2491.

20. Estrella V, Pustilnik T, Claret FX, Gallick GE, Mills GB, and Wiener JR. Lysophosphatidic acid induction of urokinase plasminogen activator secretion requires activation of the p38^{MAPK} pathway. Submitted 2000.

21. Imai A, Furui T, Tamaya T, and Mills GB. A gonadotropin-releasing hormone-responsive phosphatase hydrolyses lysophosphatidic acid within the plasma membrane of ovarian cancer cells J. Clin Endrocrinol Metab 2000; 85:3370-3375.

22. Erickson JR, Espinal G, and Mills GB. Analysis of the Edg2 receptor based on the structure/activity relationship of LPA. Annals of the New York Academy of Science 2000; 905:279-81.

23. Furui T, LaPushin R, Mao M, Kahn H, Watt SR, Watt MV, Lu Y, Fang XJ, Tsutusi S, Siddik Z, Bast R, and Mills GB. Overexpression of Edg-2/vzg-1 induces apoptosis and anoikis in ovarian cancer cells in a lysophosphatidic acid independent manner. Clinical Cancer Research 1999; 5:4308-4318.

24. Spiegel S. Sphingosine 1-phosphate: a ligand for the EDG-1 family of G-protein-coupled receptors. Ann N Y Acad Sci 2000; 905:54-60.

25. Zebrowski BK, Liu W, Ramirez K, Akagi MD, Mills GB, Ellis LM. Markedly elevated levels of vascular endothelial growth factor in malignant ascites: Ann Surg Oncol 1999; 6:373-8.

26. Goetzl EJ, Dolezalova H, Kong Y, Hu YL, Jaffe RB, Kalli KR, Conover CA. Distinctive expression and functions of the type 4 endothelial differentiation gene-encoded G protein-coupled receptor for lysophosphatidic acid in ovarian cancer. Cancer Res 1999; 59:5370-5375.

27. Shi Y, Wang R, Sharma A, Gao C, Wasfy G, Collins M, Penn L, and Mills GB. Dissociation of cytokine signals for proliferation and apoptosis J Immunol 1997; 159:5318-5328.

28. Goetzl EJ, Lee H, Dolezalova H, Kalli KR, Conover CA, Hu YL, Azuma T, Stossel TP, Karliner JS, Jaffe RB.Mechanisms of lysolipid phosphate effects on cellular survival and proliferation. Ann N Y Acad Sci 2000; 905:177-87.

29. Erickson JR, Wu JJ, Goddard JG, et al. Edg-2/Vzg-1 couples to the yeast pheromone response pathway selectively in response to lysophosphatidic acid. J Biol Chem 1998; 273(3):1506-10.

30. Bandoh K, Aoki J, Hosono H, Kobayashi S, Kobayashi T, Murakami-Murofushi K, Tsujimoto M, Arai H, Inoue K. Molecular cloning and characterization of a novel human G-protein-coupled receptor, Edg7, for lysophosphatidic acid. J Biol Chem 1999; 274:1-10.

31. Bandoh K, Aoki J, Taira A, Tsujimoto M, Arai H, Inoue K. Lysophosphatidic acid (LPA) receptors of the EDG family are differentially activated by LPA species. Structure-activity relationship of cloned LPA receptors. FEBS Lett 2000; 478(1-2):159-65.

32. Holtsberg FW, Steiner MR, Bruce-Keller AJ, Keller JN, Mattson MP, Moyers JC, Steiner SM.Lysophosphatidic acid and apoptosis of nerve growth factor-differentiated PC12 cells. J Neurosci Res 1998; 53(6):685-96.

33. Laffargue M, Raynal P, Yart A, Peres C, Wetzker R, Roche S, Payrastre B, Chap H. An epidermal growth factor receptor/Gab1 signaling pathway is required for activation of phosphoinositide 3-kinase by lysophosphatidic acid. J Biol Chem 1999; 274(46):32835-41.

34. Prenzel N, Zwick E, Daub H, Leserer M, Abraham R, Wallasch C, Ullrich A. EGF receptor transactivation by G-protein-coupled receptors requires metalloproteinase cleavage of proHB-EGF. Nature 1999; 402(6764):884-88.

35. Goppelt-Struebe M, Fickel S, Reiser CO. The platelet-derived-growth-factor receptor, not the epidermal-growth-factor receptor, is used by lysophosphatidic acid to activate p42/44 mitogen-activated protein kinase and to induce prostaglandin G/H synthase-2 in mesangial cells. Biochem J 2000; 345(Pt 2):217-24.

36. Goetzl EJ, Dolezalova H, Kong Y, Zeng L. Dual mechanisms for lysophospholipid induction of proliferation of human breast carcinoma cells. Cancer Research 1999; 59:4732-37.

37. Herrlich A, Daub H, Knebel A, Herrlich P, Ullrich A, Schultz G, Gudermann T. Ligand-independent activation of platelet-derived growth factor receptor is a necessary intermediate in lysophosphatidic, acid-stimulated mitogenic activity in L cells. Proc natl Acad Sci USA 1998; 95:8985-90.

38. Chua CC, Hamdy RC, Chua BHL. Upregulation of endothelin-1 production by lysophosphatidic acid in rat aortic endothelial cells. Biochimica et Biophysica Acta 1998; 1405:29-34.

39. Luttrell LM, Hawes BE, van Biesen T, Luttrell DK, Lansing TJ, Lefkowitz RJ. Role of c-Src tyrosine kinase in G protein-coupled receptor- and Gβγ subunit-mediated activation of mitogen-activated protein kinases. J Biol Chem 1996; 271(32):19443-50.

40. Nakano T, Raines EW, Abraham JA, Klagsbrun M, Ross R. Lysophosphatidylcholine upregulates the level of heparin-binding epidermal growth factor-like growth factor mRNA in human monocytes. Proc Natl Acad Sci USA 1994; 91:1069-73.

41. Guo Z, Liliom K, Fischer DJ, et al. Molecular cloning of a high-affinity receptor for the growth factor-like lipid mediator lysophosphadic acid from Xenopus oocytes. Proc Natl Acad Sci USA 1996; 93(25):14367-72.

42. Hecht JH, Weiner JA, Post SR, et al. Ventricular zone gene-1 (vzg-1) encodes a lysophosphatadic acid receptor expressed in neurogenic regions of the developing cerebral cortex. J Cell Biol 1996; 135(4):1071-83.

43. Fukushima N, Kimura Y, Chun J. A single receptor encoded by vzg-1/lpA1/edg-2 couples to G proteins and mediates multiple cellular responses to lysophosphatic acid. Proc Natl Acad Sci USA 1998; 95:6151-6.

44. Lee MJ, Thangada S, Liu CH, et al. Lysophosphatidic acid stimulates the G-protein-coupled receptor EDG-1 as a low affinity agonist. J Biol Chem 1998; 273: 22105-12.

45. Graler MH, Bernhardt G, Lipp M. EDG6, a Novel G-Protein-Coupled Receptor Related to Receptors for Bioactive Lysophospholipids, Is Specifically Expressed in Lymphoid Tissue. Genomics 1998; 53:164-169.

46. Lee MJ, Van Brocklyn JR, Thangada S, et al. Sphingosine-1-phosphate as a ligand for the G protein-coupled receptor EDG-1. Science 1998; 279(5356):1552-5.

47. Fischer DJ, Liliom K, Guo Z, et al. Naturally Occurring Analogs of Lysophosphatidic Acid Elicit Different Cellular Responses through Selective Activation of Multiple Receptor Subtypes. Mol Pharmocol 1998; 54:979-988.

48. An S, Bleu T, Zheng Y, et al. Recombinant Human G Protein-Coupled Lysophosphatidic Acid Receptors Mediate Intracellular Calcium Mobilization. Mol Pharmocol 1998; 54:881-888.

49. Im DS, Heise CE, Harding MA, George SR, O'Dowd BF, Theodorescu D, Lynch KR. Molecular cloning and characterization of a lysophosphatidic acid receptor, Edg-7, expressed in prostate. Mol Pharmacol 2000; 57:753-9.

50. Im DS, Heise CE, Ancellin N, O'Dowd BF, Shei GJ, Heavens RP, Rigby MR, Hla T, Mandala S, McAllister G, George SR, Lynch KR.Characterization of a novel sphingosine 1-phosphate receptor, Edg-8. J Biol Chem 2000; 275(19):14281-6.

51. Ancellin N, Hla T.Differential pharmacological properties and signal transduction of the sphingosine 1-phosphate receptors EDG-1, EDG-3, and EDG-5. J Biol Chem 1999; 274(27):18997-9002.

52. Windh RT, Lee MJ, Hla T, An S, Barr AJ, Manning DR.Differential coupling of the sphingosine 1-phosphate receptors Edg-1, Edg-3, and H218/Edg-5 to the G(i),G(q), and G(12) families of heterotrimeric G proteins. J Biol Chem 1999; 274(39):27351-8.

53. Okamoto H, Takuwa N, Yatomi Y, Gonda K, Shigematsu H, Takuwa Y.EDG3 is a functional receptor specific for sphingosine 1-phosphate and sphingosylphosphorylcholine with signaling characteristics distinct from EDG1 and AGR16. Biochem Biophys Res Commun 1999; 260(1):203-8.

54. Okamoto H, Takuwa N, Gonda K, Okazaki H, Chang K, Yatomi Y, Shigematsu H, Takuwa Y.EDG1 is a functional sphingosine-1-phosphate receptor that is linked via a Gi/o to multiple signaling pathways, including phospholipase C activation, Ca2+ mobilization, RAS-mitogen-activated protein kinase activation, and adenylate cyclase inhibition. J Biol Chem 1998; 273(42):27104-10.

55. Sato K, Kon J, Tomura H, Osada M, Murata N, Kuwabara A, Watanabe T, Ohta H, Ui M, Okajima F. Activation of phospholipase C-Ca2+ system by sphingosine 1-phosphate in CHO cells transfected with Edg-3, a putative lipid receptor. FEBS Lett 1999; 443(1):25-30.

56. Beer MS, Stanton JA, Salim K, Rigby M, Heavens RP, Smith D, Mcallister G. EDG receptors as a therapeutic target in the nervous system. Ann N Y Acad Sci 2000; 905:118-31.

57. Chun J, Weiner JA, Fukushima N, Contos JJ, Zhang G, Kimura Y, Dubin A, Ishii I, Hecht JH, Akita C,Kaushal D.Neurobiology of receptor-mediated lysophospholipid signaling. From the first lysophospholipid receptor to roles in nervous system function and development. Ann N Y Acad Sci 2000; 905:110-7.

58. Peyruchaud O, Mosher DF. Differential stimulation of signaling pathways initiated by Edg-2 in response to lysophosphatidic acid or sphingosine-1-phosphate. Cell Mol Life Sci 2000; 57:1109-16.

59. Roche S, Downward J, Raynal P, Courtneidge SA. A function of phosphatidylinositol 3-kinase β (p85α -p110β) in fibroblasts during mitogenesis: requirement for insulin- and lysophosphatidic acid-mediated signal transduction. Molecular and Cellular Biology 1998; 18:7119-7129.

60. Xu Y, Shen Z, Wiper DW, Wu M, Morton RE, Elson P, Kennedy AW, Belinson J, Markman M, Casey G. Lysophosphatidic acid as a potential biomarker for ovarian and other gynecologic cancers. JAMA 1998; 280(8):719-723.

61. Shen Z, Belinson J, Morton RE, et al. Phorbol 12-myristate 13-acetate stimulates lysophosphatidic acid secretion from ovarian and cervical cancer cells but not from breast or leukemia cells. Gyneco Oncol 1998; 71:364-8.

62. Gerrard, J.M. and Robinson, P. Identification of the molecular species of lysophosphatidic acid produced when platelets are stimulated by thrombin. Biochimica et Biophysica Acta 1989; 1001:282-285.

63. Wang A, Dennis EA. Review mammalian lysophospholipases. Biochimica et Biophysica Acta 1999; 1439:1-16.

64. Fourcade O, Simon MF, Viode C, Rugani N, Leballe F, Ragab A, Fournie B, Sarda L, Chap H. Secretory phospholipase A_2 generates the novel lipid mediator lysophosphatidic acid in membrane microvesicles shed from activated cells. Cell 1995; 80:919-27.

65. Sato T, Aoki J, Nagai Y, Dohmae N, Takio K, Doi T, Arai H, Inoue K. Serine phospholipid-specific phospholipase A that is secreted from activated platelets. A new member of the lipase family. J Biol Chem. 1997; 272:2192-8.

66. Waite M. The PLD superfamily: insights into catalysis. Biochim Biophys Acta 1999; 1439:187-97.

67. Tokumura A, Nishioka Y, Yoshimoto O, Shinomiya J, Fukuzawa K. Substrate specificity of lysophospholipase D which produces bioactive lysophosphatidic acids in rat plasma. Biochim Biophys Acta 1999; 1437(2):235-45.

68. Sugimoto H, Yamashita S. Purification, characterization, and inhibition by phosphatidic acid of lysophospholipase transacylase from rat liver. J Biol Chem 1994; 269(8):6252-58.

69. Schmidt A, Wolde M, Thiele C, Fest W, Kratzin H, Podtelejnikov AV, Witke W, Huttner WB, Soling HD. Endophilin I mediates synaptic vesicle formation by transfer of arachidonate to lysophosphatidic acid. Nature 1999; 401(6749):133-41.

70. Wang A, Deems RA, Dennis EA. Cloning, expression, and catalytic mechanism of murine lysophospholipase I. J Biol Chem 1997; 272(19):12723-29.

71. Xu J, Love LM, Singh I, Zhang QX, Dewald J, Wang DA, Fischer DJ, Tigyi G, Berthiaume LG, Waggoner DW, Brindley DN. Lipid phosphate phosphatase-1 and Ca2+ control lysophosphatidate signaling through EDG-2 receptors. J Biol Chem 2000; 275:27520-30.

72. Goetzl EJ, Kong Y, Mei B. Lysophosphatidic acid and sphingosine 1-phosphate protection of T cells from apoptosis in association with suppression of Bax. J Immunol 1999; 162(4):2049-56.

73. Aoki J, Bandoh K, Inoue K A novel human G-protein-coupled receptor, EDG7, for lysophosphatidic acid with unsaturated fatty-acid moiety. Ann N Y Acad Sci 2000; 905:263-6

74. Mills, G.B., May, C., McGill, M., Roifman, C., and Mellors, A. A putative new growth factor in ascitic fluid from ovarian cancer patients: Identification, characterization and mechanism of action. Cancer Research 1988; 48:1066-71.

75. Mills, G.B., May, C., Hill, M., Campbell, S., Shaw, P., and Marks A. Ascitic fluid from human ovarian cancer patients contains growth factors necessary for intraperitoneal growth of human ovarian cancer cells. J Clin Invest 1990; 86:851-855.

76. Westermann AM, Havik E, Postma FR, Beijnen JH, Dalesio O, Moolenaar WH, Rodenhuis S. Malignant effusions contain lysophosphatidic acid (LPA)-like activity. Ann Oncol 1998; 9(4):437-442.

77. Frisch SM and Ruoslahti E. Integrins and anoikis. Current Opinion in Cell Biol 1997; 9:701-706.

78. Valentinis B, Reiss K, Baserga R. Insulin-like growth factor-I-mediated survival from anoikis: role of cell aggregation and focal adhesion kinase. J Cell Physiol 1998; 176(3):648-657.

79. Ono A, Maines-Bandiera DL, Roskelley CD, Auersperg N. An ovarian adenocarcinoma line derived from SV40/E-cadherin-transfected normal human ovarian surface epithelium. Int J Cancer 2000; 85:430-437.

80. Hong G, Baudhuin LM, Xu Y. Sphingosine-1-phosphate modulates growth and adhesion of ovarian cancer cells. FEBS Lett 1999; 460(3):513-18.

81. Yoshida A, Ueda H. Activation of Gi1 by lysophosphatidic acid receptor without ligand in the bacculovirus expression system. Biochem Biophys Res Commun 1999; 259(1):78-84.

82. Xu Y, Zhu K, Hong G, Wu W, Baudhuin LM, Xiao Y, Damron DS. Sphingosylphosphorylcholine is a ligand for ovarian cancer G-protein-coupled receptor 1. Nat Cell Biol 2000; 2(5):261-7.

83. Xu Y, Casey G. Identification of human OGR1, a novel G protein-coupled receptor that maps to chromosome 14. Genomics. 1996; 35(2):397-402.

84. An S, Tsai C, Goetzl EJ. Cloning, sequencing and tissue distribution of two related G protein-coupled receptor candidates expressed prominently in human lung tissue. FEBS Lett. 1995; 375(1-2):121-4.

85. Xiao Y, Chen Y, Kennedy AW, Belinson J, Xu Y. Evaluation of plasma lysophospholipids for diagnostic significance using electrospray ionization mass spectrometry (ESI-MS) analyses. Ann N Y Acad Sci 2000; 905:242-59.

86. Sasagawa T, Suzuki K, Shiota T, Kondo T, Okita M. The significance of plasma lysophospholipids in patients with renal failure on hemodialysis. J Nutr Sci Vitamionol (Tokyo) 1998; 44(6):809-818.

87. Sasagawa T, Okita M, Murakami J, Kato T, Watanabe A. Abnormal serum lysophospholipids in multiple myeloma patients. Lipids 1999; 34(1):17-21.

88. Bast, R.C., Xu, F., Yu, Y., Barnhill, S., Zhang, Z., and Mills G.B. CA125: The past and the future. International Journal of Biological Markers 1998; 13:179-87.

89. Santos WL, Rossi JA, Boggs SD, MacDonald TL. The molecular pharmacology of lysophosphatidate signaling. Ann N Y Acad Sci 2000; 905:232-41.

Chapter 13

EXPRESSION OF CSF-1 AND ITS RECEPTOR CSF-1R IN NON-HEMATOPOIETIC NEOPLASMS

Barry Kascinski
Department of Therapeutic Radiology, YaleUniversity School of Medicine
New Haven, CT 06520

1. INTRODUCTION

In 1984, long before anyone had even conceived of the possibility of DNA microarray analyses of gene expression in histologic sections, we employed a rather cumbersome and laborious *in situ* hybridization analysis of cDNAs to tissue RNA in serial sections of ovarian, endometrial, and breast carcinomas (in which autoradiographic grains were counted and data calculated in terms of cDNA hybrids/square micron of tissue). Our purpose was to ascertain whether the levels of transcript expression of any of 20 genes under study correlated with tumor grade and clinical stage (which even in the year 2000 remain the best overall predictors of prognosis in patients with these three neoplasms). Out of over 20 genes studied, only the levels of the transcript of the fms oncogene, which had at that time recently been shown to encode the receptor for CSF-1 (CSF-1R) correlated strongly with both grade (p <0.001) and stage (p <0.04) and thus, indirectly, with clinical outcome [1].

At the time, this observation was considered puzzling since CSF-1R was then known to be important only in the physiology of hematopoeitic cells and not other cell types. To better understand the significance of our results, we needed to determine whether our ISH observations were the consequence of tumor epithelial cell expression of the fms gene (which appeared to be the case from the ISH autoradiograms) or the consequence of heavy infiltration by tumor infiltrating macrophages [2,3].

CSF-1, the first cytokine purified to homogeneity over 20 years ago, has been shown to exist in both membrane-bound and soluble forms (resulting from alternative transcript splicing); and nearly all cells which express CSF-1 (which include many epithelial cells, fibroblasts, and many cells of the immune system) express both forms. Its receptor, CSF-1R, found to be encoded by a mutated feline c-fms gene transduced by a feline retrovirus, has been shown to be a tyrosine kinase growth factor receptor very similar in overall structure to both the B-type receptor for PDGF and to the c-kit encoded receptor for stem cell factors. The extracellular portion of the receptor is composed of five heavily glycosylated IgG-like domains which are responsible for ligand binding. These are linked to a hydrophobic transmembrane domain, and an intracellular domain which includes an ATP binding site, a spacer domain which includes a variety of sites where the receptor binds to other intracellular proteins and second messengers and a tyrosine kinase domain. Upon binding of the dimeric ligand, two identical receptor monomers dimerize and autophosphorylate each other on several different tyrosines. Since only one or two of the known sites of tyrosine phosphorylation appears able to be directly phosphorylated by the kinase domain of the opposite dimer, other intracellular kinases must participate in this process. The fully activated receptor is phosphorylated on at least 6 tyrosines and a variety of serines and threonines. By binding and interaction with other intracellular kinases, phosphatases, and second messengers, the receptor activates many different intracellular signal transduction pathways altering cellular motility, gene expression, progression through the cell cycle, and apoptosis [2,3,7,9, 14, 16, 20, 22, 25, 26, 27, 32, 33].

Immunohistochemical studies carried out with an anti-CSF-1R mouse monoclonal antibody on the same specimens confirmed that the CSF-1R antigen was strongly expressed by neoplastic epithelial cells as well as by tissue macrophages in many ovarian and endometrial carcinomas. In breast carcinomas, the same anti-CSF-1R antibody stained tissue macrophages and histologically invasive carcinoma strongly, *in situ* carcinoma weakly, and benign resting ductal epithelium and fibroblasts not at all [1,4,19]. In breast carcinomas, a polyclonal anti-CSF-1 antibody stained the membranes and cytoplasm of the malignant epithelial cells of breast carcinomas quite intensely along with stromal macrophages. Fibroblasts, which also synthesize some CSF-1, stain less intensely. In ovarian and endometrial carcinomas, staining with anti-CSF-1 antibodies was usually less intense and confined to the cell membrane [11, 12].

In subsequent studies, we have been able to demonstrate that staining with an anti-CSF-1R antibody with or without co-staining with anti-CSF-1 correlates with adverse prognosis. More recent studies with specific polyclonal antibodies, which we have prepared to recognize CSF-1R only when phosphorylated on specific tyrosines, demonstrate that breast and ovarian neoplasms clearly express tyrosine phosphorylated CSF-1R. The phosphorylation state of at least one of these autophosphoryaltion sites, TYR-723 appears to predict short metastasis free survival in breast cancer patients and more recently has been shown to predict short disease free and overall survival in ovarian carcinoma patients. Such results strongly suggest that activation of CSF-1R (either by binding of ligand or by transphosphorylation by other membrane bound or cytoplasmic tyrosine kinases) plays an important role in determining the biological behavior of breast and ovarian carcinomas in vivo [28, 29, 30].

2. CIRCULATING CSF-1 LEVELS IN CANCER PATIENTS

When a secreted protein such as CSF-1 is produced in quantities great enough to be readily detected by immunohistochemical staining, significant levels of the same antigen often can be found in extracellular fluid and in the circulation. In collaboration with E. R. Stanley, we measured CSF-1 concentrations in the sera of ovarian, endometrial, pulmonary, and breast carcinoma patients and in the ascites of patients with advanced ovarian carcinoma. We observed surprisingly high levels (100 ng/ml) in the sera of patients with active neoplastic disease. High ascitic fluid levels of CSF-1 also appeared to predict poor prognosis in patients with Stage III and IV disease [4, 6,9,10, 15, 24].

In ovarian carcinomas, changes in the level of CSF-1 often corresponded with changes in the level of another tumor-associated antigen CA-125. Changes in the level of each marker alone correctly correlated with or anticipated changes in neoplastic disease status 80% of the time while both together predicted changes in neoplastic disease activity 95% of the time. As such, CSF-1 appears to be a useful tumor marker complementary to CA-125 in the monitoring of disease activity in ovarian carcinoma patients. In endometrial carcinoma, CSF-1 is in fact, superior, to any other available tumor maker for disease detection and monitoring of response to therapy [4, 24]. Taken together, the above results are also intriguing because they suggest that CSF-1 and its receptor might be regulating phenotypes of ovarian, endometrial, and breast carcinoma cells similar to those which CSF-1 regulates during macrophage activation and placental implantation. However, to test this hypothesis, we required breast, ovarian, and endometrial carcinoma cell lines that express one or both of these genes.

3. EFFECTS OF CSF-1 AND CSF-1R ON BREAST, OVARIAN, AND ENDOMETRIAL CELL LINES *IN VITRO*

To find cell lines that expressed CSF-1 was not at all difficult; in fact, it is difficult to find tumor derived cell lines that do not express high levels of CSF-1. To find cell lines that expressed high levels of CSF-1Rs was more difficult, perhaps because chronic autocrine activation led to downregulation of the receptor and/or promotes apoptosis. We observed that many breast, ovarian, and endometrial cell lines expressed low, but detectable, levels of CSF-1Rs on Northern blot. In an attempt to increase the levels of expression of CSF-1R, we treated these cells with a variety of hormonal stimuli and observed that glucocorticoids, and to a lesser extent progestins, increased CSF-1R gene expression in several breast derived cell lines, in organ cultures of normal mammary alveolar epithelium, and in organ cultures of more than 80% of breast carcinomas obtained from our patient population [8, 12].

Culture of many of our breast, ovarian, and endometrial cell lines in serum free medium for 12-24 hours produced a modest 2-3 fold increase in CSF-1R transcript levels. Whereas estrogens, androgens, and mineralocorticoids had no measureable effects on CSF-1 or CSF-1R levels, progestins raised levels 5-10 fold while glucocorticoids increased CSF-1R levels in breast carcinoma cell lines 50-100 fold without obvious effects on CSF-1. Because glucocorticoids are known to play important roles in normal mammary epithelial cell differentiation, these results were not totally unexpected and we were able to exploit them to devise culture systems for further studies.

When the structure of CSF-1R transcripts in breast and endometrial carcinomas was investigated, no differences were observed from the wild-type transcripts expressed by trophoblast and macrophages. However, ovarian carcinomas appear to express several unusual transcript splice variants of the CSF-1R gene, some of which lack the second exon (which contains the translation start site for the wild-type protein). This transcript is analogous to that encoded by a fms gene variant transduced by several tumorigenic murine retroviruses that express a truncated version of the CSF-1R gene constitutively active in the absence of ligand. Overexpression of such an aberrant form of the CSF-1R which may not require ligand for activation may thus contribute to the malignant phenotype of ovarian carcinoma cells.

4. GLUCOCORTICOID REGULATION OF CSF-1R EXPRESSION IN BREAST CARCINOMA DERIVED CULTURED CELL LINES

When the effects of glucocorticoids on breast carcinoma cell lines was investigated in greater detail, as little as 10 nM dexamethasone was observed to induced a rapid increase in CSF-1R mRNA levels. This increase in transcript levels increased levels of surface receptors from 5,000 up to 50,000 per cell. Mifepristone (RU-486) which is a competitive inhibitor of binding of both glucocorticoids and progestins to their respective receptors completely abolished this increase [13, 21]. Prior to these observations, it was already known that the CSF-1R gene was transcribed from two widely separated promoters, the first of which was found to be active in trophoblastic epithelial cells, while the second was only active in hematopoietic cells. In order to determine which of these two promoters was active in mammary cells and cells of other female reproductive tract epithelia, nuclear run-on, promoter-reporter, and RNAse protection analyses were carried out. In breast carcinoma cells, nuclear run-on and promoter-reporter gene construct studies all suggested that the first promoter, active in trophoblast, was much more active in breast and other reproductive tract epithelia than the second promoter. In breast carcinoma cells, activity from this promoter was strongly stimulated by glucocorticoids which also led to a time dependent change in transcript initiation site utilization [21].

Analysis of the promoter itself revealed two glucocorticoid response elements (GREs) and one variant or negative GRE. Mutation of the second of the two GREs or of the nGRE dramatically decreased basal promoter activity and also blocked any stimulatory effects of glucocorticoids. DNAse I protection studies and electrophoretic mobility shift analyses (EMSA) revealed that the nGRE (which overlaps bHLH and AP-1 binding sites) is also important to the regulation of CSF-1R gene expression by glucocorticoids and by serum. The prevalence of certain AP-1 proteins complexed with the CSF-1R gene promoter in various cell lines tested appears to render the cells more or less responsive to glucocorticoid regulation. We are currently investigating how levels of specific AP-1 proteins, as well as steroid receptor coactivators, correlate with glucocorticoid responsiveness of the CSF-1R gene in organ cultures of primary breast carcinoma specimens. We have also observed a potent anti-sense promoter activity in the first intron of the CSF-1R gene which we believe may control the regulation of the CSF-1R gene by glucocorticoids, retinoids, and in tissues where this promoter is not normally used such as cells of hematopoietic origin)

5. CSF-1, CSF-1R AND TUMOR INVASIVENESS

CSF-1R regulates urokinase expression and thus invasion by macrophages and trophoblasts. To determine whether activation of breast carcinoma CSF-1R stimulates the expression of urokinase or its ability to invade basement membrane analogs, we have employed both matrigel and an amniotic membrane invasion systems often employed in studies of leukocytes and macrophages. These assay systems revealed that the basal level of invasiveness of these cells was low but markedly stimulated by the addition of CSF-1 [13, 34].

Using a mouse mammary epithelial cell line HC11, we were able to find that transfection of this cell line (which is non-tumorigenic and non-invasive) with the CSF-1R gene rendered the cells locally invasive and able to produce metastatic tumors after intravascular injection. Transfection of the cell line with mutant CSF-1Rs in which specific sites of TYR phosphorylation were mutated to PHE revealed that two of the sites of TYR phosphorylation, TYR-723 and TYR-809 were relevant to the phenotype of the cells. Mutations which abolished phosphorylation at TYR-809 rendered the cells incapable of local invasion or protease production and more sensitive to ionizing radiation but did not affect anchorage independent growth or metastatic tumorigenicity. Mutations at TYR-723 rendered the cells incapable of anchorage independent growth or metastatic tumorigenicity but they had no effect on local invasiveness or sensitivity to ionizing radiation [25, 33].

When we employed the antibodies described above which could recognize

CSF-1R only if phosphorylated on TYR-723 or on TYR-809, we found that the phosphorylation state of the former correlated with short metastasis free survival. When these antibodies were employed to study tyrosine phosphorylation of CSF-1R in a variety of cell lines, they revealed, much to our surprise, that not all sites of phosphorylation were evident in all cell lines. These results suggest that either all sites are phosphorylated but some are rapidly dephosphorylated after receptor activation or that intermediate kinases are involved in phosphorylation of many of the sites of tyrosine phosphorylation and not all cell lines contain all of the same intermediate kinases [28, 30].

6. SUMMARY

CSF-1 and its receptor appear to be important in the physiology of several different neoplasms including those of the breast and female reproductive tract. Levels of CSF-1 and CSF-1R expression appear to correlate with tumor cell invasiveness and an adverse clinical prognosis and may be modulated by hormones involved in normal lactogenic differentiation. Also, it appears that CSF-1R activates several different signal transduction pathways but only some of these appear to have direct bearing on tumor cell phenotypes and the activation of pathways in specific cell types may depend on factors above and beyond the receptor itself.

REFERENCES

1. Kacinski BM, Carter D, Mittal K, Kohorn EI, Bloodgood RS, Donahue J, Donofrio L, Edwards R, Schwartz PE, Chambers JT, Chambers SK. High Level Expression of FMS Proto-oncogene mRNA is Observed in Clinically Aggressive Human Endometrial Adenocarcinomas. Int J Radiat Oncol Biol Phys 1988;15:823-829.
2. Stanley ER, Guilbert LJ. Methods for the purification, assay, characterization and target cell binding of a colony-stimulating factor, CSF-1 J. Immunol. Methods 1989; 42: 53-284.
3. Taylor GR, Reedijk M, Rothwell V., Rohrschneider L, Pawson T. The unique insert of cellular and viral fms protein kinase is indispensable for enzymatic and transforming activity. EMBO J 1989; 8: 2029-2037.
4. Kacinski BM, Stanley ER, Carter D, Chambers JT, Chambers SK, Kohorn EI, Schwartz PE. Circulating Levels of CSF-1 (M-CSF), a Lymphohematopoietic Cytokine, May Be a Useful Marker of Disease Status in Patients with Malignant Ovarian Neoplasms. Int J Radiat Oncol Biol Phys 1989; 17:159-164.
5. Kacinski BM, Carter D, Kohorn EI, Mittal K, Bloodgood RS, Donahue J, Kramer CA, Fischer D, Edwards R, Chambers SK, Chambers JT, Schwartz PE. Oncogene Expression in vivo by Ovarian Adenocarcinomas and Mixed-mullerian Tumors. Yale J Biol Med 1989; 62:379-392.
6. Kacinski BM, Bloodgood RS, Schwartz PE, Carter DC, Stanley ER. The macrophage colony stimulating factor CSF-1 is produced by human ovarian and endometrial adenocarcinoma-derived cell lines and is present at abnormally high levels in the plasma of ovarian carcinoma patients with active disease. Molecular Diagnostics of Human Cancer, Ca. Cells 7, Cold Spring Harbor Press, Cold Spring Harbor, NY, pp 333-337, 1989.

7. Tapley P, Kazlauskas A, Cooper JA, Rohrschneider LR. Macrophage colony stimulating factor induced tyrosine phosphorylation of c-fms protein expressed in FDC-P1 and Balb/c T3 cells. Mol Cell Biol 1990; 10: 2538-2558.

8. Kacinski BM, Carter D, Mittal K, Yee LD, Scata KA, Donofrio L, Chambers SK, Wang KI, Yang-Feng T, Rohrschneider LR, Rothwell V. Ovarian Adenocarcinomas Express fms-complementary Transcripts and Antigen, Often With Co-expression of CSF-1. Am J Pathol 1990; 137:135-147.

9. Kacinski BM, Chambers SK, Stanley ER, Carter DC, Tseng P, Scata KA, Chang DHY, Pirro MH, Nguyen JT, Ariza A, Rohrschneider LR, Rothwell V. The Cytokine CSF-1 (M-CSF), Expressed by Endometrial Carcinomas in vivo and in vitro, May Also Be a Circulating Tumor Marker of Neoplastic Disease Activity in Endometrial Carcinoma Patients. Int J Radiat Oncol Biol Phys 1990; 19:619-626.

10. Kacinski BM, Chambers SK, Carter D, Filderman AE, Stanley ER. The Macrophage Colony Stimulating Factor CSF-1, an Auto- and Paracrine Tumor Cytokine, is also a Circulating "Tumor Marker" in Patients with Ovarian, Endometrial and Pulmonary Neoplasms. In: "The Physiological and Pathological Effects of Cytokines", Dinarello, C.A., et al., eds., New York, Wiley-Liss, Prog Leuk Biol 10B:393-400, 1990.

11. Tang R, Kacinski BM, Validire P, Beuvon F, Sastre X, Benoit P, de la Rochefordiere A, Mosseri V, Pouillart P, Scholl S. Oncogene amplification correlates with dense lymphocyte infiltration in human breast cancers: a role for hematopoieitic growth factor release by tumor cells? J Cell Biochem 1990; 44:189-198.

12. Kacinski BM, Scata KA, Carter D, Yee LD, Sapi E, King BL, Chambers SK, Jones MA, Pirro 3MH, Stanley ER, Rohrschneider LR. FMS (CSF-1 receptor) and CSF-1 transcripts and protein are expressed by human breast carcinomas in vivo and in vitro. Oncogene 1991; 6:941-952.

13. Filderman AE, Bruckner A, Kacinski BM, Deng N, Remold HG. Macrophage colony-stimulating factor (CSF-1) enhances invasiveness in CSF-1 receptor-positive carcinoma cell lines. Cancer Res 1992; 52(13):3661-3669.

14. Pellici G. Lauframcone I. Grignani F. McGlade J, Cavallo F. Forni G, Nicolletti I, Grignani F Pawson T, Pellici PG. A novel transforming protein SHC with an SH2 domain is implicated in mitogenic signal transduction. Cell 1992; 70: 93-104.

15. Price FV, Chambers SK, Chambers JT, Carcangiu ML, Schwartz PE, Kohorn EI, Stanley ER, Kacinski BM. Colony-stimulating factor-1 in primary ascites of ovarian cancer is a significant predictor of survival. Am J Obstet Gynecol 1993; 168:520-527.

16. Courtneidge SA , Dhand R, Pilat D, Twalmley GM, Waterfield MD, Roussel MD. Activation of Src kinases by CSF-1 and their association with its receptor. EMBO J 1993; 12: 943-950.

17. Bauknecht T, Kiechle-Schwarz M, duBois A, Wölfle J, Kacinski BM. Expression of transcripts for CSF-1 and for the "macrophage" and "epithelial" isoforms of the CSF-1R transcripts in human ovarian carcinomas. Cancer Detect Prev 1994; 18:231-239.

18. Chambers SK, Wang Y, Gilmore-Hebert M, Kacinski BM. Post-transcriptional regulation of c-fms proto-oncogene expression by dexamethasone and of CSF-1 in human breast carcinomas in vitro. Steroids 1994; 59:514-522.

19. Kommoss F, Wölfle J, Bauknecht T, Pfisterer J, Kiechle-Schwartz M, Pfleiderer A, Sauerbrei W, Kiehl R, Kacinski BM. Co-expression of M-CSF transcripts and protein, FMS (M-CSF receptor) transcripts and protein, and steroid receptor content in adenocarcinomas of the ovary. J Pathol 1994; 174:111-119.

20. Carlberg K. Rohrscheider L. The effect of inactivating mutations on dimerization, tyrosine phosphorylation, and internalization of the macrophage colony stimulating factor. Mol Cell Biol 1994; 5: 81-95.

21. Sapi E, Flick MB, Gilmore-Hebert M, Rodov S, Kacinski BM. Transcriptional regulation of the c-fms (CSF-1r) proto-oncogene in human breast carcinoma cells by glucocorticoids. Oncogene 1995; 10:529-542.

22. Troilaris S. Smola U, Chang J-H, Parsons SJ, Niemann H. Tamura T. Tyrosine 807 of the v-

fms oncogene product controls cell morphology and association with p120rasGAP. J Virol 1995; 69: 6010-6020.

23. Chambers SK, Wang Y, Gertz RE, Kacinski BM. Macrophage colony stimulating factor mediates invasion of ovarian cancer cells through urokinase. Cancer Res 1995; 55:1578-1585.

24. Hakala A, Kacinski BM, Stanley ER, Kohorn E, Puistola U, Risteli J, Risteli L, Tomas C, Kauppila A. Macrophage-colony stimulating factor 1, a clinically useful tumor marker in endometrial adenocarcinoma; comparison with CA-125 and aminoterminal propeptide of type III procollagen. Am J Obstet Gynecol 1995; 173:112-119.

25. Sapi E, Flick MB, Rodov S, Gilmore-Hebert M, Kelley M, Rockwell S, Kacinski BM. Independent regulation of invasion and anchorage-independent growth by different autophosphorylation sites of the macrophage colony-stimulating factor 1 receptor. Cancer Res 1996;56:5704-12.

26. van der Geer, Hunter T. Mutation of Tyr697, a GRB2 binding site and TYR-721, a PI-3 kinase binding site, abrogates signal transduction by the murine CSF-1 receptor expressed in Rat-2 fibroblasts. EMBO J 1996; 12: 5161-5172.

27. Hamilton J.A. CSF-1 signal transduction. J. Leukocyte Biology 1997; 62: 145-155.

28. Flick MB, Sapi E, Perrotta L, Maher MG, Halaban R, Carter D, Kacinski BM. Recognition of activated CSF-1 receptor in breast carcinomas by a tyrosine 723 phosphospecific antibody. Oncogene 1997; 14:2553-2561.

29. Chambers SK, Kacinski BM, Ivins CM, Carcangiu ML. Overexpression of epithelial CSF-1 and CSF-1 receptor: a poor prognostic factor in epithelial ovarian cancer; contrasted to a protective effect of stromal CSF-1. Clin Cancer Res 1997; 3:999-1007.

30. Maher MG, Sapi E, Turner B, Gumbs A, Perrotta PL, Carter D, Kacinski BM, Haffty B. CSF-1R expression correlates with local recurrence in breast cancer patients. Clinical Cancer Research 1998; 4:1851-1856.

31. Sapi E, Flick MB, Rodov S, Carter D, Kacinski BM. Expression of CSF-1 and CSF-1 receptor by normal lactating mammary epithelial cell. J Soc Gynecol Invest 1998; 5:94-101.

32. Sapi E, Flick MB, Rodov S, Kacinski BM. Ets-2 transdominant mutant abolishes anchorage-independent growth and CSF-1-stimulated invasion by BT20 breast carcinoma cells. Cancer Res 1998; 58: 1027-1033.

33. Kacinski BM, Rodov S, Sapi E. Signal Transduction Pathways Regulated by CSF-1 Receptors Modulate the In Vitro Radiosensitivity of Mammary Epithelial Cells. Int. J. Radiation Oncology Biol Phys 1999; 45(4):969-973.

34. Sapi E, Flick M, Tartaro K, Kim S, Rakhlin Y, Rodov S, Kacinski BM. Effect of All-trans-Retinoic Acid on c-fms Proto-oncogene [Colony-stimulating Factor 1 (CSF-1) Receptor] Expression and CSF-1-induced Invasion and Anchorage-independent Growth of Human Breast Carcinoma Cells. Cancer Research 1999; 59:5578-5585.

Chapter 14

ROLE OF INHIBINS AND ACTIVINS IN OVARIAN CANCER

Teresa K. Woodruff
Department of Neurobiology and Physiology, Northwestern University and Department of Medicine, Northwestern University Medical School, Evanston, IL 60208

1. INTRODUCTION

Ovarian cancer strikes 1 in 70 women and is usually fatal. The frank mortality associated with this disease is largely due to the lack of effective diagnostics and a poor understanding of the molecular basis of the disease. Few factors have been directly correlated with the tissue-specific onset of cancer, however, recent work on inhibins and activins may provide clues to ovarian cancer onset and progression.

During the course of each reproductive cycle, the somatic cells of the follicle (the granulosa cells) proliferate at a rate more rapid than any other cell in the body. The control of granulosa cell proliferation is not completely understood, however, many of the hormones and local growth factors that regulate the granulosa cell cycle have been identified. At the time of ovulation, the surface epithelial cells auto-destruct to allow the release of a mature oocyte. The epithelial cells are then required to clear cellular debris, repair damaged cells, and proliferate rapidly to seal the wound on the surface of the ovary. The epithelial cells then become dormant until the next month (in the human) when the process is repeated. Sometimes the processes of cellular proliferation and repair do not proceed with absolute fidelity. Damaged cells accumulate mutations that may result in a neoplasia.

Because the ovarian cells are programmed for proliferation, ovarian cancer is particularly deadly. It strikes 1 in 100 women and is usually fatal. Mortality associated with ovarian cancer is largely due to the lack of effective diagnostics and a poor understanding of the molecular basis of the disease. It is the goal of a number of studies in a variety of labs to address the molecular basis of ovarian cancer and to identify key events that result in poor survival of women with the disease.

One hypothesis regarding the onset of ovarian cancer is that the biological regulators of normal ovarian granulosa and epithelial cell proliferation

294

become the vehicles of uncontrolled cell growth. We have studied the TGFβ superfamily ligands, activin and inhibin, in the context of normal ovarian function and recent advances in inhibin and activin biology suggest that these multi-functional proteins are associated with ovarian neoplasias. Inhibin and activin are ovarian-derived dimeric proteins and are related through a common β-subunit. During a normal reproductive cycle, pituitary follicle-stimulating hormone (FSH) stimulates ovarian granulosa cell inhibin and activin production. Inhibin and activin are required for the normal progression of granulosa cells through the stages of follicle maturation. Recent studies indicate that an inappropriate inhibin signal may participate in the onset and progression of granulosa- and epithelial-cell tumorigenesis. How a normal growth factor, inhibin, may become a cancer potentiator is an interesting question that must be addressed.

2. INHIBIN IS A CENTRAL REGULATOR OF GONADAL FUNCTION

Inhibin is an ovarian-derived disulfide-linked dimeric glycoprotein composed of an α-subunit and a β-subunit [1]. One gene encodes the α-subunit, while the b-subunit is found as independent isoforms encoded by at least four different genes. The four mammalian β-subunits (β_A, β_B, β_c, β_E) are expressed in restricted cellular sites. The β_A and b_B subunits are co-expressed with α-subunits in the ovary leading to the biosynthesis of an inhibin molecule [2]. In the female, the inverse relationship between FSH and inhibin forms a classic endocrine feedback system that is established in the prepubertal years leading to the first ovulation. This feedback loop is maintained in a cycle-dependent manner during the reproductive lifespan, and is lost following follicular exhaustion in the postmenopausal years [3]. In addition, inhibin regulates follicle growth in a paracrine manner [4]. Inhibin stimulates theca cell androgen production and promotes follicle growth [5-6]. Inappropriate inhibin signals in the primate result in an imbalance between LH and FSH, a delay in the follicular phase, and luteal phase deficiency [7-8]. Absence of inhibin in animals genetically deficient in the ligand, results in unopposed FSH and abnormal follicle growth leading to tumor formation [1,9].

Activin is a homodimer of the inhibin β-subunits. It was originally identified as a functional antagonist to inhibin, however, the cellular systems that respond to activin are more diverse than the systems that are regulated by inhibin. Activin regulates hormonogenesis (FSH, GH, ACTH, insulin), cellular homeostasis (divide or die pathways), and differentiation programs (developmentally and in adult cells) [1]. The cellular mechanisms that integrate an activin signal into a physiological response include a binary receptor complex and tandem serine threonine kinases, intracellular signal mediators, and nuclear transcription factors [9-11]. Correct intracellular execution of an activin cue regulates functions as fundamental as embryonic mesoderm development, neuronal survival, hematopoietic function, and reproductive cyclicity. Absent or incorrect activin signaling results in phenotypes as catastrophic as embryonic lethality, tumor formation, and infertility [1,3,11].

3. THE INHIBIN RECEPTOR AND SIGNAL TRANSDUCTION PATHWAYS

Cellular response to most TGFβ ligands is transduced through two single membrane spanning serine-threonine kinase subunits [9-11]. The activin receptor was the first receptor in the superfamily to be identified. Subsequently, a whole class of receptor serine-threonine receptor subunits have been identified that have structural characteristics similar to those described for the activin receptor. Each ligand in the TGFβ superfamily binds to a receptor in a ligand discriminant way. Generally speaking, ligand binds a type II receptor (70-75kDa) which transphosphorylates a type I receptor (50-55kDa). The holo-receptor complex is then competent to initiate intracellular signaling cascades [12]. Within the activin receptor family, two ligand binding type II receptor genes have been identified (RII and RIIB) and four alternatively spliced variants of the type IIB receptor have been cloned [13]. The receptor isoforms differ by changes in an extracellular proline-rich region immediately preceding the transmembrane domain and in a region between the transmembrane domain and serine-threonine kinase domain. The specific roles of all 6 ligand binding receptor subunits has not been clearly delineated. The receptors differ in affinity and may be expressed differentially to engage different aspects of intracellular signaling cascade components.

Target cytoplasmic substrates for activated TGFβ, activin, and other superfamily receptors have been identified using *Drosophila melanogaster*, *Caenorhabditis elegans*, *Xenopus laevis*, and mouse genetic systems. Complementation studies in *Drosophila* were used to identify a family of genes, now referred to as Smad, that are downstream of the fly TGFβ signal [14]. A family of seven Smad homologues have been identified and each Smad has specificity for different ligands of the TGFβ family. Smad1 is a BMP associated co-factor [24-27]. Smad2 is activin and TGFβ specific [15-21]. Smad3 is TGFβ and activin specific [22]. Smad4 was identified as a deleted gene product in spontaneous arising pancreatic cancers that were TGFβ-insensitive [22-26]. This tumor suppressor gene (also known as a member of the *dwarfin* gene family) is required for both activin and TGFβ activity. Both Smad2 and Smad4 reside on human chromosome 18q21, which is a region deleted in human pancreatic and colorectal cancers [20,22]. Smad6 and Smad7 have recently been identified [27-28]. Smad6 and Smad7 are gene products unique to vascular endothelial cells subjected to laminar fluid stress shear. These Smads, unlike the previously described activating Smad proteins, are antagonist to the TGFβ type I receptor and act through disruption of Smad2-Smad4 complex assembly and downstream transcriptional activities.

Smad1, Smad2, Smad3, and Smad4 have conserved domains in the N-terminus (MH1) and C-terminus (MH2) and are separated by a dissimilar serine-threonine hinge region. C-terminal serines have been defined as phosphorylation targets and phosphorylation is required for concentration of Smads into the nucleus [30]. Excision of the C-terminal domain of the Smads confers transcriptional activation on synthetic targets suggesting that the Smads are present in the cytoplasm as inactive, latent proteins. Within the nucleus, the Smads are functional co-activators or co-repressors of DNA-binding proteins and activin/ TGFβ-dependent gene transcription. Assembly of specific heterodimeric and homodimeric Smad proteins has been demonstrated following receptor activation by activin, BMP, and TGFβ indicating that intracellular specificity of response is dependent on the type of Smad activated by ligand [19,22]. Naturally occurring mutations of Smad2 and Smad4 exist in the carboxy-terminal domain and disrupt Smad activity through increased association of the C- with N-terminal inhibitory domain. This 'gain of autoinhibitory function' is a novel and important mechanism specific to the TGFβ superfamily. The crystal structure of the activating C-terminal domain of Smad4 has been solved (2.5A resolution) and it is a protein trimer [29]. Mutations in amino acids disrupting protein-protein interface regions (such as those found in tumor tissues) cause inactivation of the protein [30].

The implication that these cytoplasmic regulators of TGFβ and activin action act as tumor suppressors may be an important clue in the study of the etiology of human cancer. Indeed, loss of function at any level of the inhibin/activin/TGFβ-dependent cell regulation can result in abnormal cellular function. Smad4 was identified as a loss of function gene in spontaneously arising pancreatic cancers [22-26]. Further, cell lines that are TGFβ-insensitive or activin-insensitive have been studied and they lack either an intact receptor system or intracellular Smad [31]. Conversely, overexpression of Smad4 causes cell cycle arrest in some cells [25]. Similarly, imbalance in the local inhibin/activin milieu and the consequential activation of Smads also results in tumor development. This result led to the assignment of α-inhibin subunit as a tumor suppressor gene. Clearly, the study of inhibin and receptor targets as mediators of cancers phenotypes merits further analysis.

4. INHIBIN, ACTIVIN, AND THE ETIOPATHOLOGY OF GRANULOSA CELL TUMORS

Alteration in inhibin and activin subunit protein levels or expression and translation of products from abnormal cellular locations, mutations or aberrant expression of receptor, and mutations in the signaling Smad molecules have all been identified in various types of cancer. One form of ovarian cancer originates in a cell type that normally produces estrogen, the granulosa cell. In a normal ovary, granulosa cell growth is regulated by a pituitary hormone called follicle stimulating hormone (FSH). This hormone binds to receptors on the surface of the cell and causes the production of paracrine acting inhibin and activin. Inhibin and activin are required for normal follicle function and are inappropriately regulated in ovarian tumors. Granulosa cell tumors account for 10% of primary ovarian cancer and the mechanisms leading to unrestrained granulosa cell growth are not fully understood. One hypothesis is that the tumors arise from unregulated FSH action on the cells leading to an increase in the hormones inhibin and activin which cause granulosa cell accumulation.

A powerful model used to delineate the physiological relevance of inhibin and activin is the genetic deletion of subunit sequences through homologous recombination (also known as the 'knock-out' mouse model). In a mouse line deficient in the inhibin α-subunit, 100% of the animals develop sex cord stroma tumors [32]. The development of ovarian tumors in the absence of inhibin α-subunit led to the hypothesis that inhibin a-subunit is a tumor suppressor gene. Further studies demonstrated that the animals lacking inhibin α-subunit produce activins at supraphysiological levels, suggesting the possibility that tumor development may have been primarily activin-driven [34]. This possibility was partially addressed when compound homozygous knockout animals deficient in both the inhibin α-subunit and the activin receptor were found to develop ovarian tumors (although the animals survived much longer due to the elimination of cachexia symptoms caused by activin) [33]. This experiment does not completely eliminate the effect of activin on ovarian tumor pathogenesis because the ovary expresses more than one activin receptor that would not have been eliminated through the genetic strategy employed in the double knockout. Moreover, activin is able to bind the TGFβ receptor when in the concentration predicted by hormone measurements in the animals. Secondary to the loss of inhibin negative feedback and amplification of activin positive stimulation, animals lacking an inhibin α-subunit also produce supraphysiological levels of FSH [32].

The tumors have a second important phenotype - they express inhibin receptor. The physiology of inhibin predicts that the receptor should be restricted to the ovary and pituitary. Therefore, over-expression of inhibin receptor in gonadal tumor might be a molecular target, similar to the current anti-Her2/neu therapeutic option, for some types of ovarian cancer.

5. THE ETIOPATHOLOGY OF EPITHELIAL CELL-DERIVED OVARIAN TUMORS: ASSOCIATION OF DISEASE WITH INHIBIN AND ACTIVIN-DEPENDENT PATHWAYS

The majority of ovarian neoplasia (approximately 90%) arise from the epithelial cell [33]. The ovarian epithelial cell is the target of a series of proteolytic events during ovulation that allows the release of an oocyte. The epithelial cells must then rapidly proliferate to close the surface wound. There is a direct correlation between ovulation number and cancer incidence suggesting that the rapid repair mechanisms employed by the epithelial cells may lead to increased opportunity for genetic mutations. Four subtypes of epithelial ovarian neoplasia are recognized based on immunohistochemical markers and include serous, mucinous, endometrioid, and clear cell carcinomas. Inhibin is a FSH-regulated ovarian-derived dimeric protein hormone that suppresses pituitary FSH secretion in a classic endocrine feedback loop and regulates ovarian follicle development in a paracrine manner [1]. Inhibin serum concentration is inversely correlated to circulating FSH throughout the normal menstrual cycle and the balance between inhibin and FSH is key to the maintenance of reproductive cyclicity [35]. Inhibin is elevated in serum from patients with mucinous ovarian cancer (82% positive), a population that represents 15% of ovarian cancer patients [36]. Inhibin serum concentration declines following surgical ablation of the tumor, suggesting that the tumors are the source of the inhibin. In a retrospective study of a cohort of postmenopausal women with primary epithelial ovarian carcinoma inhibins and activins were measured to determine whether the presence of either ligand predicted outcomes in these patients. Interestingly, preoperative serum inhibin A concentration was an important independent predictor of survival in a multivariate analysis which included the traditional measures of prognosis of stage, grade, age and residual disease. Univariate analysis of inhibin A levels greater than the median were associated with a 5 year DFS of 10% compared to 43% for those with levels below the median. More recently, we have examined inhibin binding to epithelial ovarian tumors and find that some of the variant cell lines are enriched for inhibin binding sites. Thus, inhibin may act directly on ovarian cancer to increase tumor progression.

Taken together, the data point to a role for inhibin in the etiopathology and progression of ovarian cancer. Inhibin is a product of the normally cycling ovary. In granulosa-cell and postmenopausal epithelial ovarian tumors, there is a gain of inhibin expression, a gain of inhibin receptor, or mutations in signaling components of the inhibin/activin/TGFβ pathway. Because inhibin functionally antagonizes activin, the shift toward inhibin growth promoting pathways may also disrupt TGFβ/activin growth suppression pathways.

One of the important issues in any study of cancer phenotypes is to define the potential participants in the pathology. We have correlated inhibin with ovarian cancer and can therefore begin to analyze the loci of inhibin involvement in the disease (Figure 1). One of the first suspects in the disease is Smad. As previously mentioned, Smad4 mutations account for 50% of spontaneous pancreatic tumors. Thus, and examination of this transcription factor in ovarian disease would be of interest. The abnormal expression of the inhibin subunits in the epithelial compartment, is another facet to this complex disease that may contribute to the progression of the cells from normal to neoplastic. We have clearly shown elevated inhibin subunits and serum levels in granulosa cell tumors. Whether inhibin has anything to do with the granulosa cell tumor itself is not presently known. More importantly, we have identified the oncogenic epithelial cell as a site of expressed inhibin. During development, the granulosa cell and surface epithelial cell share a common stem cell, therefore, it is possible that the neoplastic epithelial cell no longer retains is fully differentiated phenotype and instead is 'reset' to a more primitive stage. The change in growth factor expression may lead to alterations in cell phenotypes. These may include a change in the types of extracellular matrix proteins, the ability of the cells to migrate, the induction of angiogenic factors, or a change in the rate of cell division. Loss of cell cycle regulation is known to contribute to cancers of many types. The relative contibution of inhibin to the overall insensitively of cancer cells to proliferative signals is not known. Last, receptor loss of function is a point of disjuncture in the course of many cancers and it is possible that receptors (such as the inhibin receptor, activin receptor, or FSH receptor) underlie this disease. Illumination of these questions will provide new insight into the hypothesis that a gain of inhibin function through ligand upregulation or Smad mutation in the postmenopausal ovary results in abnormal cell function leading to neoplasia. The next few years of discovery should be exciting relative to inhibin biology.

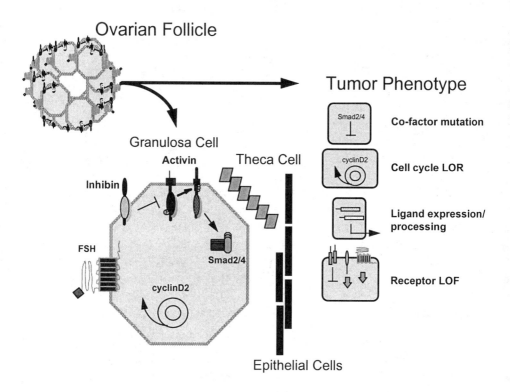

Figure 1: *A representation of the molecules that function in the normal follicle and the potential abnormalities that may lead to neoplasia. These factors may include co-factor mutation, cell cycle loss of regulation, ligand expression/processing and receptor loss of function.*

REFERENCES

1. Woodruff TK Regulation of Cellular and System Function by Activin. Biochemical Pharmacology 1997; 55:953-963.
2. Vale W, Rivier C, Hsueh A, Campen C, Meunier H, and Bicsak T. Chemical and biological characterization of the inhibin family of protein hormones. Recent Progress in Hormone Research 1988; 44:1-34.
3. Woodruff, T., D'Agostino, J., Schwartz, N., Mayo, K. Dynamic changes in inhibin messenger RNAs in rat ovarian follicles during the reproductive cycle. Science 1988; 239:1296-1299.
4. Woodruff, T., Mather, J. Inhibin, activin and the female reproductive axis. Ann Rev Physiol 1995; 57:219-244.
5. Woodruff, T.K., Lyon, R.J., Hansen, S.E., Rice, G.C., Mather, J.P. Inhibin and activin locally regulate rat ovarian folliculogenesis. Endocrinology. 1990; 127:3196-3205.
6. Hillier, S., Yong, E., Illingworth, P., Baird, D., Schwall, R., Mason, A. Effect of recombinant inhibin on androgen synthesis in cultured human thecal cells. Mol Cell Endocrinol 1991; 75:R1-R6.
7. Stouffer, R.L., Dahl, K.D., Hess, D.L., Woodruff, T.K., Mather, J.P., Molkness, T.A. Systemic and intraluteal infusion of inhibin A and activin A in rhesus monkeys during the luteal phase of the menstrual cycle. Biol Reprod 1994; 50:888-895.
8. Molskness, T., Woodruff, T.K., Hess, D., Dahl, K., Stouffer, D. Recombinant human inhibin A administered early in the menstrual cycle alters concurrent pituitary and follicular, plus subsequent luteal, function in rhesus monkeys. J Clin Endocrinol Met 1996; 81:4002-4006.
9. Massague, J. TGF signaling: receptors, transducers, and MAD proteins. Cell 1996; 85:947-950.
10. Massague J, Cheifetz S, Laiho M, Ralph D, Weis F, and Zentella A. Transforming growth factor-beta. Cancer Surveys. 1992; 12: 81-103.
11. Mathews, L. Activin receptors and cellular signaling by the receptor serine kinase family. Endocrine Reviews. 1994; 15:310-325.
12. Mathews, L.S., Vale, W.W. Expression cloning of an activin receptor, a predicted transmembrane serine kinase. Cell 1991; 65: 973-982.
13. Attisano, L., Wrana, J., Cheifetz, S., Massague, J. Novel activin receptors: Distinct genes and alternative mRNA splicing generate a repertoire of serine threonine kinase receptors. Cell 1992; 86:97-108.
14. Sekelsky J, Newfeld S, Raftery L, Chartoff E, and Gelbart W. Genetic characterization and cloning of mothers against dpp, a gene required for decapentaplegic function in Drosophila melanogaster. Genetics 1995; 139:1347-1358.
15. Graff J, Bansal A, and Melton D. Xenopus Mad proteins transduce distinct subsets of signals for the TGFB superfamily. Cell 1996; 85:479-487.
16. Derynck R, Gelbart WM, Harland RM, Heldin CH, Kern SE, Massague J, Melton DA, Mlodzik M, Padgett RW, Roberts AB, Smith J, Thomsen GH, Vogelstein B, and Wang XF. Nomenclature: vertebrate mediators of TGFbeta family signals. Cell 1996; 87:173-175.
17. Hoodless P, Haerry T, Abdollah S, Stapleton M, O'Connor M, Attisano L, and Wrana J. MADR1, a MAD-related protein that functions in BMP2 signaling pathways. Cell 196; 85:489-500.
18. Liu F, Hata A, Baker J, Doody J, Carcamo J, Harland R, and Massague J. A human Mad protein activin as a BMP-regulated transcriptional activator. Nature 1996; 381:620-623.
19. Lagna G, Hata A, Hemmati-Brivanlou A, and Massague J. Partnership between DPC4 and SMAD proteins in TGF-beta signalling pathways. Nature 1996; 383: 832-836.

20. Eppert K, Scherer S, Ozcelik J, Perone R, Hoodless P, Kim H, Tsui L, Bapat B, Gallinger S, Andrulis I, Thomsen G, Wrana J, and Attisano L. Madr2 maps to 18q21 and encodes a TGFb-regulated MAD-related protein that is functionally mutated in colorectoal carcinoma. Cell 1996; 86: 543-552.

21. Macias-Silva M, Abdollah S, Hoodless PA, Pirone R, Attisano L, and Wrana JL. MADR2 is a substrate of the TGFbeta receptor and its phosphorylation is required for nuclear accumulation and signaling. Cell 1996; 87:1215-24.

22. Wu T-Y, Zhang Y, Feng X, and Derynck R. Heteromeric and homomeric interactions correlate with signaling activity and functional cooperativity of smad3 and smad4/dpc4. Molecular and Cellular Biology 1997; 17:2521-2528.

23. Hahn SA, Schutte M, Hoque AT, Moskaluk CA, da Costa LT, Rozenblum E, Weinstein CL, Fischer A, Yeo CJ, Hruban RH, and Kern SE. DPC4, a candidate tumor suppressor gene at human chromosome 18q21.1. Science 1996; 271:350-353.

24. Schutte M, Hruban RH, Hedrick L, Cho KR, Nadasdy GM, Weinstein CL, Bova GS, Isaacs WB, Cairns P, Nawroz H, Sidransky D, Casero RA Jr, Meltzer PS, Hahn SA, and Kern S. DPC4 gene in various tumor types. Cancer Research 1996; 56:2527-2530.

25. Yingling JM, Das P, Savage C, Zhang M, Padgett RW, Wang XF. Mammalian dwarfins are phosphorylated in response to transforming growth factor beta and are implicated in control of cell growth. Proceedings of the National Academy of Sciences of the United States of America 1996; 93:8940-8944.

26. Riggins GJ, Thiagalingam S, Rozenblum E, Weinstein CL, Kern SE, Hamilton SR, Willson JK, Markowitz SD, Kinzler KW, and Vogelstein B. Mad-related genes in the human. Nature Genetics 1996; 13:347-349.

27. Imamura T, Takase M, Nishihara A, Oeda E, Hanai J, Kawabata M, Miyazono K. Smad6 inhibits signalling by the TGF-beta superfamily. Nature 1997; 389:622-626.

28. Nakao A, Afrakhte M, Moren A, Nakayama T, Christian JL, Heuchel R, Itoh S, Kawabata M, Heldin NE, Heldin CH, ten Dijke P. Identification of Smad7, a TGFbeta-inducible antagonist of TGF-beta signalling. Nature 1997; 389:631-635.

29. Shi Y, Hata A, Lo RS, Massague J, Pavletich NP. A structural basis for mutational inactivation of the tumour suppressor Smad4. Nature 1997; 388:87-93.

30. Hata A, Lo RS, Wotton D, Lagna G, Massague J. Mutations increasing autoinhibition inactivate tumour suppressors Smad2 and Smad4. Nature 1997; 388: 82-87.

31. Kalkhoven E, Roelen BA, de Winter JP, Mummery CL, van den Eijnden-van Raaij AJ, van der Saag PT, and van der Burg B. Resistance to transforming growth factor beta and activin due to reduced receptor expression in human breast tumor cell lines. Cell Growth & Differentiation 1995; 6:1151-1161.

32. Matzuk MM, Kumar TR, Shou W, Coerver KA, Lau AL, Behringer RR, and Finegold MJ. Transgenic models to study the roles of inhibins and activins in reproduction, oncogenesis, and development. Recent Progress in Hormone Research 1996; 51:123-154.

33. Blaustein A. Surface germinal epithelium and related ovarian neoplasms. Pathology Annuals 1981; 16:247-294.

34. Coerver, K, Woodruff, TK, Finegold, M, Mather, J, Bradley, A, Matzuk, M. Molec Endocrinol 1996; 10:534-538.

35. Groome NP, Illingworth PJ, O'Brien M, Pai R, Rodger FE, Mather JP, and McNeilly AS. J Clin Endocrinol Metabol 1996; 81:1401-1405.

36. Healy, D, Burger, H, Mamers, P, Jobling, T, Bangah, M, Quinn, M. New Eng J Med 1996; 329:1539-1342.

II.   RESEARCH

C. Cellular Regulation and Metastasis

Chapter 15

ADHESION MOLECULES

Amy P.N. Skubitz
Department of Laboratory Medicine and Pathology, University of Minnesota Medical School, Minneapolis, MN 55455

1. BACKGROUND

This chapter will focus on the role of adhesion molecules in ovarian carcinoma. Specifically, we will focus on the interactions that occur between ovarian carcinoma cells and peritoneal mesothelial cells as well as their associated extracellular matrices (ECM). Cell-cell and cell-ECM interactions play an important role in cancer cell adhesion, migration, invasion, growth, survival, and programmed cell death (apoptosis). By better understanding the molecules involved in ovarian carcinoma cell adhesion, it may be possible to identify reagents that can prevent the dissemination of ovarian carcinoma *in vivo*.

Ovarian cancer is the fifth leading cause of cancer death in women in the U.S. with over 25,000 new cases diagnosed each year in the U.S. [1]. In 80-90% of the cases, ovarian cancer originates in the surface epithelium of the ovary and is termed "ovarian carcinoma" [2] (which will be the focus of this chapter), while the remaining 10-20% of the cases originate in the germ or stromal cells. Epithelial ovarian cancer is an aggressive malignancy. Since the disease is often asymptomatic, it is usually diagnosed in advanced stages with peritoneal dissemination and distant metastases, resulting in a poor prognosis for the patients. At the time of diagnosis, the cancer has spread beyond the ovary in 75% of patients, and in 60% of the patients the cancer has spread beyond the pelvis [3,4].

In ovarian carcinoma, cancer cells of epithelial origin are shed from the ovary into the peritoneal fluid. The cancer cells attach to the single layer of mesothelial cells that line the inner surface of the peritoneal cavity. After adhesion to mesothelial cells and their associated ECM, the ovarian cancer cells may migrate through the layer of mesothelial cells and the ECM, invade the local organs, and metastasize to distant sites. Metastases are most frequently found at sites within the peritoneum, omentum, bowel surfaces, and retroperitoneal lymph nodes. This multi-step process of cancer cell adhesion, migration, and invasion eventually results in the death of the patient. Curing advanced ovarian cancer is difficult because of both the inability to completely resect diffuse tumor involvement on the peritoneal surface and the eventual resistance of the cancer cells to chemotherapy [5,6].

Although an early step of metastasis involves the adhesion of ovarian carcinoma cells to mesothelial cells and their associated ECM, few studies have focused on this interaction. Several families of adhesion molecules that are involved in cell-cell and cell-ECM interactions have been described in other cell systems. These adhesion molecules may also be important in the interaction of ovarian carcinoma cells with mesothelial cells and their associated ECM. Surface adhesion molecules are categorized into families based on structural similarities. They are grouped into at least five structural classes [7-10], consisting of proteoglycans, integrins, cadherins, selectins, and the immunoglobulin superfamily. In this chapter, we will focus on the proteoglycan CD44, integrins, and E-cadherin, since these molecules have been most widely studied with respect to ovarian carcinoma.

2. CD44

The CD44 proteoglycans, a member of the hyaladherin family (also known as Hermes, H-CAM, Pgp-1, ECMR III, HUTCH-1, gp85, and In(Lu)-related) are expressed by a wide variety of cell types, including epithelial cells and hematopoietic cells [11], and play a role in cell-cell and cell-matrix adhesion [12]. Due to alternative splicing and differential glycosylation, there are many variants of CD44. One isoform of CD44 (denoted CD44H or CD44s) is expressed by most normal cell types. CD44H binds the ECM molecule hyaluronan and is 80-95 kD in size. CD44E is predominantly expressed on epithelial cells. CD44 with attached chondroitin sulfate binds to ECM molecules including fibronectin and collagen types I, IV, and VI. In addition, CD44 can also bind the cytokine osteopontin and heparin-binding growth factors.

CD44 exists in a variety of forms with different molecular sizes ranging from 85 to 169 kDa. The 85 kDa protein is the predominant form in leukocytes and is thought to be important in homing to lymphocyte organs and sites of inflammation. The larger (150-160 kDa) CD44 isoform is found on epithelial cells and mesenchymal cells and appears to function as the major receptor for hyaluronan. CD44 also functions in cell adhesion to stromal elements and as a co-stimulatory molecule. Signaling through CD44 induces cytokine release and T-cell activation.

2.1. Hyaluronan Serves as a Ligand for CD44

Hyaluronan (also known as hyaluronic acid or hyaluronate), a ligand for CD44, is the simplest of the glycosaminoglycans. It consists of repeating sequences of up to 25,000 nonsulfated disaccharide units, which are not attached to a protein core, to form a proteoglycan. Hyaluronan is found in variable amounts in all tissues and fluids of adult animals. It is extruded directly from the cell surface by an enzyme complex embedded in the plasma membrane. Hyaluronan varies in size between 100 – 5,000 kDa, and occupies a great deal of space in aqueous solution. It is highly viscous and functions in molecular exclusion, flow resistance, tissue osmosis, and matrix integrity. The smallest functional unit of hyaluronan has been shown to be a hexasaccharide, which can compete for the binding of native hyaluronan to its receptor [13]. In contrast, the binding of hyaluronan to other ECM macromolecules such as cartilage proteoglycan and link protein, requires a minimum hyaluronan oligosaccharide sequence of 10-12 monosaccharides for competition [14-16]. *In vitro* studies using chondrocytes have shown that the assembly of a pericellular matrix can be blocked by the addition of hyaluronan hexasaccharides [17,18] and that the pericellular matrix can be displaced from the cell surface in 2 hr by the addition of hyaluronan hexasaccharides [17].

In animal studies, hyaluronan has been show to have a variety of effects. It has been shown to reduce the formation of adhesions after peritoneal surgery [19] by forming a viscous solution that coats the peritoneal surfaces and forms a barrier to tissue apposition [20]. Furthermore, depending upon the molecular weight and source of hyaluronan, it can enhance or suppress the function of macrophages, neutrophils, and lymphocytes [21-28]. Some studies report that injection of hyaluronan into the peritoneal cavity of mice stimulates the migration of inflammatory cells and induces the recruitment of a population of stimulating macrophages [29]. In these studies, up to 4% hyaluronan (40 mg/ml) was injected into the peritoneal cavities of mice. After 24 hr, a 3.3-fold increase in granulocytes (predominantly neutrophils) was observed, and at 72 hr, the peritoneal macrophage count doubled [29]. In contrast, other studies suggest that macrophages "disappear" from the peritoneal cavity following the intraperitoneal injection of hyaluronan into normal mice; however this clearance has been attributed to an increased adhesion of macrophages to the cells lining the peritoneal cavity [26]. Finally, native hyaluronan has been shown to inhibit the vascularization of chick embryo [30], while degradation products of hyaluronan have been shown to induce angiogenesis [31].

The half-life of hyaluronan has been reported to be ~3 hr when trace amounts (12 ug/ml) were injected into the peritoneal cavity of rabbits; its half-life could be extended to ~29 hr when higher concentrations (2 mg/ml) of hyaluronan was injected [32]. The rapid removal of hyaluronan was attributed to a local uptake, most likely receptor-mediated, and its subsequent degradation in the tissue [32]. It is possible that hyaluronan may be removed from the peritoneal cavity by flow, and that the higher concentration of hyaluronan was cleared at a ten-time slower rate due to the higher viscosity of the solution [32].

2.2. Role of CD44 and Hyaluronan in Cancer

In support of a role for CD44 and hyaluronan in cancer, there is increasing evidence that CD44-hyaluronan interactions may enhance tumor growth and metastasis. A wide range of malignancies of epithelial and mesenchymal origin express high levels of CD44H (the standard CD44 isoform which does not contain variant exon products) and a variety of variant isoforms of CD44 [33]. CD44 variant expression has been shown to be a common feature in epithelial ovarian cancer [34], and tumor cell-associated hyaluronan has been shown to be an unfavorable prognostic factor in colorectal cancer [35]. In some experimental systems, an increase in CD44 expression correlates with increased adhesion to hyaluronan, which then has been postulated to cause an increase in metastatic potential. Murine studies with melanoma and lymphoma cell lines have shown marked effect on tumor growth by transfection with CD44 [36,37], interaction with soluble CD44-Ig fusion protein [36-38], or subcutaneous injection of hyaluronan oligomers [33]. However, other studies have shown that invasiveness of certain tumors coincides with down-regulation of CD44 expression [39], or that hyaluronan does not appear to be involved in tumor progression [40]. In summary, the growth and/or metastasis of some, but not all, tumors may be altered by CD44-hyaluronan interactions. The interactions between CD44 and hyaluronan that effect tumor growth may be cell type specific and will require further investigation for a complete understanding.

2.3. Expression of CD44 and Hyaluronan in Ovarian Carcinoma

An immunohistochemical study using formalin-fixed paraffin embedded samples of primary ovarian tumors and peritoneal metastasis reported that CD44 expression was detected in only about 10% of the samples [41]. The authors concluded that CD44 is not involved in the metastatic spread of ovarian cancer [41]. In contrast, another study has shown that the expression of CD44 on human ovarian carcinoma cells differs depending upon the source of cells [42]. In 15 of 16 samples (94%) derived from ovarian carcinoma solid tumor implants, CD44 expression was noted [42]. In contrast, only 2 of 8 (25%) of the specimens derived from ascites expressed CD44 [42]. This contradiction of results could be attributed to differences in the fixation procedures as well as differences in the antibodies against CD44 that were used in the two studies.

In our studies, we have shown that SKOV3 and NIH:OVCAR5 ovarian carcinoma cell lines express high levels of CD44, when analyzed by flow cytometry [43,44]. Other groups have also shown that many ovarian carcinoma cell lines and normal ovarian surface epithelium express high levels of CD44 [42,45-47]. In a study of the expression of CD44s and variant isoforms in 43 human ovarian cancer cells lines, it was shown that 60% of the cell lines expressed CD44s [48].

Our group has extended these studies by showing that a cell-associated matrix, also termed a "pericellular matrix", comprised of hyaluronan surrounds ovarian carcinoma cell lines. In our study, SKOV3 and NIH:OVCAR5 ovarian carcinoma cell lines were grown for 24 hr and a pericellular matrix was visualized by a particle exclusion assay using fixed goat red blood cells [44]. The NIH:OVCAR5 cells exhibited a large pericellular matrix, which could be removed by enzymatic treatment with hyaluronidase. The pericellular matrix surrounding the NIH:OVCAR5 cells was slightly enlarged by incubation with exogenous rat chondrosarcoma proteoglycan. This is consistent with the presence of hyaluronan bound to the cell surface, which then binds the exogenous proteoglycan, and excludes the red blood cells more effectively. In contrast, SKOV3 cells did not exhibit a pericellular matrix until exogenous rat chondrosarcoma proteoglycan was added. These results suggest that SKOV3 cells do not produce as much hyaluronan and/or an associated proteoglycan as do the NIH:OVCAR5 cells. Thus, it is possible that each cell line, and potentially each patient's ovarian carcinoma cells that are present in the peritoneal fluid, may secrete different levels of hyaluronan.

Several studies have examined the levels of various isoforms of CD44 in the ascites fluid and serum samples of patients with ovarian carcinoma. In one study, circulating CD44 isoforms were detected in the sera of 6 of 8 patients, and 12 of 16 ascitic fluid samples [49]. In addition, all six CD44 positive sera samples were also positive for variant CD44 [49]. In another study, the preoperative levels of sera from 51 patients with ovarian carcinoma were analyzed and found to contain soluble CD44s and splice variants v5 and v6 [50]. Low levels of the variant forms were associated with advanced, poorly differentiated tumors and with large residual disease [50]. This study was confirmed by another group, whereby the serum levels of 96 ovarian carcinoma patients were analyzed for soluble CD44 [51]. A high pretreatment serum level of soluble CD44 isoform v5 was shown to be associated with a favorable clinical outcome [51].

2.4. Characterization of CD44 and Hyaluronan on Mesothelial Cells

Studies have shown that CD44 on the surface of ovarian carcinoma cells is important in the binding to mesothelium-associated hyaluronan [45]. For example, it has been demonstrated that hyaluronan resides in a pericellular matrix around the mesothelial cells that can be destroyed by aspirating the mesothelial cells' medium, or by treating the mesothelial cells with hyaluronidase [52].

Our group and others have performed particle exclusion assay to show that a pericellular matrix surrounds the mesothelial cells [44,52]. As described above for the ovarian carcinoma cell lines, the pericellular matrix of the LP9 mesothelial cell line was visibly removed by enzymatic treatment with hyaluronidase. The pericellular matrix surrounding the mesothelial cells was enlarged by incubation with exogenous rat chondrosarcoma proteoglycan. This is consistent with the presence of hyaluronan bound to the mesothelial cell surface, which then binds the exogenous proteoglycan, and excludes the red blood cells more effectively. Furthermore, we have shown that the LP9 mesothelial cell line expresses high levels of CD44 when analyzed by flow cytometry [43,44]. Other groups have shown that the L3 and L9 mesothelial cell lines, as well as normal mesothelial cells also express high levels of CD44 [42,46].

2.5. Role of CD44 and Hyaluronan in the Adhesion of Ovarian Carcinoma Cells to Mesothelial Cells

Recently, Cannistra et al. [42] isolated both mesothelial cells and ovarian carcinoma cells from the peritoneal cavity of patients, and performed *in vitro* adhesion assays with the cells. They found that clone 515, a CD44 monoclonal antibody (mAb), was able to partially inhibit the adhesion of these two cell types, and concluded that CD44 on the surface of ovarian cancer cells may mediate binding to mesothelium-associated hyaluronan [42]. This group also showed that 94% of ovarian carcinoma samples derived from solid tumor implants expressed CD44, and these CD44-positive cells adhered to monolayers of mesothelial cells [42]. In contrast, only 25% of the specimens derived from ascites were positive, and these cells adhered poorly to monolayers of mesothelial cells [42]. Furthermore, Cannistra's group inhibited the intra-abdominal spread of human ovarian cancer xenograft in nude mice using the same CD44 mAb [53]. Taken together, these studies and others [47] suggest that CD44 and hyaluronan play an important role in the adhesion of ovarian carcinoma cells to mesothelial cell during peritoneal implantation. However, since the CD44 mAb did not cause complete inhibition in either the *in vitro* or the *in vivo* studies, it is likely that other cell surface molecules also contribute to the adhesion of ovarian carcinoma cells to mesothelial cells.

Our group has performed similar *in vitro* assays to quantitate the adhesion of ovarian carcinoma cells to mesothelial cells [43,44]. In our assay, mesothelial cells were grown as confluent monolayers. Radiolabeled human ovarian carcinoma cell lines were allowed to adhere to the mesothelial cell monolayers, washed, and quantitated. We have shown that pretreatment of NIH:OVCAR5 ovarian carcinoma cells with a mAb (clone IM7) against the hyaluronan-binding site of CD44 significantly inhibited NIH:OVCAR5 cell adhesion to mesothelial cells by about 40%, whereas a blocking mAb against the β1 integrin subunit (clone P5D2) failed to cause significant inhibition. The inhibitory effect of the mAb against CD44 varied depending upon the ovarian carcinoma cell line used, since it did not inhibit the adhesion of the SKOV3 ovarian carcinoma cell line, as described below.

Our group has also demonstrated that the adhesion of NIH:OVCAR5 cells to LP9 mesothelial cells is dependent upon the availability of mesothelial-associated hyaluronan. In this assay, confluent monolayers of LP9 cells were treated with hyaluronidase to remove their cell-associated hyaluronan [44]. Removal of hyaluronan resulted in a decrease in NIH:OVCAR5 cell adhesion to mesothelial cells, which suggests that the cell-cell adhesion was partly dependent upon the presence of mesothelial cell hyaluronan.

The presence of hyaluronan on NIH:OVCAR5 ovarian carcinoma cells, and the high levels of expression of CD44 by mesothelial cells, suggest that a second type of CD44-hyaluronan interaction contributes to the cell-cell adhesion. Namely, CD44 and hyaluronan may be present on both the mesothelial cells and the NIH:OVCAR5 cells, resulting in a dual interaction of these adhesion molecules.

In preliminary studies, we have observed that adhesion of ovarian carcinoma cells to mesothelial cells can be partially inhibited by oligomers of hyaluronan. NIH:OVCAR5 cells were preincubated with intact hyaluronan or oligomers of hyaluronan, added to monolayers of mesothelial cells, and allowed to adhere. We found that the oligomers of hyaluronan inhibited cell-cell adhesion in a concentration-dependent manner, whereas intact hyaluronan had no effect. It is likely that these oligomers of hyaluronan (which are comprised of hyaluronan hexasaccharides) are able to occupy the CD44 receptors on the ovarian carcinoma cells and thus block the adhesion of the ovarian carcinoma cells to the hyaluronan present on the pericellular matrix surrounding the mesothelial cells.

In addition, CD44 and hyaluronan appear to be involved in the migration of ovarian carcinoma cell lines. We have shown that hyaluronan, hyaluronan oligomers, and a mAb against CD44 can inhibit the migration of NIH:OVCAR5 and SKOV3 cells toward ECM proteins [54]. Furthermore, the interaction between CD44 and the repeat domain of ankyrin has been shown to promote hyaluronan-mediated migration of SKOV3 cells [55].

3. INTEGRINS

Integrins are a widely expressed family of cell surface adhesion receptors that are comprised of an α subunit noncovalently associated to a β subunit [56,57]. Together, these two integrin subunits confer specificity to ECM proteins or other cell surface molecules. For example, the integrins $\alpha1\beta1$, $\alpha2\beta1$, $\alpha3\beta1$, $\alpha6\beta1$, and $\alpha6\beta4$ serve as receptors for laminin. Certain integrins function as receptors for ECM proteins such as fibronectin, collagen, and laminin. In many cases, individual integrin heterodimers may interact with more than one ECM protein [58]. Other integrins participate in cell-cell adhesion; for instance, the $\alpha4\beta1$ integrin on leukocytes recognizes and binds to VCAM-1 molecules expressed on the endothelial surface. Some integrins can serve in both capacities; for example, the $\alpha4\beta1$ integrin can also bind to fibronectin [7].

Integrins have been shown to be involved in signal transduction, whereby "inside-out" and "outside-in" signaling occurs via integrins interacting with a variety of extracellular and intracellular molecules [reviewed in 59-61], many of which still remain to be elucidated. Due to the transmembrane structure of integrins, they are capable of linking the ECM components to intracellular molecules and mediating the attachment, spreading, and migration of cells. Since integrins also interact with the signal transduction apparatus, the engagement of integrins results in the release of lipid second messengers, activation of protein kinases, and changes in intracellular calcium and pH. Integrin signaling can therefore also regulate cell proliferation, gene expression, differentiation, and apoptosis. The exact mechanism by which integrins are capable of sending signals and how cells integrate these signals with others from their environmental milieu remains to be determined.

3.1. Role of Integrins in Cancer

The receptors that cells use to adhere to ECM molecules have been characterized in a variety of cell types [62,63]. Previous studies have shown that integrins may be involved in the invasion and metastasis of a variety of tumor cells [64]. Furthermore, the malignant transformation of cells has been associated with an alteration in the expression and structure of several integrin subunits.

Immunofluorescence studies have been conducted using anti-integrin antibodies (Abys) to localize the various integrin subunits in normal and cancerous tissues. For example, the $\alpha6\beta4$ complex has been localized in hemidesmosomes [65] and the basal surface of epithelial cells [66], indicating that it plays an important role in the adhesion of epidermal cells to the basement membrane. Interestingly, alterations in integrin expression and localization have been noted in several types of cancer, including ovarian carcinoma. In comparing normal human skin to nodular basal cell carcinomas and squamous cell carcinomas, different patterns of distribution for $\beta1$, $\alpha2$, $\alpha3$, and $\alpha5$ integrin subunits were observed [67]. Other studies have shown that there is a progressive decrease in the expression of $\alpha6$ and $\beta1$ subunits, but not the $\beta4$ subunit, when comparing benign, malignant, and metastatic human melanocytic lesions [68]. Additional studies have shown an increase in the expression of $\alpha v\beta3$ and $\alpha4\beta1$ as human melanoma cell lines of increasing invasive and metastatic properties were compared [69]. Still other studies report a correlation between the expression of various integrin subunits and increased metastatic potential [70-72].

Expression of the $\alpha6\beta4$ integrin on normal epithelial cells compared to cells of primary tumors or metastatic cells is still somewhat of a controversy and seems to differ between various types of tumors as well as between various studies. In normal epithelium, $\alpha6\beta4$ is localized to the basal surface of cells, where the cells are in contact with the basement membrane [73]. However, in some cases of carcinoma, for example squamous cell carcinoma of the skin [74,75], $\alpha6\beta4$ expression is no longer polarized to the basal surface of the cell, instead $\alpha6\beta4$ is diffusely distributed over the entire surface of the cell. Other immunohistochemical studies have shown that $\alpha6\beta4$ expression in carcinoma tissues compared to their normal tissue counterpart appears to be decreased [73-78], increased [79,80], or not changed [78,81,82]. Our studies, described below, show that the expression of $\alpha6$ and $\beta4$ integrins in serous ovarian carcinoma correlates with expression of the basement membrane protein laminin [83].

Many studies have been designed to investigate the role of different adhesion molecules in the hematogenous spread of cancer cells. For instance, VLA-4 ($\alpha4\beta1$ integrin) on cancer cells facilitates cell-to-cell interactions with vascular cell adhesion molecule-1 (VCAM-1) on endothelial cells. It has been shown that an increased expression of VLA-4 in renal cell cancer is proportional to the percentage of metastatic renal cell carcinoma [84]. Furthermore, adhesion of VLA-4 positive renal cell carcinoma cell lines to human umbilical vein endothelial cells (HUVECs) was inhibited by antibodies against VLA-4 or VCAM-1, suggesting that VLA-4/VCAM-1 interactions are involved in the adhesion between renal cell carcinoma cells and HUVECs [84].

3.2. Extracellular Matrix Molecules Serve as Ligands for Integrins

Basement membranes are thin layers of ECM components that surround epithelial tissues, nerves, fat cells, and smooth, striated, and cardiac muscle [85]. Basement membranes are responsible for proper maintenance and compartmentalization of tissue architecture [86]. Their status modulates repair after injury by providing the scaffolding that maintains normal tissue form during regeneration and growth [85,86]. In addition, basement membranes may provide anchorage for adjacent cells and thus maintain their polarized and differentiated state [86]. Furthermore, basement membranes regulate cell migration and invasion, and serve as selective barriers against the filtration of macromolecules in capillaries and glomeruli [86]. There are indications from various systems that basement membrane molecules modify the growth and phenotype of both normal and malignant cells.

The basement membrane plays a key role in the metastasis of tumor cells [87]. During the complex, multi-step process of metastasis, tumor cells disseminate from the primary tumor mass, migrate through the epithelial cell basement membrane, enter the bloodstream or lymphatic system, arrest in a capillary bed or elsewhere, adhere to a secondary site where they must degrade and migrate through another basement membrane, proliferate, and become vascularized. The basement membrane serves as a barrier through which the tumor cells must invade to be metastatic. In cases of ovarian carcinoma, the tumor cells first tend to seed the peritoneal cavity, whereby ovarian tumor cells disseminate, attach, grow, and ultimately locally invade at various sites. Ovarian carcinoma invasion through the submesothelial basement membrane may be mediated by a variety of enzymes, including matrix metalloproteinases [88-94].

Basement membrane and ECM components, in particular laminin, type IV collagen, and fibronectin are important in the phenotypic modulation of various normal and malignant cells. These three proteins are relatively large, complex molecules, each having multiple subunits. Each glycoprotein has several domains with functional properties ascribed to them, including: domains that promote cell adhesion, spreading, and/or migration; domains that promote neurite extension from neurons; and domains that bind glycosaminoglycans, such as heparin [85]. These functional domains have been localized by a variety of techniques, including: digestion of the proteins with proteolytic enzymes followed by purification of fragments, use of Abys against specific domains to inhibit functional activity, chemical synthesis of peptides from functionally active domains, production of recombinant polypeptides, and site-directed mutagenesis studies [95,96].

In addition, these three ECM proteins also play an important role in tumor cell metastasis, since they potentiate the adhesion, spreading, migration, and invasiveness of a variety of cell types. They also can modify the *in vitro* growth, morphology, survival, and differentiation of various cells [87]. Pretreatment of a number of different tumor cell types with fragments of these molecules or specific peptides derived from them, can inhibit the experimental metastasis seen after tail vein injection in mice [97-99].

3.3. Role of Integrins and Extracellular Matrix Molecules in Ovarian Cancer

Our group investigated the role of laminin and integrins in ovarian carcinoma [83]. We have identified the cell surface integrin receptors by which ovarian carcinoma cells adhere to laminin. Our studies show that ovarian carcinoma cell lines derived from the ascites fluid of patients express very low levels of the α6 and β4 integrin subunits, which serve as laminin receptors. These results suggest that the ovarian carcinoma cells present in the ascites fluid may adhere poorly to laminin and would therefore be released from the basement membrane on the surface of the ovary. In addition, we have determined the expression of integrin subunits on the surface of four ovarian carcinoma cell lines (SKOV3, OVCA-429, OVCA-433, and NIH:OVCAR5) by flow cytometry using mAbs against specific integrin subunits [54,83,100]. We found that the cell lines express very high levels of the α2, α3, and β1 integrin subunits, which suggests the ability to adhere to type IV collagen and other ECM proteins. They express low levels of the α6 and β4 integrin subunits, and no CD11 or β2 (CD18). Other groups have observed similar results with these and other ovarian carcinoma cell lines, including 36M2 and CAOV-3 [46,101].

Our group has identified β1 integrins as the cell adhesion molecules responsible for the adhesion of ovarian carcinoma cells to ECM molecules. We have observed that four ovarian carcinoma cell lines adhere to the ECM molecules laminin, fibronectin, and type IV collagen in a time- and concentration-dependent manner [44,100]. In addition, we have shown that each of these cell lines uses the β1 integrin to mediate their adhesion to the ECM molecules [44,100].

Several immunohistochemical studies have focused on the expression of integrin subunits in ovarian carcinoma. For example, the expression of a variety of α and β integrin subunits was described for a series of normal ovaries, serous ovarian tumors, and ascites cytospins [102]; however, the study did not correlate the integrin expression with the presence or absence of a basement membrane in these tissues. The expression of the α3 or α6 integrin subunits was studied in a variety of histological types and grades of ovarian cancer [103,104]. To date, the exact role that integrin subunits play in the progression of ovarian carcinoma is not clearly defined.

We performed immunohistochemical studies to localize laminin and integrin subunits *in situ* in tissue sections of normal ovaries and ovarian carcinomas [83]. Laminin was present in the basement membrane underneath the single layer of epithelial cells on the surface of normal ovaries. The single layer of epithelial cells on the surface of normal ovaries expresses the integrin subunits: $\alpha2$, $\alpha3$, $\alpha6$, $\beta1$, and $\beta4$, which can serve as laminin receptors. Ovarian carcinoma cells that have invaded into the stroma of the ovary also express $\alpha2$, $\alpha3$, and $\beta1$ integrin subunits. Interestingly, ~40% of the ovarian carcinoma cells that form nest-like groupings are surrounded by laminin and express $\alpha6$ and $\beta4$ integrin subunits where they interact with laminin. Furthermore, ovarian carcinoma cells derived from the ascites of the same patients are deficient in the $\alpha6$ and $\beta4$ integrin subunits. Expression of the $\alpha6$ and $\beta4$ integrin subunits appears to be regulated by laminin expression, since we have observed a loss of the $\alpha6$ and $\beta4$ integrin subunits in ovarian carcinoma tissues that were also lacking expression of laminin.

Our results are in partial agreement with an immunohistochemical study that examined normal ovaries, serous ovarian solid tumors, and ascites cytospins for the expression of integrin subunits [102]. The major difference between this study and our results was in the expression of the $\alpha6$ and $\beta4$ integrin subunits. The other group noted a basal staining pattern for the $\alpha6$ and $\beta4$ integrin subunits for all of their tumor specimens, whereas we noted $\alpha6$ and $\beta4$ integrin subunit staining to be strongly positive in ~50% of the cases, weak or patchy in ~25% of the cases, and negative in ~25% of the cases. Furthermore, they noted a loss of expression of the $\alpha6$ and $\beta4$ integrin subunits in six out of nine ascites cytospin samples, whereas we noted this loss of $\alpha6$ and $\beta4$ integrin subunit expression in all of our ascites cytospin cases. In another immunohistochemical study, a newly characterized mAb against the $\alpha6$ integrin subunit was tested and the staining pattern was shown to correlate with the degree of ovarian carcinoma tumor differentiation [104]; our results, however, did not show such a correlation. In another review article, $\alpha6\beta4$ is reported to be absent from normal epithelial cells of the ovary, although no data is presented [73]. Therefore, the expression levels of the $\alpha6$ and $\beta4$ integrin subunit, and their role in the progression of ovarian carcinoma are still controversial.

The immunohistochemistry results we observed with our anti-$\alpha3$ integrin mAbs are not in complete agreement with a previous study that examined the expression of the $\alpha3$ integrin subunit in serous ovarian carcinoma [103]. In our study, the epithelial cells of all of the tissues that we examined stained positively for the $\alpha3$ integrin subunit. In contrast, Bartolazzi *et al.* [103]

found 3 of the 18 cases of serous ovarian carcinoma in which the epithelial cells did not stain positively for the anti-α3 integrin subunit. However, our two studies are in agreement with the observation that there is a correlation between the presence of a putative "basement membrane" (as detected by peripheral immunohistochemistry staining of the tumor cell nests for laminin and type IV collagen) and the basal/lateral localization of the α3 integrin subunit. Differences in results could be attributed to differences in tissue preparation and antibodies against the α3 integrin subunit.

3.4. Characterization of Extracellular Matrix Proteins and Adhesion Molecules of Mesothelial Cells

Since an important step in the progression of ovarian carcinoma involves the adhesion of the ovarian carcinoma cells to monolayers of mesothelial cells that line the peritoneal cavity, it is also important to understand the adhesion molecules expressed by mesothelial cells. Mesothelial cell lines have been shown to express fibronectin, laminin, vitronectin, and collagens types I, III, and IV; however, the ECM molecules that are expressed from one cell line to another vary [105-108]. Mesothelial cells have been reported to express cell adhesion molecules [46,109], secrete ECM components [109], and promote the adhesion of ovarian carcinoma cells [110,111]. In a recent study [109], it was found that mesothelial cells synthesize the ECM molecule fibronectin and that ovarian cancer cells express integrins. However, the study did not provide evidence that integrins play a role in the interaction of ovarian carcinoma cells with mesothelial cells. Recently, it has been shown that cultured mesothelial cells produce fibronectin and that fibronectin promotes the migration of ovarian carcinoma cells [112].

By flow cytometry, we have determined that the human mesothelial cell line LP-9 expresses very high levels of the α3, αV, and β1 integrin subunits [43,44]. They express low levels of the α1, α5, and α6 integrin subunits, and no α2, α4, CD11, β2 (CD18), β3, or β4 integrins. Other groups have shown that normal mesothelial cells express high levels of β1, α5, and αvβ3 integrin subunits, but no α4 integrin subunits [42,46].

Our group has also examined the expression of ECM proteins by LP9 human mesothelial cells [43,44]. We tested for the presence of ECM molecules on the mesothelial cell monolayer by designing an ELISA in which mesothelial cells were incubated with polyclonal antibodies against the ECM molecules: fibronectin, laminin, vitronectin, and collagens types I, III, and IV. Fibronectin was detected at a much higher level than any of the other ECM molecules. To confirm these results, proteins that were either extracted from the mesothelial cell layer or secreted into the medium were immunoprecipitated using polyclonal antibodies to ECM molecules [44]. The mesothelial LP9 cells were found to express the following ECM molecules on their surface: fibronectin, laminin, type I collagen, type III collagen, and type IV collagen. No vitronectin was detected in the mesothelial cell surface extract. Autoradiographs of the immunoprecipitated radiolabeled material secreted into the media by LP9 cells showed that fibronectin, laminin, and collagen types I, III, and IV were synthesized and secreted by the LP9 cells. The relative amounts of these ECM components were similar to that seen in the cell extract.

Recently, we have examined the ability of ECM molecules to mediate ovarian carcinoma cell migration [54]. We found that laminin, fibronectin, and type IV collagen promote the adhesion of NIH:OVCAR5 and SKOV3 ovarian carcinoma cells in a concentration-dependent manner. In contrast, hyaluronan had no effect on ovarian carcinoma cell migration.

3.5. Role of the β1 Integrin in the Adhesion of Ovarian Carcinoma Cells to Mesothelial Cell Monolayers

Our group and others have developed *in vitro* assays to quantitate the adhesion of ovarian carcinoma cells to mesothelial cells [43,44], as described above. We have shown that pretreatment of SKOV3 ovarian carcinoma cells with the mAb against the ß1 integrin subunit (clone P5D2) significantly decreased SKOV3 cell adhesion to mesothelial cells in a concentration-dependent manner. However, the CD44 mAb did not cause significant inhibition. In contrast, pretreatment of NIH:OVCAR5 ovarian carcinoma cells with the CD44 mAb inhibited NIH:OVCAR5 cell adhesion to mesothelial cells by about 40%, whereas the mAb against the β1 integrin subunit did not cause significant inhibition. These studies showed that different cell lines may have different mechanisms for adhering to mesothelial cells, even though the level of expression of CD44 and the β1 integrin subunit are high in both cell lines. An earlier study contradicted our results by stating that CD44, not the β1 integrin subunit, was utilized by ovarian carcinoma cells to adhere to mesothelial cells [42]. However, the group recently confirmed our results that the β1 integrin subunit plays a role in mediating the adhesion of ovarian carcinoma cells to mesothelial cells [101]. They now report that mAb clone 4B4 against the β1 integrin subunit that they had used in their earlier study [42] was not effective as a neutralizing mAb, whereas an alternative mAb against the β1 integrin subunit (clone MAB13) did inhibit ovarian carcinoma cell adhesion to mesothelial cell monolayers [101].

Interestingly, we observed that when SKOV3 or NIH:OVCAR5 ovarian carcinoma cells were preincubated with a mAb against the β1 integrin subunit, then were added to monolayers of mesothelial cells that were pretreated with hyaluronidase to remove their matrix-associated hyaluronan, cell adhesion decreased [44]. Removal of hyaluronan from the pericellular matrix of mesothelial cells may expose other ECM molecules that are expressed by the mesothelial cells, which permits the ovarian carcinoma cells to adhere, primarily via their β1 integrin subunit, to the exposed ECM molecules.

3.6. Association of the β1 Integrin Subunit of Ovarian Carcinoma Cell Lines with Protein Kinase Activity

Phosphorylation is an important mechanism of regulating protein function in a variety of systems, including the functioning of integrin subunits [59-61]. Recently, integrin-mediated cell adhesion has been shown to result in tyrosine phosphorylation of focal adhesion kinase, which then may initiate a series of phosphorylation events including the binding of Src [59]. Integrin-mediated cell adhesion may also result in the phosphorylation of the intracellular proteins tensin, paxillin, and p130 [113-115]. Integrins, cytoskeletal proteins, and kinases have been localized at focal adhesion sites, where cells are in contact with the ECM. In particular, focal adhesion kinase, protein kinase C, and cSrc have been implicated as important kinases activated by integrins to mediate a variety of cell functions including cell proliferation, cell differentiation, and apoptosis [59]. In addition, protein kinase activity has been found to be associated with a variety of membrane proteins involved in signal transmission [116-119]. Recent studies have demonstrated the existence of large detergent resistant complexes in cell extracts that contain important signaling molecules, including protein kinases and membrane proteins capable of transmitting signals [120,121].

To address whether the β1 integrin subunit is associated with protein kinase activity, five ovarian cancer cell lines (OVCA 433, SKOV3, CAOV-3, PA-1, and SW626) were screened for the expression of β1 integrin and for integrin associated protein kinase activity [122]. When the β1 integrin was immunoprecipitated from the solubilized cells, protein serine kinase activity associated with the integrin was detected. Although protein kinase C (PKC) activity was present in these cells, it was not detected in the β1 integrin immunoprecipitates. The data suggest that phosphorylation of cellular proteins by an associated serine kinase, other than PKC, may affect signal transduction by β1 integrins. In addition, studies using gel filtration chromatography demonstrated that most of the cell surface β1 integrin, as well as the associated kinase activity, was present in large detergent resistant complexes.

Although the exact role of protein kinase activity in ovarian cancer is not known, a variety of scenarios could be postulated whereby an imbalance in the maintenance of proper regulation of phosphorylation could ultimately result in the transformation of normal epithelial ovarian cells to cancer cells. The surface of the ovary is comprised of a monolayer of epithelial cells that adhere to an underlying basement membrane, presumably in a tightly controlled "inside out" and "outside in" signaling manner. During the progression of cancer, some alteration in signaling may occur such that these epithelial cells no longer adhere to the basement membrane. Perhaps the cells are signaled to secrete more proteolytic enzymes and thereby degrade components of the basement membrane, resulting in cells that are now capable of invading into the stroma of the ovary. Alternatively, or in conjunction, the cancerous epithelial cells may alter their synthesis of basement membrane components. This may then signal the cells via "outside in" signaling to alter their expression of integrin receptors for these basement membrane components. The net result would be that the epithelial cells would no longer be anchored to the basement membranes. The cells may be released from the surface of the ovary to reside in the ascites fluid of the peritoneal cavity. When the epithelial cells lose contact with a basement membrane, their expression of integrin receptors may change, and their invasive capacity may be affected as well.

4. E-CADHERIN

Cadherins are members of a family of transmembrane glycoproteins that mediate cell-cell adhesion [reviewed in 123-125]. Cadherin adhesion is usually homophilic, although a heterotypic interaction between E-cadherin (E denotes epithelial) and the integrin $\alpha E\beta 7$ has been shown [126]. Cadherins mediate intercellular cell-cell adhesion in adherens junctions and desmosomes. The extracellular regions of cadherins contain calcium-binding domains; cell-cell adhesion via cadherins is calcium dependent. The cytoplasmic tails of cadherins are able to cluster and interact with catenins (β-catenin or plakoglobin and others) which then interact with α-catenin and actin [123]. Cadherins have also been implicated in signal transduction, and the E-cadherin-catenin complex is important for the regulation of cancer invasion [125].

4.1. Role of E-cadherin in Cancer

The E-cadherin complex has been shown to be altered in most human cancers. E-cadherin is expressed early in development and is found in most embryonic and adult epithelia [125]. In most tissues, E-cadherin is expressed at the highest levels in normal epithelia, then expressed at lower levels in differentiated carcinomas, and finally is down-regulated or non-functional as cancer cells become undifferentiated and invasive [127]. Altered cadherin expression has been correlated with low histological differentiation, increased risk of local invasion and metastasis, and poor prognosis [128,129].

4.2. Expression of E-cadherin in Ovarian Carcinoma

The pattern of expression of E-cadherin in normal ovarian surface epithelia, ovarian carcinoma solid tumors, and ascites cells remains controversial. Some groups maintain that E-cadherin expression in normal ovarian surface epithelia is rare [130-134], while others demonstrate that E-cadherin is present [83,128,135]. In our studies [83], E-cadherin followed a similar pattern of expression compared to the α2, α3, and β1 integrin subunits. We observed E-cadherin on the surface of normal ovary epithelial cells, ovarian carcinoma epithelial cells in solid tumor nests, and epithelial ovarian carcinoma cells isolated from the ascites fluid. These results were confirmed by others who detected E-cadherin along the lateral membranes of epithelial cells in normal ovary tissues and ovarian tumors [128]. In contrast to our results, other groups did not observe expression of E-cadherin on ovarian epithelial cells or on cultured human ovarian surface epithelium [102,133]. However, another group has reported the positive expression of E-cadherin in solid ovarian carcinoma tumors [136]. They observed a decreased expression of E-cadherin on the surface of ascites cells compared to the solid tumor counterpart from the same patient [136]. Additional studies utilizing standardized sample preparation protocols and antibodies will be needed to clarify these differences.

5. SUMMARY

The exact mechanisms by which serous ovarian cancer cells invade through their underlying basement membrane or are released from the surface of the ovary have yet to be elucidated. This process undoubtedly has a complex molecular basis that most likely involves multiple cell surface receptors, basement membrane components, intercellular adhesion molecules, and signaling from the cell [137]. One possible mechanism by which ovarian carcinoma tumor cells may alter their basement membrane is by the synthesis and secretion of proteolytic enzymes that degrade their basement membranes [88-94,138]. Alternatively, metastatic ovarian carcinoma cells may decrease their synthesis and/or secretion of ECM molecules.

Additional studies are required to determine whether the more aggressive behavior of malignant ovarian carcinoma cells, compared to normal ovarian epithelial cells, is related to an altered cellular response towards ECM molecules, perhaps due to alterations in adhesion molecules/receptors. A further elucidation of the mechanisms by which serous ovarian carcinoma cells regulate their expression of ECM molecules and adhesion molecules/receptors will help in our understanding of the invasion and metastasis of tumor cells.

Members of several families of adhesion molecules have been described that seem to be important in the progression of ovarian carcinoma, including CD44, integrins, and E-cadherin. Due to the complexity of this disease, it is likely that other adhesion molecules will also be implicated in the adhesion, migration, invasion, growth, proliferation, and apoptosis of ovarian carcinoma cells.

Our group and others have shown that CD44 and the $\beta1$ integrin subunit play fundamental roles in the adhesion and migration of ovarian carcinoma cells to mesothelial cells and their associated pericellular matrix. Subsequent to the initial adhesion, the ovarian carcinoma cells may migrate through the layer of mesothelial cells, penetrate through the underlying basement membrane, invade into the tissue, and establish a secondary site of growth.

Further studies will be required in order to fully understand the relationship of each adhesion molecule and their ligand(s) in the progression of this disease. Once the adhesion molecules and their ligand(s) for each step of the progression of this disease have been identified, it should be possible to develop reagents that can inhibit these interactions. Then, when ovarian carcinoma cells can no longer interact with mesothelial cells and their associated ECM, the dissemination of ovarian carcinoma cells *in vivo* may be prevented.

ACKNOWLEDGMENTS

Funding was provided by the Minnesota Medical Foundation (Grant #SMF-2078-99), and the Office of the Vice President for Research and Dean of the Graduate School of the University of Minnesota. Funding was also provided by the Department of the Army, Grant #DA/DAMD17-99-1-9564. The content of the information does not necessarily reflect the position of the Government.

REFERENCES

1. Landis SH, Murray T, Bolden SH, Wingo PA. Cancer statistics. Ca: Cancer J Clin 1999; 49:8-31.
2. Dietl J, Marzusch K. Ovarian surface epithelium and human ovarian cancer. Gynecol Obstet Invest 1993; 35:129-135.
3. Teneriello MG, Park RC. Early detection of ovarian cancer. CA - Cancer J Clin 1995; 45:71-87.

4. Kataosha A, Nishida T, Sugiyama T, Ushijima K, Ohta S, Kumagai S, Yakushiji M, Kojiro M, Morimatsu M. A study on the distribution of metastases at autopsy in 70 patients with ovarian cancer. Nippon Sanka 1994; 46:337-344.

5. Cannistra SA. Why should the clonogenic cell assay be prognostically important in ovarian cancer? J Clin Oncol 1994; 9:368-370.

6. Omura GA, Brady MF, Homesley HD, Yordan E, Major FJ, Buchsbaum HJ, Park RC Long-term follow-up and prognostic factor analysis in advanced ovarian carcinoma: the Gynecologic Oncology Group experience. J Clin Oncol 1991; 9(7):1138-1150.

7. Albelda SM. Role of cell adhesion molecules in tumor progression and metastasis. In: Wegner CD, ed. Adhesion Molecules, San Diego, CA: Academic Press, pp. 71-88, 1994.

8. Albelda SM, Buck CA. Integrins and other cell adhesion molecules. FASEB J 1990; 4: 2868-2879.

9. Faassen AE, Drake SL, Iida J, Knutson JR, McCarthy JB. Mechanisms of normal cell adhesion to the extracellular matrix and alterations associated with tumor invasion and metastasis. In: Weinstein RS, Graham AR, Anderson RE, et al., ed. Advances in Pathology and Laboratory Medicine, Chicago, IL: Mosby Year Book Inc., pp.229-259, 1992.

10. Honn KV, Tang DG. Adhesion molecules and tumor cell interaction with endothelium and subendothelial matrix. Cancer Met Rev 1994; 11:353-375.

11. Haynes BF, Liao HX, Patton KL. The transmembrane hyaluronate receptor (CD44): multiple function, multiple forms. Cancer Cells 1991; 3:347-350.

12. Pigott R, Power C. The adhesion molecule facts book, Academic Press, London, pp. 1-190, 1993.

13. Knudson W, Knudson CB. Assembly of a chondrocyte-like pericellular matrix on non-chondrogenic cells: Role of the cell surface hyaluronan receptors in the assembly of a pericellular matrix. J Cell Sci 1991; 99:227-235.

14. Solursh M, Hardingham TE, Hascall VC, Kimura JH. Separate effects of exogenous hyaluronic acid on proteoglycan synthesis and deposition in pericellular matrix by cultured chick embryo limb chondrocytes. Dev Biol 1980; 75:121-129.

15. Kimura JH, Hardingham TE, Hascall VC, Solursh M. Biosynthesis of proteoglycans and their assembly into aggregates in cultures of chondrocytes from the Swarm rat chondrosarcoma. J Biol Chem 1979; 254:2600-2609.

16. Hascall VC, Heinegard D. Aggregation of cartilage proteoglycans. J Biol Chem 1974; 249:4242-4249.

17. Knudson CB, Keuttner KE. A role for hyaluronate in chondrocyte pericellular matrix assembly. Orthoped Trans 1990; 14:370.

18. Knudson CB, Coombs LJ, Kuettner KE. Chondrocyte pericellular matrix assembly and displacement mediated via hyaluronate. Orthoped Trans 1991; 15: 307.

19. Rodgers KE, Campeau J, Johns DB, diZerega GS, Girgis W. Reduction of adhesion formation with hyaluronic acid after peritoneal surgery in rabbits. Fertil Steril 1997; 67:553-558.

20. Morris ER, Rees DA, Welsh EJ. Conformation and dynamic interactions in hyaluronate solution. J Mol Biol 1983; 138:383-386.

21. Darzynkiewicz A, Balazs EA. Effect of connective tissue intracellular matrix on lymphocyte stimulation. I. Suppression of lymphocyte stimulation by hyaluronic acid. Exp Cell Res 1971; 66:113-117.

22. Balazs EA, Darzynkiewicz A. The effect of hyaluronic acid on fibroblasts, mononuclear phagocytes and lymphocytes. In: Kulonen E, Pikkarainen J, eds. Biology of the Fibroblast, New York, pp. 237-249, 1973.

23. Pessac B, Defendi V (1972) Cell aggregation: role of acid mucopolysaccharides. Science 172:898-903.

24. Hakansson L, Hallgren R, Venge P. Regulation of granulocyte function by hyaluronic acid in vitro and in vivo effects phagocytosis, locomotion and metabolism. J Clin Invest 1980; 66:298-304.

25. Forrester V, Balazs EA. Inhibition of phagocytosis by high molecular weight hyaluronate. Endocrinology 1980; 40:435-442.
26. Shannon BT, Love SH, Myroik QN. Participation of hyaluronic acid in the macrophage disappearance reaction. Immunol Commun 1980; 9:735-746.
27. Ahgren T, Jarstrand C. Hyaluronic acid enhances phagocytosis of human monocytes in vitro. J Clin Immunol 1984 ; 4:246-252.
28. Hakansson L, Venge P. The molecular basis of the hyaluronic acid-mediated stimulation of the granulocyte function. J Immunol 1987; 138:4347-4351.
29. Ponzin D, Vacchia P, Toffano G, Giordano C, Bruni A. Characterization of macrophages elicited by intraperitoneal injection of hyaluronate. Agents and Actions 1986; 18:544-546.
30. Feinberg RN, Beebe DC. Hyaluronate in vasculogenesis. Science 1983 220:1177-1179.
31. West DC, Hampson IN, Arnold F, Kumar S. Angiogenesis induced by degradation products of hyaluronic acid. Science 1985; 228:1324-1326.
32. Edelstam GAB, Laurent UBG, Lundkvist OE, Fraser JRE, Laurent TC. Concentration and turnover of intraperitoneal hyaluronan during inflammation. Inflammation 1992; 16:459-469.
33. Zeng C, Toole BP, Kinney SD, Kuo J, Stamenkovic I. Inhibition of tumor growth in vivo by hyaluronan oligomers. Int J Cancer 1998; 77:396-401.
34. Cannistra SA, Abu-Jawdeh G, Niloff J, Strobel T, Swanson L, Andersen J, Ottensmeier C CD44 variant expression is a common feature of epithelial ovarian cancer: lack of association with standard prognostic factors. J Clin Oncol 1995; 13(8):1912-1921.
35. Ropponen K, Tammi M, Parkkinen J, Eskelinen M, Tammi R, Lipponen P, Agren U, Alhava E, Kosma VM. Tumor cell-associated hyaluronan as an unfavorable prognostic factor in colorectal cancer. Cancer Res 1998; 58(2):342-347.
36. Sy M, Guo Y, Stamenkovic I. Inhibition of tumor growth in vivo with soluble CD44-immunoglobulin fusion protein. J Exp Med 1992; 176:623-627.
37. Bartolazzi A, Peach R, Aruffo A, Stamenkovic I. Interaction between CD44 and hyaluronate is directly implicated in regulation of tumor development. J Exp Med 1994; 180:53-66.
38. Zahalka M, Okon E, Gosslar U, Holzmann B, Naor D. Lymph node (but not spleen) invasion by murine lymphoma is both CD44- and hyaluronate-dependent. J Immunol 1995; 154:5345-5355.
39. Salmi M, Gron-Virta K, Sointu P, Grenman R, Kalimo H, Jalkanen S. Regulated expression of exon v6 containing isoforms of CD44 in man: downregulation during malignant transformation of tumors of squamocellular origin. J Cell Biol 1993; 122:431-442.
40. Sleeman J, Arming S, Moll J, Hekele A, Rudy W, Sherman L, Kreil G, Ponta H, Herrlich P. Hyaluronate-independent metastatic behavior of CD44 variant-expressing pancreatic carcinoma cells. Cancer Res 1996; 56:3134-3141.
41. Speiser P, Wanner C, Breitenecker G, Kohlberger P, Kainz C. CD-44 is not involved in the metastatic spread of ovarian cancer in vivo. Anticancer Res 1995; 15(6B):2767-2769.
42. Cannistra SA, Kansas GS, Niloff J, DeFranzo B, Kim Y, Ottensmeier C. Binding of ovarian cancer cells to peritoneal mesothelium in vitro is partly mediated by CD44H. Cancer Res 1993; 53:3830-3838.
43. Lessan K, Skubitz APN. Binding of an ovarian carcinoma cell line to peritoneal mesothelial cells in vitro is partially inhibited by an antibody against the β1 integrin subunit. FASEB J 1998; 12:A377.
44. Lessan K, Aguiar DJ, Oegema T, Siebenson L, Skubitz APN. CD44 and the β1 integrin mediate ovarian carcinoma cell adhesion to peritoneal mesothelial cells. Amer J Path 1999; 154:1525-1537.
45. Gardner MJ, Catterall JB, Jones LM, Turner GA. Human ovarian tumour cells can bind hyaluronic acid via membrane CD44: a possible step in peritoneal metastasis. Clin Exp Met 1996; 14(4):325-334.

46. Gardner MJ, Jones LMH, Catterall JB, Turner GA. Expression of cell adhesion molecules on ovarian tumour cell lines and mesothelial cells, in relation to ovarian cancer metastasis. Cancer Lett 1995; 91:229-234.

47. Cannistra SA, DeFranzo B, Niloff J, Ottensmeier C. Functional heterogeneity of CD44 molecules in ovarian cancer cell lines. Clin Cancer Res 1995; 1:333-342.

48. Stickeler E, Runnebaum IB, Möbus VJ, Kieback DG, Kreienberg R. Expression of CD44 standard and variant isoforms v5, v6 and v7 in human ovarian cancer cell lines. Anticancer Res 1997; 17:1871-1876.

49. Taylor DD, Gercel-Taylor C, Gall SA. Expression and shedding of CD44 variant isoforms in patients with gynecologic malignancies. J Soc Gynecol Invest 1996; 3:289-294.

50. Gadducci A, Ferdeghini M, Fanucchi A, Annicchiarico C, Cosio S, Prontera C, Bianchi R, Genazzani AR. Serum assay of soluble CD44 standard (sCD44-st), CD44 splice variant v5 (sCD44-v5), and CD44 splice variant v6 (sCD44-v6) in patients with epithelial ovarian cancer. Anticancer Res 1997; 17:4463-4466.

51. Zeimet AG, Widschwendter M, Uhl-Steidl M, Mueller-Holzner E, Daxenbichler G, Marth C, Dapunt O. High serum levels of soluble CD44 variant isoform v5 are associated with favourable clinical outcome in ovarian cancer. Brit J Cancer 1997; 76(12):1646-1651.

52. Jones LMH, Gardner MJ, Catterall JB, Turner GA. Hyaluronic acid secreted by mesothelial cells: a natural barrier to ovarian cancer cell adhesion. Clin Exp Met 1995; 13:373-380.

53. Strobel T, Swanson L, Cannistra SA. In vivo inhibition of CD44 limits intra-abdominal spread of a human ovarian cancer xenograft in nude mice: A novel role for CD44 in the process of peritoneal implantation. Cancer Res 1997; 57:1228-1232.

54. Casey RC, Skubitz APN. CD44 and $\beta1$ integrins mediate ovarian carcinoma cell migration toward extracellular matrix proteins. Clin Exp Metastatis, 2000; in press.

55. Zhu D, Bourguignon LYW. Interaction between CD44 and the repeat domain of ankyrin promotes hyaluronic acid-mediated ovarian tumor cell migration. J Cell Physiology 2000; 183:182-195.

56. Newham P, Humphries MJ. Integrin adhesion receptors: structure, function and implications for biomedicine. Mol Med Today 1996; 2(7):304-313.

57. Sheppard D. Epithelial integrins. Bioessays 1996; 18(8):655-660.

58. Tozer EC, Hughes PE, Loftus JC. Ligand binding and affinity modulation of integrins. Biochem Cell Biology 1996; 74(6):785-798.

59. LaFlamme SE, Auer KL. Integrin signalling. Sem Cancer Biol 1996; 7:111-118.

60. Dedhar S, Hannigan GE. Integrin cytoplasmic interactions and bidirectional transmembrane signalling. Curr Opin Cell Biol 1996; 8:657-669.

61. Schwartz MA, Schaller MD, Ginsberg MH. Integrins: emerging paradigms of signal transduction. Annu Rev Cell Dev Biol 1995; 11:549-599.

62. Kramer RH, Enenstein J, Waleh NS. Integrin Structure and Ligand Specificity in Cell-Matrix Interactions. Edited by Rohrbach DH, Timpl R. Molecular and Cellular Aspects of Basement Membranes. San Diego, Academic Press, Inc., pp. 239-265, 1993.

63. Mercurio AM. Laminin: multiple forms, multiple receptors. Curr Opin Cell Biol 1990; 2:845-849.

64. Dedhar S, Saulnier R, Nagle R, Overall CM. Specific alterations in the expression of $\alpha3\beta1$ and $\alpha6\beta4$ integrins in highly invasive and metastatic variants of human prostate carcinoma cells selected by in vitro invasion through reconstituted basement membrane. Clin Exp Metastasis 1993; 11:391-400.

65. Sonenberg A, Calafat J, Janssen H, Daams H, van der Raaij-Helmer LMH, Falcioni R, Kennel SJ, Aplin JD, Baker J, Loizidou M, Garrod D. Integrin $\alpha6/\beta4$ complex is located in hemidesmosomes, suggesting a major role in epidermal cell-basement membrane adhesion. J Cell Biol 1991; 113:907-917.

66. Sonnenberg A, Linders CJT, Daams JH, Kennel SJ. The $\alpha6\beta4$ protein complexes: tissue distribution and biochemical properties. J Cell Sci 1990; 96:207-217.

326

67. Peltonen J, Larjava H, Jaakkola S, Gralnick H, Akiyama SK, Yamada SS, Yamada KM. Localization of integrin receptors for fibronectin, collagen, and laminin in human skin. Variable expression in basal and squamous cell carcinomas. J Clin Invest 1990; 84:1916-1923.
68. Natali PG, Nicotra MR, Cavaliere R, Giannarelli D, Bigotti A. Tumor progression in human malignant melanoma is associated with changes in α6/β1 laminin receptor. Int J Cancer 1991; 49:168-172.
69. Gehlsen KR, Davis GE, Sriramarao P. Integrin expression in human melanoma cells with differing invasive and metastatic properties. Clin Exp Metastasis 1992; 10:111-120.
70. Liebert M, Lee HS, Carey TE, Grossman HB. Loss of association of the α6β4 integrin and collagen VII in invasive bladder cancer. Proc Am Assoc Cancer Res 1992; 33:33.
71. Bao L, Tarin D. Correlation of VLA-4 integrin expression with metastatic potential in various human tumour cell lines. Proc Am Assoc Cancer Res 1992; 33:69.
72. Kramer RH, Waleh N, Vu MP, Cheng YF, Ramos RM. Reduced levels of the laminin-binding α7β1 integrin correlate with increased metastatic potential in malignant melanoma. Proc Am Assoc Cancer Res 1992; 33:197.
73. Quaranta V, Tamura RN, Collo G, Cooper HM, Hormia M, Rozzo C, Gaietta G, Starr L Distinctive functions of α6β4 and other integrins in epithelial cells. Edited by Cheresh DA, Mecham RP. Integrins: Molecular and Biological Responses to the Extracellular Matrix. San Diego, Academic Press, pp. 141-161, 1994.
74. Rossen K, Dahlstrom KK, Mercurio AM, Wewer UM. Expression of the α6β4 integrin by squamous cell carcinomas and basal cell carcinomas: Possible relation to invasive potential? Acta Derm Venereol (Stockh) 1994; 74:101-105.
75. Savoia P, Trusolino L, Pepino E, Cremona O, Marchisio PC. Expression and topography of integrin and basement membrane proteins in epidermal carcinomas: basal but not squamous cell carcinomas display loss of α6β4 and BM-600/nicein. J Invest Dermatol 1993; 101:352-358.
76. Stallmach A, Lampe BV, Matthes H, Bornhöft G, Riecken EO. Diminished expression of integrin adhesion molecules on human colonic epithelial cells during the benign to malign tumour transformation. Gut 1992; 33:342-346.
77. Koukoulis GK, Virtanen I, Korhonen M, Laitinen L, Quaranta V, Gould VE. Immunohistochemical localization of integrins in the normal, hyperplastic, and neoplastic breast. Am J Pathol 1991; 139:787-799.
78. Costantini RM, Falcioni R, Battista P, Zupi G, Kennel SJ, Colasante A, Venturo I, Curcio CG, Sacchi A. Integrin (α6/β4) expression in human lung cancer as monitored by specific monoclonal antibodies. Cancer Res 1990; 50:6107-6112.
79. Kimmel KA, Carey TE. Altered expression in squamous carcinoma cells of an orientation restricted epithelial antigen detected by monoclonal antibody A9. Cancer Res 1986; 46:3614-3623.
80. Wolf GT, Carey TE, Schmaltz SP, McClatchey KD, Poore J, Glaser L, Hayashida DJS, Hsu S. Altered antigen expression predicts outcome in squamous cell carcinoma of the head and neck. J Natl Cancer Inst 1990; 82:1566-1572.
81. Lee EC, Lotz MM, Steele GD, Mercurio AM. The integrin α6β4 is a laminin receptor. J Cell Biol 1992; 117:671-678.
82. Hall PA, Coates P, Lemoine NR, Horton MA. Characterization of integrin chains in normal and neoplastic human pancreas. J Pathology 1991; 165:33-41.
83. Skubitz APN, Bast RC Jr, Wayner EA, Letourneau PC, Wilke MS. Expression of α6 and β4 integrin in serous ovarian carcinoma correlates with expression of the basement membrane protein laminin. Am J Path 1996; 148:1445-1461.
84. Tomita Y, Saito K. Possible significance of VLA-4 (alpha 4 beta 1) for hematogenous metastasis of renal cell carcinoma. Nippon Rinsho 1995; 53:1666-1671.
85. Martin GR, Timpl R. Laminin and other basement membrane components. Ann Rev Cell Biol 1987; 3:57-85.

86. Timpl R, Dziadek M. Structure, development, and molecular pathology of basement membranes. Int Rev Exp Path 1986; 29:1-112.
87. Liotta LA, Rao CN, Wewer UM. Biochemical interactions of tumor cells with the basement membrane. Ann Rev Biochem 1986; 55:1037-1057.
88. Ellerbroek, SM, Fishman DA, Kearns AS, Bafetti LM, Stack MS. Ovarian carcinoma regulation of matrix metalloproteinase-2 and membrane type 1 matrix metalloproteinase through β1 integrin. Cancer Res 1999; 59:1635-1641.
89. Moser TL, Pizzo SV, Bafetti LM, Fishman DA, Stack MS. Evidence for preferential adhesion of ovarian epithelial carcinoma cells to type I collagen mediated by the α2β1 integrin. Int J Cancer 1996; 67:695-701.
90. Auersperg N, Maines-Bandiera SL, Kruk PA. Human surface epithelium: growth patterns and differentiation. In: Sharp F, Mason P, Blacket T, Berek J (eds), Ovarian Cancer III, London: Chapman & Hall, pp. 157-169, 1994.
91. Stack MS, Ellerbroek SM, Fishman DA. The role of proteolytic enzymes in the pathology of epithelial ovarian carcinoma. Int J Oncol 1998; 12:569-576.
92. Afzel S, Lalani EN, Poulsom R, Stubbs A, Rowlinson G, Sato H, Seiki M, Stamp GW. MT1-MMP and MMP-2 mRNA expression in human ovarian tumors: possible implications for the role of desmoplastic fibroblasts. Hum Pathol 1998; 29:155-165.
93. Fishman DA, Bafetti LM, Stack MS. Membrane-type matrix metalloproteinase expression and matrix metalloproteinase-2 activation in primary human ovarian epithelial carcinoma cells. Inv Metastasis 1996; 16:150-159.
94. Moser TL, Young TN, Rodriguez GC, Pizzo SV, Bast RC, Stack MS. Secretion of extracellular matrix-degrading proteinases is increased in epithelial ovarian carcinoma. Int J Cancer 1994 ; 56:552-559.
95. Schwarzbaur JE. Identification of the fibronectin sequences required for assembly of a fibrillar matrix. J Cell Biol 1991; 113:1463-1473.
96. Nagai T, Yamakawa N, Aota S, Yamada SS, Akiyama SK, Olden K, Yamada KM. Monoclonal antibody characterization of two distant sites required for function of the central cell-binding domain of fibronectin in cell adhesion, cell migration, and matrix assembly. J Cell Biol 1991; 114:1295-1305.
97. Iwamoto Y, Robey FA, Graf J, Sasaki M, Kleinman HK, Yamada Y, Martin GR. YIGSR, a synthetic laminin pentapeptide, inhibits experimental metastasis formation. Science 1987; 238:1132-1134.
98. McCarthy JB, Skubitz AP, Palm SL, Furcht LT. Metastasis inhibition of different tumor types by purified laminin fragments and a heparin-binding fragment of fibronectin. J Natl Cancer Inst 1988; 80(2):108-116.
99. Humphries MJ, Olden K, Yamada KM. A synthetic peptide from fibronectin inhibits experimental metastasis of murine melanoma cells. Science 1986; 233:467-469.
100. Skubitz APN, Grossman PE, Wayner EA, Bast RC Jr. Role of integrins in the interaction of ovarian carcinoma cell lines with laminin. Mol Biol Cell 1993; 4:283a.
101. Strobel T, Cannistra SA. β1-Integrins partly mediate binding of ovarian cancer cells to peritoneal mesothelium in vitro. Gynecol Oncol 1999; 73:362-367.
102. Bridges JE, Englefield P, Boyd IE, Roche WR, Thomas EJ. Expression of integrin adhesion molecules in normal ovary and epithelial ovarian tumors. Int J Gynecol Cancer 1995; 5:187-192.
103. Bartolazzi A, Kaczmarek J, Nicolo G, Risso AM, Tarone G, Rossino P, Defilippi P, Castellani P. Localization of the α3ß1 integrin in some common epithelial tumors of the ovary and in normal equivalents. Anticancer Res 1993; 13:1-12.
104. Bottini C, Miotti S, Fiorucci S, Facheris P, Menard S, Colnaghi MI. Polarization of the α6β4 integrin in ovarian carcinomas. Int J Cancer 1993; 54:261-267.
105. Kumano K, Schiller B, Hjelle JT, Moran J. Effects of osmotic solutes on fibronectin mRNA expression in rat peritoneal mesothelial cells. Blood Purif 1996; 14(2):165-169.

328

106. Yen CJ, Fang CC, Chen YM, Lin RH, Wu KD, Lee PH, Tsai TJ. Extracellular matrix proteins modulate human peritoneal mesothelial cell behavior. Nephron 1997; 75(2):188-195.
107. Harvey W, Amlot PL. Collagen production by human mesothelial cells in vitro. J Pathol 1983; 139(3):337-347.
108. Perfumo F, Altieri P, Degl'Innocenti ML, Ghiggeri GM, Caridi G, Trivelli A, Gusmano R. Effects of peritoneal effluents on mesothelial cells in culture: cell proliferation and extracellular matrix regulation. Nephrol Dialysis Transplant 1986; 11(9):1803-1809.
109. Cannistra SA, Ottensmeier C, Niloff J, Orta B, DiCarlo J. Expression and function of β1 and αvβ3 integrins in ovarian cancer. Gynecol Oncol 1995; 58:216-225.
110. Niedbala MJ, Crickard K, Bernacki RJ. Interactions of human ovarian tumor cells with human mesothelial cells grown on extracellular matrix. Exp Cell Res 1985; 160:499-513.
111. Catterall JB, Gardner MJ, Jones LMH, Thompson GA, Turner GA. A precise, rapid and sensitive in vitro assay to measure the adhesion of ovarian tumour cells to peritoneal mesothelial cells. Cancer Lett 1984; 87:199-203.
112. Rieppi M, Vergani V, Gatto C, Zanetta G, Allavena P, Taraboletti G, Giavazzi R. Mesothelial cells induce the motility of human ovarian carcinoma cells. Int J Cancer 1999; 80:303-307.
113. Bockholt SM, Burridge K. Cell spreading on extracellular matrix proteins induces tyrosine phosphorylation of tensin. J Biol Chem 1993; 268:14565-14567.
114. Burridge K, Turner CE, Romer LH. Tyrosine phosphorylation of paxillin and pp125FAK accompanies cell adhesion to extracellular matrix: a role in cytoskeletal assembly. J Cell Biol 1992; 119:893-903.
115. Petch LA, Bockholt SM, Bouton A, Parsons JT, Burridge K. Adhesion-induced tyrosine phosphorylation of the p130 src substrate. J Cell Sci 1995; 108:1371-1379.
116. Skubitz KM, Ahmed K, Campbell KD, Skubitz APN. CD50 (ICAM-3) is phosphorylated on tyrosine kinase activity in human neutrophils. J Immunol 1995; 154:2888-2895.
117. Skubitz KM, Campbell KD, Ahmed K, Skubitz APN. CD66 family members are associated with tyrosine kinase activity in human neutrophils. J Immunol 1995; 155:5382-5390.
118. Skubitz KM, Campbell KD, Iida J, Skubitz APN. CD63 associates with tyrosine kinase activity and CD11/CD18, and transmits an activation signal in neutrophils. J Immunol 1996; 157:3617-3626.
119. Stefanova I, Horejsi V, Ansotegui IJ, Knapp W, Stockinger H. GPI-anchored cell-surface molecules complexed to protein tyrosine kinase. Science 1991; 254:1016-1019.
120. Cinek T, Horejsí V. The nature of large noncovalent complexes containing glycosyl-phosphatidylinositol-anchored membrane glycoproteins and protein tyrosine kinases. J Immunol 1992; 149:2262-2270.
121. Dráberová L, Amoui M, Dráber P. Thy-1-mediated activation of rat mast cells: the role of Thy-1 membrane microdomains. Immunology 1996; 87:141-148.
122. Skubitz APN, Campbell KD, Goueli S, Skubitz KM. Association of β1 integrin with protein kinase activity in large detergent resistant complexes. FEBS Letters 1998; 426:386-391.
123. Vleminckx K, Kemler R. Cadherins and tissue formation: integrating adhesion and signaling. BioEssays 1999; 21:211-220.
124. Steinberg MS, McNutt PM. Cadherins and their connections: adhesion junctions have broader functions. Curr Opin Cell Biol 1999; 11:554-560.
125. Noë V, Chastre E, Bruyneel E, Gespach C, Mareel M. Extracellular regulation of cancer invasion: the E-cadherin-catenin and other pathways. Biochem Soc Symp 1999; 65:43-62.
126. Higgins JM, Mandlebrot DA, Shaw SK, Russell GJ, Murphy EA, Chen YT, Nelson WJ, Parker CM, Brenner MB. Direct and regulated interaction of integrin alphaEbeta7 with E-cadherin. J Cell Biol 1998; 140:197-210.
127. Birchmeier W. E-cadherin as a tumor (invasion) suppressor gene. BioEssays 1995; 17:97-99.

128. Dara E, Leblanc M, Walker-Combrouze F, Bringuier A-F, Madelenat P, Scoazec JY. Expression of cadherins and CD44 isoforms in ovarian endometrial cysts. Human Reprod 1998; 13(5):1346-1352.

129. Dara E, Scoazec J-Y, Walker-Combrouze F, Mlika-Cabanne N, Feldmann G, Madelenat P, Potet F. Expression of cadherins in benign, borderline, and malignant ovarian epithelial tumors: A clinicopathologic study of 60 cases. Hum Pathol 1997; 28: 922-928.

130. Ong A, Maines-Bandiera SL, Roskelley CD, Auersperg N. An ovarian adenocarcinoma line derived from SV40/E-cadherin-transfected normal human ovarian surface epithelium. Int J Cancer 2000; 85:430-437.

131. Maines-Bandiera SL, Auersperg N. Increased E-cadherin expression in ovarian surface epithelium: an early step in metaplasia and dysplasia? Int J Gynecol Pathol 1997; 16:250-255.

132. Sundfeldt K, Piontkewitz Y, Ivarsson K, Nilsson O, Hellberg P, Bronnstrom M, Janson P-O, Enerboeck S, Hedin L. E-cadherin expression in human epithelial ovarian cancer and normal ovary. Int J Cancer 1997; 74:275-280.

133. Wong AST, Maines-Bandiera SL, Rosen B, Wheelock MJ, Johnson KR, Leung PCK, Roskelley CD, Auersperg N. Constitutive and conditional cadherin expression in cultured human ovarian surface epithelium: influence of family history of ovarian cancer. Int J Cancer 1999; 81: 180-188.

134. Davies BR, Worsley SD, Ponder BAJ. Expression of E-cadherin, α-catenin and β-catenin in normal ovarian surface epithelium and epithelial ovarian cancers. Histopath 1998; 32:69-80.

135. Dara E, Scoazec J-Y. Expression of cadherins and CD44 proteins in ovarian tumors: Physiopathology and diagnosis interest. Eur J Obst Gynecol Reprod Biol 1999; 86:131-133.

136. Veatch AL, Carson LF, Ramakrishnan S. Differential expression of the cell-cell adhesion molecule E-cadherein ascites and solid human ovarian cancer cells. Int J Cancer 1994; 58:393-399.

137. Ashkenas J, Damsky CH, Bissell MJ, Werb Z. Integrins, signaling, and the remodeling of the extracellular matrix. In: Integrins: Molecular and Biological Responses to the Extracellular Matrix, Cheresh DA, Mecham RP, eds. San Diego, Academic Press, pp. 79-109, 1994.

138. Campo E, Merino MJ, Tavassoli FA, Charonis AS, Stetler-Stevenson WG, Liotta LA . Evaluation of basement membrane components and the 72 kDa type IV collagenase in serous tumors of the ovary. Am J Surg Pathol 1992; 16:500-507.

Chapter 16

OVARIAN CANCER- ASSOCIATED PROTEINASES

Supurna Ghosh, Yi Wu and M. Sharon Stack
Departments of Cell & Molecular Biology and Obstetrics & Gynecology,
Northwestern University Medical School, Chicago, IL, 60611

1. INTRODUCTION

Ovarian carcinoma is the leading cause of death from gynecologic malignancies and the fourth most common cause of cancer related deaths among North American women. Approximately one out of every 70 women is estimated to develop ovarian cancer and one in 100 will die from the disease. A major cause of the high mortality of ovarian cancer is the lack of proper diagnostic tools for early detection when the tumor is still confined to the ovaries (FiGO stage I). Approximately 75% of patients are diagnosed with pre-existing disseminated intra-abdominal metastases (FIGO stage III or IV). Although the 5-year survival rate for cancer localized to the ovary can be as high as 90%, women with distant metastases have a less than 20% survival rate (Hoskins, 1995). Thus, a more detailed understanding of the factors that control ovarian cancer invasion and metastasis may have a significant impact on patient survival.

In contrast to most other cancers, dissemination of ovarian cancer is thought to occur through direct exfoliation into the peritoneal cavity from the primary tumor, followed by spread through the peritoneal fluid, leading to implantation, invasion, and growth at a secondary site. Exfoliated tumor cells also obstruct peritoneal lymphatics, leading to malignant ascites that further facilitates spread of micro-metastases (Hoskins, 1995). As dissemination of ovarian cancer is largely contained within the peritoneal cavity, dysregulated cellular adhesion (both cell-cell and cell-matrix), intraperitoneal invasion and migration likely contribute predominantly to the pathobiology of the disease. Consequently, investigation of the factors that regulate these biological processes will likely provide better tools for diagnosis and treatment.

The mammalian body is composed of interdependent tissue compartments that are separated from each other by a specialized extracellular matrix (ECM). In addition to providing mechanical support, the ECM also acts as a barrier to prevent cellular invasion across tissue boundaries. However, a distinguishing characteristic of neoplastic cells is their ability to invade tissue barriers and establish secondary tumors. Hematogenously metastasizing tumor cells are thought to require proteolytic breakdown of ECM for metastasis (Liotta *et al.*, 1986). Relatively little is known about the requirement of proteinases for the intraperitoneal metastasis of ovarian cancer. However, proteolytic degradation may play an important role in disruption of the mesothelial cell layer during invasion of the implanted tumor through the peritoneal submesothelial basement membrane into visceral organ stroma and for subsequent tumor-mediated angiogenesis.

2. OVARIAN CANCER-ASSOCIATED PROTEINASES

Malignant cells express a number of proteinases to facilitate invasion of the ECM. Predominant among these are serine proteases in the plasminogen activator (PA) family and matrix metalloproteinases (MMPs) (Andreasen *et al.*, 1997; Rabbani *et al.*, 1998). This review will primarily focus on the regulation and the clinical relevance of these two proteinase families in ovarian cancer invasion and metastasis, and will further assess their potential utility as diagnostic/prognostic indicators and therapeutic targets.

PAs are a class of serine proteinases that efficiently catalyze the hydrolysis of the Arg^{560}-Val^{561} bond of plasminogen, an inactive plasma zymogen, leading to the formation of catalytically active plasmin. There are two physiological PAs, urinary type PA (uPA or urokinase), and tissue-type PA (tPA) (Figure 1). A uPA-specific receptor (uPA receptor or uPAR) has been identified on many normal and neoplastic cells (Andreason *et al.*, 1997). Colocalization of uPAR and plasminogen facilitates pericellular plasminogen activation. There are several PA inhibitors (PAI), with PAI-1 being the most abundantly expressed. PAI-1 inactivates both soluble and receptor-bound uPA, forming a 1:1 covalent, inactive enzyme-inhibitor complex.

Nascent uPA is expressed as a single chain 411 amino acid zymogen (designated scuPA) that is proteolytically processed at Lys^{158}-Ile^{159} to a two chain, active enzyme. The A chain has an epidermal growth factor-like domain that mediates binding of uPA to uPAR, whereas the B chain contains the catalytic domain (Andreason *et al.*, 1997). uPAR is a glycosyl phosphatidyl-inositol (GPI)-anchored cell surface receptor that plays an important role in the regulation of pericellular plasminogen activation by focalizing enzyme activity at the invading edge of migrating cells. In addition, uPAR also functions to downregulate uPA activity by internalization of the uPA-uPAR-PAI-1 complex. Internalized uPA is subsequently degraded, while free receptor is recycled back to the cell surface (Conese and Blasi 1995; Mondino *et al.*, 1999). The plasmin generated as a result of plasminogen activation is a broad-spectrum serine proteinase that can degrade a number of ECM components such as fibronectin, laminin, and vitronectin. In addition, plasmin can also process various other zymogens present in the extracellular environment to their active forms and thus initiate a proteolytic cascade resulting in the degradation of ECM barriers. Plasmin activity is also regulated by proteinacious inhibitors including α2-antiplasmin and α2-macroglobulin (Andreason *et al.*, 1997).

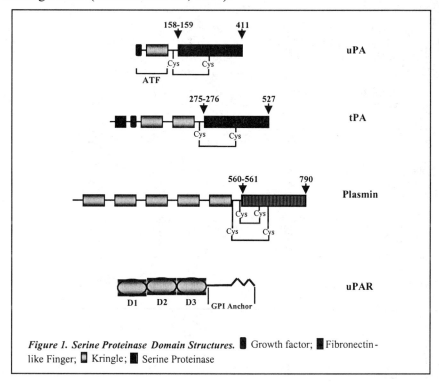

Figure 1. Serine Proteinase Domain Structures. ▌ Growth factor; ▪ Fibronectin-like Finger; ▢ Kringle; ▪ Serine Proteinase

Although plasmin can mediate the degradation of some matrix protein components, interstitial collagen, which is rich in peritoneum, is resistant to plasmin cleavage. MMPs are a family of zinc-dependent metalloendo-peptidases that function in the degradation or processing of collagen, gelatin and other extracellular matrix macromolecules. According to their substrate specificity and protein structure, members of MMP family can be categorized into the subgroups of gelatinases, collagenases, stromelysins, membrane type MMPs (MT-MMPs) and other MMPs. Structurally, most MMPs share several well-conserved domains (Figure 2), including an amino-terminal propeptide, a catalytic domain, a hinge region, and a hemopexin-like domain at or near the carboxyl-terminal (reviewed in Nagase and Woessner, 1999). The MT-MMPs contain an additional transmembrane and cytoplasmic domain. Like uPA and plasmin, the majority of MMPs are also synthesized

334

and secreted as zymogens and this represents a major control point for regulation of proteinase activity. The catalytic activity of MMPs is dependent upon an essential Glu residue and a zinc cation that interacts with an highly conserved sequence motif within the catalytic domain (HEXXHXXGXXH). The latency of MMP zymogens is maintained via ligation of the catalytically essential zinc cation by an unpaired Cys residue in the propeptide domain. MMP zymogen activation requires disruption of the Cys-zinc interaction, followed by propeptide cleavage. In addition to zymogen activation, the matrix-degrading activity of MMPs is also tightly regulated by a family of natural inhibitors designated tissue inhibitors of metalloproteinases (TIMPs). TIMPs form a 1:1 non-covalent enzyme:inhibitor complex with their their target proteinases, resulting in loss of catalytic activity (Massova *et al.*, 1998; Nagase and Woessner, 1999).

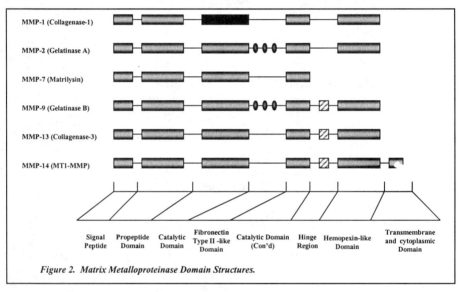

Figure 2. Matrix Metalloproteinase Domain Structures.

3. ROLE OF PAs AND MMPs IN OVARIAN CANCER

Growth of ovarian tumors requires the formation of a fibrin-fibronectin matrix around the tumor that is subsequently replaced by a mature stroma (Wilhelm *et al.*, 1988). Initial studies reported elevated levels of fibrin degradation products resulting from proteolysis of the provisional stroma in the sera of patients with advanced ovarian cancer, as well as high fibrinolytic activity in ascitic fluid (Astedt *et al.*, 1971; Hafter *et al.*, 1984; Crickard *et al.*, 1989). These reports implicated the PA/plasmin system in ovarian cancer pathology. The relationship between ovarian cancer and the fibrinolytic serine proteases has been subsequently supported by numerous experimental analyses. The majority of these studies utilized ovarian carcinoma-derived cell lines or tumor tissue samples *in vitro*. Early reports demonstrated that ovarian cancer cells produce proteinases in both the PA and MMP classes to disrupt mesothelial monolayers as well as to degrade biosynthetically labeled ECM *in vitro*. Inhibitors of both serine and metallo-proteinases efficiently blocked the invasion of reconstituted basement membranes by cultured ovarian cancer cells, further supporting the relevance of these enzymes in ovarian cancer metastasis (Kanemoto *et al.*, 1991). The following sections summarize current knowledge regarding the role of PAs and MMPs in the invasive and metastatic behavior of ovarian cancer cells.

3.1. The PA System in Ovarian Cancer

An early report in which 10 ovarian cancer cell lines were systematically evaluated for PA expression revealed preferential expression of uPA relative to tPA (Karlan *et al.*, 1988). Subsequent studies have supported a role for uPA as a prominent ovarian cancer-associated proteinase. Relative to normal ovarian epithelium, malignant ovarian epithelial cells express 17-38-fold higher uPA (Young *et al.*, 1994). Moreover, cell surface-associated uPA is indicative of uPAR expression as well. This finding is supported by data demonstrating that ovarian cancer cells contain more uPA binding ability than normal ovarian epithelium (Casslen *et al.*, 1991). A qualitative immunohisto-chemical analysis of uPA and uPAR expression in normal ovarian epithelium and ovarian carcinoma tissues demonstrated that, although both normal and malignant cells stain positively for uPAR, the receptor is occupied only in the carcinoma specimens. Enhanced uPAR immunoreactivity is also localized at the invasive edge of primary tumors (Young *et al.*, 1994). Together these data suggest that production of uPA by either tumor or stromal cells followed by binding to uPAR on tumor cell surface may result in an enhanced pericellular proteolysis. This is further supported by the observation that antisense oligonucleotides that block uPA synthesis by ovarian carcinoma cells efficiently reduce both *in vitro* invasion and *in vivo* colonization of intra-peritoneally injected cancer cells in nude mice (Wilhelm *et al.* 1995).

In addition to promoting invasion and matrix degradation, uPA has also been reported to have other distinct biological effects on ovarian carcinoma cells that may promote disease progression. For example, the amino terminal fragment (ATF) of uPA (amino acids 1-143) or the whole uPA molecule can function as a mitogen for ovarian carcinoma cells (Fischer et al., 1998; Fishman *et al.*, 1999) . In addition, ovarian cancer cells can induce release of the ATF from uPA in a serine proteinase-catalyzed reaction, suggesting the presence of an autocrine regulatory loop to control cellular proliferation (Fishman *et al.*, 1999). Although the mechanism by which ATF binding to a GPI-anchored receptor can regulate cellular growth control is currently unclear, recent studies have demonstrated that uPA-uPAR interaction can initiate a signaling cascade in ovarian cancer cells that induces rapid expression of c-fos. Moreover, such signaling promotes uPA-induced migration of ovarian cancer cells *in vitro*, and both motility and c-fos induction are dependent upon tyrosine kinase activation. Furthermore, disruption of the uPA-uPAR interaction or inhibition of tyrosine kinase signaling abolishes uPA-mediated locomotion and c-fos expression (Dumler *et al.*, 1994; Mirshahi *et al.*, 1997). These studies support the intriguing conclusion that, in addition to induction of pericellular proteolysis, uPA can also promote the growth and migration of ovarian tumor cells in a proteinase-independent manner. A detailed understanding of these mechanisms will require further investigation.

3.2. The MMP System in Ovarian Cancer

A number of MMPs, including MMP-1 (collagenase-1), -2 (gelatinase A), -7 (matrilysin), -9 (gelatinase B), -13 (collagenase-3) and –14 (MT1-MMP; Figure 2), have been linked to ovarian cancer (Moser *et al.*, 1994; Fishman *et al.*, 1997; Kanamori *et al.*, 1999; Tanimoto *et al.*, 1999; Johansson *et al.*, 1999; Shigemasa *et al.*, 2000). Expression of MMPs known to be involved in proteolysis of the basement membrane components type IV collagen and laminin-1, such as MMP-2 and MMP-9, has been the most extensively studied. Analysis of a panel of cultured ovarian carcinoma cell lines revealed abundant expression of either MMP-2 or MMP-9 whereas these proteinases were not produced in detectable amounts by normal ovarian epithelium (Moser *et al.*, 1994). Moreover, MMP secretion correlates with the ability to degrade native sub-endothelial ECM and invade reconstituted basement membrane (Young *et al.*, 1996). Examination of MMP expression by short-term primary cultures of ovarian cancer cells showed that MMP-2 is present in both latent and activated forms, indicating that primary ovarian cancer cells catalyze proMMP-2 activation. This was confirmed by immunohistochemistry and immunoprecipitation studies that demonstrated the expression of MT1-MMP, a transmembrane MMP that functions in the activation of proMMP-2 (Fishman *et al.*, 1996). It is important to note that, in addition to catalyzing proMMP-2 activation, MT1-MMP has the potential to process a broad spectrum of ECM substrates *in vitro* (d'Ortho *et al.*, 1997; Ohuchi *et al.*, 1997), suggesting that it may directly participate in the proteolysis of extracellular proteins. Furthermore, ovarian cancer cells bind activated MMP-2 and enhance the catalytic capacity of the mature enzyme (Young *et al.*, 1995), providing an additional mechanism by which tumor cells may focalize cell surface proteolytic potential. In addition to MMP-2, ovarian cancer cells also express MMP-9 and studies with primary cultures suggest that expression of MMP-9 is controlled by the *in vivo* microenvironment

(Fishman *et al.*, 1997). Additional studies using anti-catalytic MMP-9 antibodies to block *in vitro* invasion further support a crucial role of MMP-9 in ECM degradation (Ellerbroek *et al.*, 1998, Ellerbroek *et al.*, 2001). As discussed below, these studies using cultured cancer cells are consistent with immunohistochemical and *in situ* hybridization analyses of ovarian tumor specimens.

In addition to MMPs, TIMPs are also prevalent in ovarian cancer specimens. TIMP-2 expression co-localizes with MMP-2 staining patterns in high grade ovarian tumors, with enhanced staining observed at the invasive front as well as in regions of vessel penetration (Naylor *et al.*, 1994 and Afzal *et al.*, 1996). Conflicting data exist on TIMP-1 expression, as downregulation of TIMP-1 has been reported in malignant ovarian tumors (Miyagi *et al.*, 1995), while increased expression is observed in borderline and invasive tumors (Kikkawa *et al.*, 1997), suggesting that TIMP-1 may play a dual role in ovarian tumor progression.

4. PROTEINASE REGULATION IN OVARIAN CANCER
4.1. Regulation by Soluble Factors

Relatively little information is available regarding potential mechanisms by which proteinase production is regulated in ovarian cancer cells. Normal ovarian epithelial cells express little or no detectable uPA, but levels are considerably enhanced in neoplastic cells. Early studies demonstrated that glucocorticoid treatment significantly reduces uPA activity and enhances PAI-1 expression in ovarian cancer cells (Karlan *et al.*, 1989). Among the cytokines and growth factors, epidermal growth factor (EGF) and transforming growth factor (TGF)α have also been reported to influence proteinase production. Overexpression of the EGF receptor family of tyrosine kinases is associated with poor prognosis for ovarian cancer patients (Barlett *et al.*, 1996; Meden *et al.*, 1994). Moreover, ovarian cancer cell lines respond to EGF treatment by an induction of uPA and MMP-9 expression. EGF also increases cellular motility and invasiveness, and these effects are blocked by anti-catalytic antibodies against both uPA and MMP-9, suggesting the involvement of both enzyme systems in ovarian cancer invasion (Ellerbroek *et al.*, 1998, Ellerbroek *et al.*, 2001). In a related study, EGF and TGFα (an alternative ligand for the EGF receptor) were shown to increase expression of uPA, stromelysin and type IV collagenase in ovarian adenocarcinoma cells. This induction led to enhanced *in vitro* migration and invasion as well as increased expression of proangiogenic factors such as platelet-derived endothelial growth factor (Ueda *et al.*, 1999).

Macrophage colony stimulating factor (CSF1) and its receptor c-fms are also overexpressed in ovarian cancer patients and the levels correlate strongly with high grade carcinoma of poor prognostic outcome. Both uPA levels and *in vitro* invasive capacity of cultured ovarian cells correlate with CSF1 production in culture (Chambers *et al.*, 1995). Interestingly, activated ras has been shown to super-induce uPA gene expression in 4 ovarian cancer cell lines via activation of ets2, a nuclear target for activated ras (Patton *et al.*, 1998). Hence, ras-activating growth factors and cytokines may be postulated to enhance uPA production in ovarian cancer cells. Moreover, phorbol myristate acetate (PMA), an activator of cellular protein kinase C (PKC), also increases the expression of both uPA and tPA in OVCA 433 cells. PMA stimulation of uPA activity is largely dependent on new synthesis of RNA and protein (Band *et al.*, 1989). Similar results are observed upon treatment of ovarian cancer cells with lysophosphatidic acid (LPA), a bioactive lipid that functions via G protein-coupled receptors to modulate intracellular signaling (Furui *et al.*, 1999). LPA induces upregulation of uPA mRNA and protein levels in ovarian cancer cells, but not normal ovarian epithelium (Pustilnik *et al.*, 1999). As LPA is prevalent in the ascites and plasma of ovarian cancer patients (Xu *et al.*, 1995 & 1995a; Xu *et al.*, 1998; Fang *et al.*, 2000), these data suggest that LPA-induced proteinase expression may contribute to ovarian cancer invasive behavior. LPA also upregulates MMP activity in ovarian cancer cells via stimulation of MT1-MMP-catalyzed proMMP-2 activation. This increased proteolytic activity results in enhanced cellular motility and invasive activity (Fishman *et al.*, 2001).

Like uPA, expression of MMP genes is transcriptionally regulated by a variety of extracellular mediators including growth factors, cytokines and pharmacological agents. In ovarian cancer patients, vascular endothelial growth factor (VEGF) levels correlate with MMP-2 elevation and aggressiveness of serous tumors (Garzetti *et al.*, 1999). Calcium influx has also been implicated in control of MMP-2 expression and activation (Kohn *et al.*, 1994). As indicated above, EGF induces expression of MMP-9 in cultured ovarian cancer cells and stimulates motility and *in vitro* invasion (Ellerbroek *et al.*, 1998). In addition to increasing MMP-9 expression, stimulation of ovarian cancer cells with EGF also promotes cell surface association of the proteinase in a PI3K-dependent manner (Ellerbroek *et al,* 2000), suggesting that EGF may function indirectly to promote pericellular proteolysis. Similarly, activation of c-erbB2 also induces MMP-9 expression, an observation consistent with the overexpression of c-erbB2 in ovarian cancer cells (Xu *et al.*, 1997). Moreover, during ovarian follicle rupture, TNFα induces expression of specific MMPs that potentiate collagenolysis, and this phenomenon has been suggested as a putative etiologic factor in ovarian cancer (Murdoch *et al.*, 2000). In addition to growth factors and cytokines, elevation of MMP-9 has been reported in response to PMA in some ovarian cancer cells, suggesting that the PKC pathway may regulate both uPA and MMP expression (Moore *et al.*, 1997).

4.2. Regulation by Cell-Cell and Cell-Matrix Contact

Interactions between malignant cells and host stromal components may also participate in the regulation of invasive behavior of tumor cells. Early studies demonstrated that ovarian carcinoma cell adhesion to peritoneal mesothelial cells induces disruption of the mesothelial monolayer and exposure of the submesothelial ECM (Niedbala *et al.*, 1987). Furthermore, adhesion of neoplastic cells to the exposed matrix is stronger than to the mesothelial layer itself. The submesothelial ECM is rich in collagens type I and III (Harvey and Amlot, 1983) and subsequent studies demonstrated that ovarian carcinoma cells preferentially adhere to collagen I (Moser *et al.*, 1994; Fishman *et al.*, 1998). Adhesion to both collagen I and vitronectin stimulates the production of PAI-1 whereas adhesion to a collagen I- and III-rich matrix induces uPA expression by ovarian cancer cell lines (Moser *et al.*, 1994). These data suggest that proteinase activity may be regulated in part by cellular interactions with the submesothelial ECM. This hypothesis is supported by additional studies demonstrating that clustering of collagen binding integrins ($\alpha2\beta1$ and $\alpha3\beta1$) on ovarian cancer cells induces expression and activation of multiple proteinases including MMP-2, MT1-MMP and uPA (Fishman *et al.*, 1998; Ellerbroek *et al.*, 1999; and Stack lab unpublished observation). Thus, it is interesting to speculate that integrin-mediated adhesion of ascites-derived tumor cells to submesothelial collagens may induce the expression of matrix degrading proteinases to facilitate intraperitoneal invasion.

Cooperation between tumor and stromal cells has also been shown to modulate proteinase expression. For example, secretion of fibronectin by human peritoneal mesothelial cells enhances MMP-9 expression via an $\alpha5$ integrin-dependent mechanism (Shibata *et al.*, 1997). Both focal adhesion kinase and c-Ras are required for fibronectin-induced MMP-9 upregulation, and increased proteinase levels correlate with enhanced invasive activity (Shibata *et al.*, 1998). Co-culture of ovarian cancer cells with normal fibroblasts or with fibroblast-conditioned medium also stimulate tumor cell invasion; however the mediating factor(s) is unknown (Westerlund *et al.*, 1997). Moreover, ovarian cancer cells promote the production of proMMP-9 by monocytic cells *in vitro* without affecting the expression of TIMP-1, suggesting that tumor cells may also induce expression of host proteinases (Leber *et al.*, 1998).

5. CLINICAL RELEVANCE OF PROTEINASES IN OVARIAN CANCER

5.1. Proteinase Expression as a Potential Diagnostic or Prognostic Indicator

Following initial characterization of the fibrinolytic products derived from the ovarian tumor stroma by amino terminal sequence analysis, plasmin activity and PA expression were implicated in ovarian tumorigenesis (Wilhelm *et al.*, 1990). Subsequently, numerous investigators have evaluated the expression of fibrinolytic proteins in ovarian cancer specimens (sera, ascites fluid, tissue) to assess the utility of expression levels as a potential diagnostic or prognostic indicator. A significant correlation between uPA protein levels in homogenized ovarian cancer tissue and the clinical tumor stage has been reported. Patients with advanced FIGO stage III metastatic tumors contain 4-fold higher uPA protein in ovarian tissue homogenates compared to samples from nonmetastatic primary tumors (FIGO stage I/II). PAI-1 levels are also elevated in metastatic tissue samples relative to their benign counterparts (Kuhn *et al.*, 1994). These results were confirmed in an additional study which reported that uPA and PAI-1 protein levels correlate significantly with malignant progression from normal to benign and borderline adenoma and finally to primary and metastatic adenocarcinoma. However, no relationship between uPA or PAI-1 levels and parameters such as disease-free interval or overall survival was noted. Later studies have found elevated blood levels of both uPA and PAI-1 in patients with benign and metastatic tumors compared to controls but the differences were not significant enough to be used as clinical tools for early diagnosis. In contrast, tPA levels were lower in metastatic tissues compared to non-metastatic specimens (Pujade-Lauraine *et al.*, 1993).

In addition to uPA and PAI-1, a soluble form of the GPI-anchored uPAR (designated suPAR) has also been detected in the ascites fluid of 11 out of 11 ovarian cancer patients tested (Pedersen *et al.*, 1993). These authors speculate that either proteolytic modification or phospholipase digestion may give rise to this truncated receptor that retains its uPA binding capacity, but loses its cell surface association. A similar truncated human uPAR was observed in experimental mice xenografted with human carcinoma, demonstrating that the suPAR was tumor-derived rather than released from stromal cells (Holst-Hansen *et al.*, 1999). In contrast to the cell-associated uPAR, which functions to promote uPA activity and cellular invasion, the suPAR appears to have a protective action by scavenging free uPA activity (Wilhelm *et al.*, 1994). This is supported by the fact that the ratio of suPAR/uPA in ascites is positively correlated with prolonged survival and disease-free interval (Chambers *et al.*, 1995). However, a potential contradiction was reported, as ovarian cancer patients with high preoperative suPAR levels exhibit lower survival compared to women with low pre-operative suPAR (Sier *et al.*, 1998). The potential for utilizing suPAR as an early detection marker is supported by related studies demonstrating a 10 fold difference in the suPAR levels between benign and malignant ovarian cysts (Wahlberg *et al.*, 1998). However additional studies are necessary to evaluate the biological significance of suPAR to differentiate whether it functions as a uPA scavenger, or alternatively prolongs proteolytic activity by preventing uPA association with cell surface-localized uPAR and subsequent PAI-1-mediated proteinase internalization and clearance.

A similar approach has been utilized to examine the potential clinical relevance of MMP expression in ovarian cancer ascites, sera, and tissues. Initial examination of ascites fluid indicated that these specimens are rich in both MMP-2 and MMP-9, although the cellular source of the proteinases could not be identified (Young *et al.*, 1996; Fishman *et al.*, 1997). Quantitation of MMP-2 levels in sera demonstrated increased expression levels in patients with malignant tumors relative to cystadenomas or borderline tumors (De Nictolis *et al.*, 1996). A related study reported that serum MMP-2 levels are significantly increased in patients with cystadeno-carcinoma in comparison to borderline tumors and cystadenomas, supporting a role for serum MMP-2 as a diagnostic marker (Garzetti *et al.*, 1996). In addition to measurement of serum proteinase levels, tissue MMP-2 may serve as a prognostic indicator in patients with FIGO stage III ovarian serous cystadenocarcinoma, as MMP-2 expression is significantly correlated with the risk of recurrence (Garzetti *et al.*, 1995). Interestingly, the localization of MMP-2 also seems to affect the prognosis of ovarian cancer. MMP-2 positivity in cancer cells is associated with recurrent disease, whereas MMP-2 negativity in fibroblasts correlates with Grade 3 Stage III-IV recurrence and refractory disease (Westerlund *et al.*, 1999). Further analysis of tumor specimens by *in situ* hybridization coupled with immunohistochemical analyses showed that staining for activated MMP-2 is associated with the malignant phenotype in adenocarcinomas, however MMP-2 mRNA is also abundantly expressed in stromal cells (Afzal *et al.*, 1998). Significant elevation of MMP-9 expression in serous and mucinous ovarian carcinomas is also detected compared with benign and borderline tumors (Huang *et al.*, 2000). In addition to gelatinases, MT1-MMP mRNA is also present in borderline and malignant tumors. Co-localization of MT1-MMP and MMP-2 in ovarian tumors suggests that MT1-MMP may be properly positioned for MMP-2 activation *in vivo* (Afzal *et al.*, 1998).

Recent studies suggest that ovarian carcinoma cells shed membrane vesicles that are rich in proteinases and these vesicles can be isolated from ascites fluid (Ginestra *et al.*,1999). A similar phenomenon was observed with cultured ovarian cancer cells. The shed vesicles contain uPA and plasmin as well as MMP-2 and -9. Further, purified vesicles catalyze degradation of Matrigel, suggesting that the shed vesicles are likely proteolytically competent *in vivo* (Dolo *et al.*, 1999). This is supported by the observation that the amount of shed vesicles correlates with tumor malignancy, as the vesicle content in ascites of patients with benign cysts, cystadenomas and fibromas is low whereas high levels of membrane vesicles are observed in the ascites of patients with malignant tumors (Ginestra *et al.*, 1999).

5.2. Clinical Trials with MMP Inhibitors

Growing experimental evidence supporting a critical role of MMPs in ovarian cancer progression has made inhibitors of MMPs an attractive target for a new class of anticancer agents. Among them, two synthetic inhibitors, Batimastat (BB-94) and Marimastat (BB-2516), inhibit a broad spectrum of MMPs and are being extensively tested for their potential therapeutic value in xenograft models and clinical trials (Rasmussen and McCann, 1997). Batimastat is a potent but reversible MMP inhibitor, however its insolubility and poor bioavailability in oral administration compromise its therapeutic potential. Nevertheless, intraperitoneal injection of Batimastat in mice with ovarian cancer xenografts supports the potential efficacy of this approach. In these studies, intraperitoneally injected ovarian cancer cells rapidly induce development of thick, mucinous ascites containing free-floating tumor cell clumps and cause death approximately 3 weeks after injection. Treatment of these animals with Batimastat results in solidification of the tumor, resolution of ascitic disease and a 5-6-fold increase in survival. These effects are directly attributable to MMP inhibition, as an inactive isomer was ineffective (Davies *et al.*, 1993). The preliminary success in xenograft studies promoted Batimastat as the first inhibitor of this class to enter clinical trials. Phase I and phase I/II trials involved patients with malignant ascites and malignant pleural effusions. In these trials, administration of Batimastat intraperitoneally or intrapleurally in suspension gave rise to a sustained plasma concentration for weeks (Beattie and Smyth, 1998; Macaulay *et al.*, 1999).

The poor bioavailability of Batimastat has encouraged the development of soluble analogs that maintain comparable inhibitory potency. A closely related compound, Marimastat, is almost completely absorbed after oral administration and has a half-life of about 15 hr. Preclinical data from animal models are lacking, however, due to rapid clearance in rodents (Rasmussen and McCann, 1997). Justified by its close inhibitory spectrum to Batimastat, Marimastat has also entered clinical trials. Phase I/II trials of Marimastat were conducted in ovarian cancer patients and the rate of rise of the serum tumor marker CA-125 was used as an assessment of drug effect (Nemunaitis et al., 1998; Malfetano *et al.*, 1997; Poole *et al.*, 1996). Although a promising decrease in the CA-125 expression rate was observed, a definitive correlation with drug efficacy can only be determined through phase III trials.

A number of other MMP inhibitors, including AG 3340, MMI 270B and BAY 12-9566, are in various stages of development and clinical trials (Nelson *et al.*, 2000). These drugs are also broad-spectrum MMP inhibitors with some engineered specificity. Ongoing and future clinical trials will establish the therapeutic value of these compounds. In addition to MMPs, other proteinases, including uPA/plasmin and cathepsins, are also implicated in ovarian tumor metastasis. Thus, use of MMP inhibitors in combination with other proteinase inhibitors may be a promising approach for future trials.

6. ROLE OF OTHER PROTEINASES

In addition to enzymes in the PA and MMP families, other proteolytic enzymes have also been implicated in ovarian cancer. For example, ectopic (i.e. non-pancreatic) expression of trypsinogen mRNA has been described in ovarian cancer cell lines as well as in ovarian cancer tissues. Western blot analysis of tumor cell conditioned medium has confirmed the synthesis of the serine protease trypsinogen by these cells (Hirahara *et al.*, 1995). Urinary trypsin inhibitor, a low molecular weight trypsin inhibitor, blocks invasion of ovarian cancer cells *in vitro* by inhibiting plasmin activity without altering adhesion or chemotactic motility (Kobayashi *et al.*, 1994 and 1994a). Levels of a related protein designated tumor-associated trypsin inhibitor are also reported to correlate with tumor grade/stage (Medl *et al.*, 1995). A membrane anchored serine protease designated hepsin has been identified in ovarian carcinomas, however the physiological substrate remains unknown (Tanimoto *et al.*, 1997). In normal cells, the enzyme appears to function in maintenance of cell growth and morphology, suggesting that overexpression of hepsin in ovarian carcinomas may contribute to dysregulation of cell growth.

An early report of a latent thiol protease similar to cathepsin B in ovarian tumors (Mort *et al.*, 1981) was later confirmed in studies demonstrating higher cathepsin B levels in membrane preparations obtained from malignant ovarian tumors than their benign counterparts (Kobayashi *et al.*, 1993). In cultured ovarian cancer cells, cathepsin B promotes cellular invasiveness by virtue of its activation of pro-uPA (Kobayashi *et al.*, 1992, Kobayashi *et al.*, 1993a). Cathepsin D levels are also reported to be higher in the cytosol of malignant tumors compared to benign tumors or normal ovarian tissue (Scambia *et al.*, 1991). Moreover, patients with high cathepsin D had poor prognosis compared to patients with low cathepsin D levels (Scambia *et al.*, 1994). These studies suggest that additional proteinases may contribute to ovarian cancer pathobiology. A more detailed understanding of the role of distinct proteolytic enzymes in modulating the adhesion, motility, invasion,

344

and growth of ovarian cancer cells may lead to the development of novel therapeutic strategies for the control of ovarian cancer invasion and metastasis.

ACKNOWLDEGEMENTS

The authors would like to acknowledge the support of research grants RO1 CA86984 from the National Cancer Institute, PO1 DE12328 from the National Institute of Dental and Craniofacial Research, training grant DAMD 17-00-1-0386 from the Department of Defense Breast Cancer Research Program, and the Stenn Fund for Ovarian Cancer Research.

REFERENCES

Afzal, S., Lalani el, N., Foulkes, W. D., Boyce, B., Tickle, S., Cardillo, M. R., Baker, T., Pignatelli, M., and Stamp, G. W. Matrix metalloproteinase-2 and tissue inhibitor of metalloproteinase-2 expression and synthetic matrix metalloproteinase-2 inhibitor binding in ovarian carcinomas and tumor cell lines. Lab Invest 1996; 74:406-21.

Afzal, S., Lalani, E. N., Poulsom, R., Stubbs, A., Rowlinson, G., Sato, H., Seiki, M., and Stamp, G. W. MT1-MMP and MMP-2 mRNA expression in human ovarian tumors: possible implications for the role of desmoplastic fibroblasts. Hum Pathol 1998; 29:155-65.

Andreasen, P. A., Kjoller, L., Christensen, L., and Duffy, M. J. The urokinase-type plasminogen activator system in cancer metastasis: a review. Int J Cancer 1997; 72: 1-22.

Astedt, B., Svanberg, L., and Nilsson, I. M. Fibrin degradation products and ovarian tumours. Br Med J 1971; 4: 458-9.

Band, V., Karlan, B. Y., Zurawski, V. R., Jr., and Littlefield, B. A. Simultaneous stimulation of urokinase and tissue-type plasminogen activators by phorbol esters in human ovarian carcinoma cells. J Cell Physiol 1989; 138:106-14.

Bartlett, J. M., Langdon, S. P., Simpson, B. J., Stewart, M., Katsaros, D., Sismondi, P., Love, S., Scott, W. N., Williams, A. R., Lessells, A. M., et al. The prognostic value of epidermal growth factor receptor mRNA expression in primary ovarian cancer. Br J Cancer 1996; 73: 301-6.

Beattie, G. J., and Smyth, J. F. Phase I study of intraperitoneal metalloproteinase inhibitor BB94 in patients with malignant ascites. Clin Cancer Res 1998; 4:1899-902.

Casslen, B., Gustavsson, B., and Astedt, B. Cell membrane receptors for urokinase plasminogen activator are increased in malignant ovarian tumours. Eur J Cancer 1991; 27: 1445-8.

Chambers, S. K., Wang, Y., Gertz, R. E., and Kacinski, B. M. Macrophage colony-stimulating factor mediates invasion of ovarian cancer cells through urokinase. Cancer Res 1995; 55: 1578-85.

Conese, M., and Blasi, F. Urokinase/urokinase receptor system: internalization/degradation of urokinase-serpin complexes: mechanism and regulation. Biol Chem Hoppe Seyler 1995; 376, 143-55.

Crickard, K., Niedbala, M. J., Crickard, U., Yoonessi, M., Sandberg, A. A., Okuyama, K., Bernacki, R. J., and Satchidanand, S. K. Characterization of human ovarian and endometrial carcinoma cell lines established on extracellular matrix. Gynecol Oncol 1989; 32: 163-73.

Davies, B., Brown, P. D., East, N., Crimmin, M. J., and Balkwill, F. R. A synthetic matrix metalloproteinase inhibitor decreases tumor burden and prolongs survival of mice bearing human ovarian carcinoma xenografts. Cancer Res 1993; 53(15): 2087-91.

De Nictolis, M., Garbisa, S., Lucarini, G., Goteri, G., Masiero, L., Ciavattini, A., Garzetti, G. G., Stetler-Stevenson, W. G., Fabris, G., Biagini, G., and Prat, J. 72-kilodalton type IV collagenase, type IV collagen, and Ki 67 antigen in serous tumors or the ovary: a clinicopathologic, immunohistochemical, and Serological study. Int J Gynecol Pathol 1996; 15: 102-9.

Dolo, V., D'Ascenzo, S., Violini, S., Pompucci, L., Festuccia, C., Ginestra, A., Vittorelli, M. L., Canevari, S., and Pavan, A. Matrix-degrading proteinases are shed in membrane vesicles by ovarian cancer cells in vivo and in vitro. Clin Exp Metastasis 1999; 17: 131-40.

d'Ortho, M. P., Will, H., Atkinson, S., Butler, G., Messent, A., Gavrilovic, J., Smith, B., Timpl, R., Zardi, L., and Murphy, G. Membrane-type matrix metalloproteinases 1 and 2 exhibit broad-spectrum proteolytic capacities comparable to many matrix metalloproteinases. Eur J Biochem 1997; 250: 751-7.

Dumler, I., Petri, T., and Schleuning, W. D. Induction of c-fos gene expression by urokinase-type plasminogen activator in human ovarian cancer cells. FEBS Lett 1994; 343: 103-6.

Ellerbroek, S.M., Halbleib, J.M., Benavidez, M., Warmka, J.K., Wattenberg, E.V., Stack, M.S., and Hudson, L.G. Phosphatidylinositol 3-kinase activity in epidermal growth factor-stimulated matrix metalloproteinase-9 production and cell surface association. Cancer Research 2001; in press.

Ellerbroek, S. M., Fishman, D. A., Kearns, A. S., Bafetti, L. M., and Stack, M. S. Ovarian carcinoma regulation of matrix metalloproteinase-2 and membrane type 1 matrix metalloproteinase through beta1 integrin. Cancer Res 1999; 59: 1635-41.

Ellerbroek, S. M., Hudson, L. G., and Stack, M. S. Proteinase requirements of epidermal growth factor-induced ovarian cancer cell invasion. Int J Cancer 1998; 78: 331-7.

Fang, X., Gaudette, D., Furui, T., Mao, M., Estrella, V., Eder, A., Pustilnik, T., Sasagawa, T., Lapushin, R., Yu, S., et al. Lysophospholipid growth factors in the initiation, progression, metastases, and management of ovarian cancer. Ann N Y Acad Sci 2000; 905:188-208.

Fischer, K., Lutz, V., Wilhelm, O., Schmitt, M., Graeff, H., Heiss, P., Nishiguchi, T., Harbeck, N., Kessler, H., Luther, T., et al. Urokinase induces proliferation of human ovarian cancer cells: characterization of structural elements required for growth factor function. FEBS Lett 1998; 438: 101-5.

Fishman, D. A., Bafetti, L. M., and Stack, M. S. Membrane-type matrix metalloproteinase expression and matrix metalloproteinase-2 activation in primary human ovarian epithelial carcinoma cells. Invasion Metastasis 1996; 16: 150-9.

Fishman, D. A., Bafetti, L. M., Banionis, S., Kearns, A. S., Chilukuri, K., and Stack, M. S. Production of extracellular matrix-degrading proteinases by primary cultures of human epithelial ovarian carcinoma cells. Cancer 1997; 80: 1457-63.

Fishman, D. A., Kearns, A., Chilukuri, K., Bafetti, L. M., O'Toole, E. A., Georgacopoulos, J., Ravosa, M. J., and Stack, M. S. Metastatic dissemination of human ovarian epithelial carcinoma is promoted by alpha2beta1-integrin-mediated interaction with type I collagen. Invasion Metastasis 1998; 18: 15-26.

Fishman, D. A., Kearns, A., Larsh, S., Enghild, J. J., and Stack, M. S. Autocrine regulation of growth stimulation in human epithelial ovarian carcinoma by serine-proteinase-catalysed release of the urinary-type- plasminogen-activator N-terminal fragment. Biochem J 1999; 341: 765-9.

Fishman, D.A., Liu, Y., Ellerbroek, S.M. and Stack, M.S. Lysophosphatidic acid promotes matrix metalloproteinase (MMP) activation and MMP-dependent invasion in ovarian cancer cells. Cancer Research 2001; in press.

Furui, T., LaPushin, R., Mao, M., Khan, H., Watt, S. R., Watt, M. A., Lu, Y., Fang, X., Tsutsui, S., Siddik, Z. H., et al. Overexpression of edg-2/vzg-1 induces apoptosis and anoikis in ovarian cancer cells in a lysophosphatidic acid-independent manner. Clin Cancer Res 1999; 5: 4308-18.

Garzetti, G. G., Ciavattini, A., Lucarini, G., Goteri, G., de e Nictolis, M., Garbisa, S., Masiero, L., Romanini, C., and Graziella, B. Tissue and serum metalloproteinase (MMP-2) expression in advanced ovarian serous cystoadenocarcinomas: clinical and prognostic implications. Anticancer Res 1995; 15: 2799-804.

Garzetti, G. G., Ciavattini, A., Lucarini, G., Goteri, G., Romanini, C., and Biagini, G. Increased serum 72 KDa metalloproteinase in serous ovarian tumors: comparison with CA 125. Anticancer Res 1996; 16: 2123-7.

Garzetti, G. G., Ciavattini, A., Lucarini, G., Pugnaloni, A., De Nictolis, M., Amati, S., Romanini, C., and Biagini, G. Expression of vascular endothelial growth factor related to 72- kilodalton metalloproteinase immunostaining in patients with serous ovarian tumors. Cancer 1999; 85: 2219-25.

Ginestra, A., Miceli, D., Dolo, V., Romano, F. M., and Vittorelli, M. L. Membrane vesicles in ovarian cancer fluids: a new potential marker. Anticancer Res 1999; 19: 3439-45.

Hafter, R., Klaubert, W., Gollwitzer, R., von Hugo, R., and Graeff, H. Crosslinked fibrin derivatives and fibronectin in ascitic fluid from patients with ovarian cancer compared to ascitic fluid in liver cirrhosis. Thromb Res 1984; 35: 53-64.

Harvey, W., and Amlot, P. L. Collagen production by human mesothelial cells in vitro, J Pathol 1983; 139: 337-47.

Hirahara, F., Miyagi, Y., Miyagi, E., Yasumitsu, H., Koshikawa, N., Nagashima, Y., Kitamura, H., Minaguchi, H., Umeda, M., and Miyazaki, K. Trypsinogen expression in human ovarian carcinomas. Int J Cancer 1995; 63: 176-81.

Holst-Hansen, C., Hamers, M. J., Johannessen, B. E., Brunner, N., and Stephens, R. W. Soluble urokinase receptor released from human carcinoma cells: a plasma parameter for xenograft tumour studies. Br J Cancer 1999; 81: 203-11.

Hoskins, W. J. Prospective on ovarian cancer: why prevent? J Cell Biochem Suppl 1995; 23:189-99.

Huang, L. W., Garrett, A. P., Bell, D. A., Welch, W. R., Berkowitz, R. S., and Mok, S. C. Differential expression of matrix metalloproteinase-9 and tissue inhibitor of metalloproteinase-1 protein and mRNA in epithelial ovarian tumors. Gynecol Oncol 2000; 77: 369-76.

Johansson, N., Vaalamo, M., Grenman, S., Hietanen, S., Klemi, P., Saarialho-Kere, U., and Kahari, V. M. Collagenase-3 (MMP-13) is expressed by tumor cells in invasive vulvar squamous cell carcinomas. Am J Pathol 1999; 154: 469-80.

Kanamori, Y., Matsushima, M., Minaguchi, T., Kobayashi, K., Sagae, S., Kudo, R., Terakawa, N., and Nakamura, Y. Correlation between expression of the matrix metalloproteinase-1 gene in ovarian cancers and an insertion/deletion polymorphism in its promoter region. Cancer Res 1999; 59: 4225-7.

Kanemoto, T., Martin, G. R., Hamilton, T. C., and Fridman, R. Effects of synthetic peptides and protease inhibitors on the interaction of a human ovarian cancer cell line (NIH:OVCAR-3) with a reconstituted basement membrane (Matrigel). Invasion Metastasis 1991; 11: 84-92.

Karlan, B. Y., Amin, W., Band, V., Zurawski, V. R., Jr., and Littlefield, B. A. Plasminogen activator secretion by established lines of human ovarian carcinoma cells in vitro. Gynecol Oncol 1988; 31: 103-12.

Karlan, B. Y., Rivero, J. A., Crabtree, M. E., and Littlefield, B. A. Different mechanisms contribute to simultaneous inhibition of urokinase and tissue-type plasminogen activators by glucocorticoids in human ovarian carcinoma cells. Mol Endocrinol 1989; 3: 1006-13.

Kikkawa, F., Tamakoshi, K., Nawa, A., Shibata, K., Yamagata, S., Yamagata, T., and Suganuma, N. Positive correlation between inhibitors of matrix metalloproteinase 1 and matrix metalloproteinases in malignant ovarian tumor tissues. Cancer Lett 1997; 120: 109-15.

Kobayashi, H., Fujie, M., Shinohara, H., Ohi, H., Sugimura, M., and Terao, T. Effects of urinary trypsin inhibitor on the invasion of reconstituted basement membranes by ovarian cancer cells, Int J Cancer 1994; 57: 378-84.

Kobayashi, H., Moniwa, N., Sugimura, M., Shinohara, H., Ohi, H., and Terao, T. Increased cell-surface urokinase in advanced ovarian cancer. Jpn J Cancer Res 1993; 84: 633-40.

Kobayashi, H., Moniwa, N., Sugimura, M., Shinohara, H., Ohi, H., and Terao, T. Effects of membrane-associated cathepsin B on the activation of receptor-bound prourokinase and subsequent invasion of reconstituted basement membranes. Biochim Biophys Acta 1993; 1178: 55-62.

Kobayashi, H., Ohi, H., Sugimura, M., Shinohara, H., Fujii, T., and Terao, T. Inhibition of in vitro ovarian cancer cell invasion by modulation of urokinase-type plasminogen activator and cathepsin B. Cancer Res 1992; 52: 3610-4.

Kobayashi, H., Shinohara, H., Ohi, H., Sugimura, M., Terao, T., and Fujie, M. Urinary trypsin inhibitor (UTI) and fragments derived from UTI by limited proteolysis efficiently inhibit tumor cell invasion. Clin Exp Metastasis 1994; 12: 117-28.

Kohn, E. C., Jacobs, W., Kim, Y. S., Alessandro, R., Stetler-Stevenson, W. G., and Liotta, L. A. Calcium influx modulates expression of matrix metalloproteinase-2 (72- kDa type IV collagenase, gelatinase A). J Biol Chem 1994; 269: 21505-11.

Kuhn, W., Pache, L., Schmalfeldt, B., Dettmar, P., Schmitt, M., Janicke, F., and Graeff, H. Urokinase (uPA) and PAI-1 predict survival in advanced ovarian cancer patients (FIGO III) after radical surgery and platinum-based chemotherapy. Gynecol Oncol 1994; 55: 401-9.

Leber, T. M., and Balkwill, F. R. Regulation of monocyte MMP-9 production by TNF-alpha and a tumour- derived soluble factor (MMPSF). Br J Cancer 1998; 78: 724-32.

Liotta, L. A., Rao, C. N., and Wewer, U. M. Biochemical interactions of tumor cells with the basement membrane. Annu Rev Biochem 1986; 55: 1037-57.

Macaulay, V. M., O'Byrne, K. J., Saunders, M. P., Braybrooke, J. P., Long, L., Gleeson, F., Mason, C. S., Harris, A. L., Brown, P., and Talbot, D. C. Phase I study of intrapleural batimastat (BB-94), a matrix metalloproteinase inhibitor, in the treatment of malignant pleural effusions. Clin Cancer Res 1999; 5: 513-20.

Malfetano, J., Teng, N., and Barter, J. Marimastat in patients with advanced cancer of the

348

ovary: A dose-finding study. Proc Am Soc Clin Oncol 1997; 16:373a.

Massova, I., Kotra, L. P., Fridman, R., and Mobashery, S. Matrix metalloproteinases: structures, evolution, and diversification. FASEB J 1998; 12: 1075-95.

Meden, H., Marx, D., Rath, W., Kron, M., Fattahi-Meibodi, A., Hinney, B., Kuhn, W., and Schauer, A. Overexpression of the oncogene c-erb B2 in primary ovarian cancer: evaluation of the prognostic value in a Cox proportional hazards multiple regression. Int J Gynecol Pathol 1994; 13: 45-53.

Medl, M., Ogris, E., Peters-Engl, C., and Leodolter, S. TATI (tumour-associated trypsin inhibitor) as a marker of ovarian cancer. Br J Cancer 1995; 71: 1051-4.

Mirshahi, S. S., Lounes, K. C., Lu, H., Pujade-Lauraine, E., Mishal, Z., Benard, J., Bernadou, A., Soria, C., and Soria, J. Defective cell migration in an ovarian cancer cell line is associated with impaired urokinase-induced tyrosine phosphorylation. FEBS Lett 1997; 411: 322-6.

Miyagi, E., Yasumitsu, H., Hirahara, F., Minaguchi, H., Koshikawa, N., Miyazaki, K., and Umeda, M. Characterization of matrix-degrading proteinases and their inhibitors secreted by human gynecological carcinoma cells. Jpn J Cancer Res 1995; 86: 568-76.

Mondino, A., Resnati, M., and Blasi, F. Structure and function of the urokinase receptor. Thromb Haemost 1999; 82 Suppl 1: 19-22.

Moore, D. H., Allison, B., Look, K. Y., Sutton, G. P., and Bigsby, R. M. Collagenase expression in ovarian cancer cell lines. Gynecol Oncol 1997; 65: 78-82.

Mort, J. S., Leduc, M., and Recklies, A. D. A latent thiol proteinase from ascitic fluid of patients with neoplasia. Biochim Biophys Acta 1981; 662: 173-80.

Moser, T. L., Young, T. N., Rodriguez, G. C., Pizzo, S. V., Bast, R. C., Jr., and Stack, M. S. Secretion of extracellular matrix-degrading proteinases is increased in epithelial ovarian carcinoma. Int J Cancer 1994; 56: 552-9.

Murdoch, W. J. Proteolytic and cellular death mechanisms in ovulatory ovarian rupture. Biol Signals Recept 2000; 9: 102-14.

Nagase, H., and Woessner, J. F., Jr.. Matrix metalloproteinases. J Biol Chem 1999; 274: 21491-4.

Naylor, M. S., Stamp, G. W., Davies, B. D., and Balkwill, F. R. Expression and activity of MMPS and their regulators in ovarian cancer. Int J Cancer 1994; 58: 50-6.

Nelson, A. R., Fingleton, B., Rothenberg, M. L., and Matrisian, L. M. Matrix metalloproteinases: biologic activity and clinical implications. J Clin Oncol 2000; 18: 1135-49.

Nemunaitis, J., Poole, C., Primrose, J., Rosemurgy, A., Malfetano, J., Brown, P., Berrington, A., Cornish, A., Lynch, K., Rasmussen, H., et al. Combined analysis of studies of the effects of the matrix metalloproteinase inhibitor marimastat on serum tumor markers in advanced cancer: selection of a biologically active and tolerable dose for longer-term studies. Clin Cancer Res 1998; 4: 1101-9.

Niedbala, M. J., Madiyalakan, R., Matta, K., Crickard, K., Sharma, M., and Bernacki, R. J. Role of glycosidases in human ovarian carcinoma cell mediated degradation of subendothelial extracellular matrix. Cancer Res 1987; 47: 4634-41.

Ohuchi, E., Imai, K., Fujii, Y., Sato, H., Seiki, M., and Okada, Y. Membrane type 1 matrix metalloproteinase digests interstitial collagens and other extracellular matrix macromolecules. J Biol Chem 1997; 272: 2446-51.

Patton, S. E., Martin, M. L., Nelsen, L. L., Fang, X., Mills, G. B., Bast, R. C., Jr., and Ostrowski, M. C. Activation of the ras-mitogen-activated protein kinase pathway and phosphorylation of ets-2 at position threonine 72 in human ovarian cancer cell lines. Cancer Res 1998; 58: 2253-9.

Pedersen, N., Schmitt, M., Ronne, E., Nicoletti, M. I., Hoyer-Hansen, G., Conese, M., Giavazzi, R., Dano, K., Kuhn, W., Janicke, F., and et al. A ligand-free, soluble urokinase receptor is present in the ascitic fluid from patients with ovarian cancer. J Clin Invest 1993; 92: 2160-7.

Poole, C., Adams, M., and Barley, V. A dose-finding study of marimastat, an oral matrix metalloproteinase inhibitor in patients with advanced ovarian cancer. Ann Oncol 1996; 7:68.

Pujade-Lauraine, E., Lu, H., Mirshahi, S., Soria, J., Soria, C., Bernadou, A., Kruithof, E. K., Lijnen, H. R., and Burtin, P. The plasminogen-activation system in ovarian tumors. Int J Cancer 1993; 55: 27-31.

Pustilnik, T. B., Estrella, V., Wiener, J. R., Mao, M., Eder, A., Watt, M. A., Bast, R. C., Jr., and Mills, G. B. Lysophosphatidic acid induces urokinase secretion by ovarian cancer cells. Clin Cancer Res 1999; 5: 3704-10.

Rabbani, S. A. Metalloproteases and urokinase in angiogenesis and tumor progression, In Vivo 1998; 12: 135-42.

Rasmussen, H. S., and McCann, P. P. Matrix metalloproteinase inhibition as a novel anticancer strategy: a review with special focus on batimastat and marimastat. Pharmacol Ther 1997; 75: 69-75.

Scambia, G., Benedetti, P., Ferrandina, G., Battaglia, F., Baiocchi, G., and Mancuso, S. Cathepsin D assay in ovarian cancer: correlation with pathological features and receptors for oestrogen, progesterone and epidermal growth factor. Br J Cancer 1991; 64: 182-4.

Scambia, G., Panici, P. B., Ferrandina, G., Salerno, G., D'Agostino, G., Distefano, M., de Vincenzo, R., Ercoli, A., and Mancuso, S. Clinical significance of cathepsin D in primary ovarian cancer. Eur J Cancer 1994; 7: 935-40.

Shibata, K., Kikkawa, F., Nawa, A., Suganuma, N., and Hamaguchi, M. Fibronectin secretion from human peritoneal tissue induces Mr 92,000 type IV collagenase expression and invasion in ovarian cancer cell lines. Cancer Res 1997; 57: 5416-20.

Shibata, K., Kikkawa, F., Nawa, A., Thant, A. A., Naruse, K., Mizutani, S., and Hamaguchi, M. Both focal adhesion kinase and c-Ras are required for the enhanced matrix metalloproteinase 9 secretion by fibronectin in ovarian cancer cells. Cancer Res 1998; 58: 900-3.

Shigemasa, K., Tanimoto, H., Sakata, K., Nagai, N., Parmley, T. H., Ohama, K., and O'Brien, T. J. Induction of matrix metalloprotease-7 is common in mucinous ovarian tumors including early stage disease. Med Oncol 2000; 17: 52-8.

Sier, C. F., Stephens, R., Bizik, J., Mariani, A., Bassan, M., Pedersen, N., Frigerio, L., Ferrari, A., Dano, K., Brunner, N., and Blasi, F. The level of urokinase-type plasminogen activator receptor is increased in serum of ovarian cancer patients. Cancer Res 1998; 58: 1843-9.

Tanimoto, H., Underwood, L. J., Shigemasa, K., Parmley, T. H., Wang, Y., Yan, Y., Clarke, J., and O'Brien, T. J. The matrix metalloprotease pump-1 (MMP-7, Matrilysin): A candidate marker/target for ovarian cancer detection and treatment. Tumour Biol 1999; 20: 88-98.

Tanimoto, H., Yan, Y., Clarke, J., Korourian, S., Shigemasa, K., Parmley, T. H., Parham, G. P., and O'Brien, T. J. Hepsin, a cell surface serine protease identified in hepatoma cells, is overexpressed in ovarian cancer. Cancer Res 1997; 57: 2884-7.

Ueda, M., Ueki, M., Terai, Y., Ueki, K., Kumagai, K., Fujii, H., Yoshizawa, K., and Nakajima, M. Biological implications of growth factors on the mechanism of invasion in gynecological tumor cells. Gynecol Obstet Invest 1999; 48: 221-8.

Wahlberg, K., Hoyer-Hansen, G., and Casslen, B. Soluble receptor for urokinase plasminogen activator in both full- length and a cleaved form is present in high concentration in cystic fluid from ovarian cancer. Cancer Res 1998; 58: 3294-8.

Westerlund, A., Apaja-Sarkkinen, M., Hoyhtya, M., Puistola, U., and Turpeenniemi-Hujanen, T. Gelatinase A-immunoreactive protein in ovarian lesions- prognostic value in epithelial ovarian cancer. Gynecol Oncol 1999; 75: 91-8.

Westerlund, A., Hujanen, E., Puistola, U., and Turpeenniemi-Hujanen, T. Fibroblasts stimulate human ovarian cancer cell invasion and expression of 72-kDa gelatinase A (MMP-2). Gynecol Oncol 1997; 67: 76-82.

Wilhelm, O., Hafter, R., Coppenrath, E., Pflanz, M. A., Schmitt, M., Babic, R., Linke, R., Gossner, W., and Graeff, H. Fibrin-fibronectin compounds in human ovarian tumor ascites and their possible relation to the tumor stroma. Cancer Res 1988; 48: 3507-14.

Wilhelm, O., Hafter, R., Henschen, A., Schmitt, M., and Graeff, H. Role of plasmin in the degradation of the stroma-derived fibrin in human ovarian carcinoma. Blood 1990; 75: 1673-8.

Wilhelm, O., Schmitt, M., Hohl, S., Senekowitsch, R., and Graeff, H. Antisense inhibition of urokinase reduces spread of human ovarian cancer in mice. Clin Exp Metastasis 1995; 13: 296-302.

Wilhelm, O., Weidle, U., Hohl, S., Rettenberger, P., Schmitt, M., and Graeff, H. Recombinant soluble urokinase receptor as a scavenger for urokinase- type plasminogen activator (uPA). Inhibition of proliferation and invasion of human ovarian cancer cells. FEBS Lett 1994; 337: 131-4.

Xu, F. J., Stack, S., Boyer, C., O'Briant, K., Whitaker, R., Mills, G. B., Yu, Y. H., and Bast, R. C., Jr. Heregulin and agonistic anti-p185(c-erbB2) antibodies inhibit proliferation but increase invasiveness of breast cancer cells that overexpress p185(c-erbB2): increased invasiveness may contribute to poor prognosis. Clin Cancer Res 1997; 3: 1629-34.

Xu, Y., Fang, X. J., Casey, G., and Mills, G. B. Lysophospholipids activate ovarian and breast cancer cells. Biochem J 1995; 309: 933-40.

Xu, Y., Gaudette, D. C., Boynton, J. D., Frankel, A., Fang, X. J., Sharma, A., Hurteau, J., Casey, G., Goodbody, A., Mellors, A., and et al. Characterization of an ovarian cancer activating factor in ascites from ovarian cancer patients, Clin Cancer Res 1995; 1: 1223-32.

Xu, Y., Shen, Z., Wiper, D. W., Wu, M., Morton, R. E., Elson, P., Kennedy, A. W., Belinson, J., Markman, M., and Casey, G. Lysophosphatidic acid as a potential biomarker for ovarian and other gynecologic cancers [see comments]. Jama 1998; 280: 719-23.

Young, T. N., Rodriguez, G. C., Moser, T. L., Bast, R. C., Jr., Pizzo, S. V., and Stack, M. S. Coordinate expression of urinary-type plasminogen activator and its receptor accompanies malignant transformation of the ovarian surface epithelium. Am J Obstet Gynecol 1994; 170: 1285-96.

Young, T. N., Rodriguez, G. C., Rinehart, A. R., Bast, R. C., Jr., Pizzo, S. V., and Stack, M. S. Characterization of gelatinases linked to extracellular matrix invasion in ovarian adenocarcinoma: purification of matrix metalloproteinase 2. Gynecol Oncol 1996; 62: 89-99.

Young, T.N., Pizzo, S.V., Stack, M.S. A plasma membrane-associated component of ovarian adenocarcinoma cells enhances the catalytic efficiency of matrix metalloproteinase-2. J Biol Chem 1995; 270: 999-1002.

Chapter 17

ANGIOGENESIS AND METASTASIS

Gregory J. Sieczkiewicz, Mahrukh Hussain, Elise C. Kohn
National Cancer Institute, Molecular Signaling Section, Laboratory of Pathology, Bethesda, MD 20892

1. INTRODUCTION

Epithelial ovarian cancer constitutes approximately 85% of all ovarian malignancies. The lack of overt symptoms and good screening strategies precludes early diagnosis and thus greater than 70% of patients present with extensive local disease and peritoneal spread (1). While the five-year survival for patients presenting with advanced disease has improved over the past decade, there has been no increase in the number or frequency of cures of advanced ovarian cancer. The symptoms of both early and late stage ovarian cancers are frequently nonspecific, including abdominal complaints, bloating, and altered bowel habits, in part due to local tumor growth confined in stages I and II to the ovaries or pelvic organs prior to serosal spread in the abdomen. With advanced stage, the peritoneum, diaphragm, and omentum are seeded with micro- and macro-metastases of tumor cells, resulting in solid tumor masses and ascites that cause further bloating, cramping, pain and bowel complaints. Unlike its solid tumor counterparts that invade blood vessels and lymphatics and metastasize early, epithelial ovarian cancer spreads initially by surface shedding. This is followed by invasive peritoneal implantation, growth and further invasion. Distant parenchymal metastases are less common at presentation but may be seen with progression of epithelial ovarian cancer. The growth of ovarian tumors is associated frequently with the development of ascites, which is rich in cytokines and growth factors.

Angiogenesis is the formation of new blood vessels from pre-existing vessels and differs from vasculogenesis, a process wherein pleuripotent precursor cells generate endothelium. When stimulated by factors synthesized by the surrounding stroma, the endothelium initially dissociates its attachments with neighboring cells and releases extracellular matrix-

354

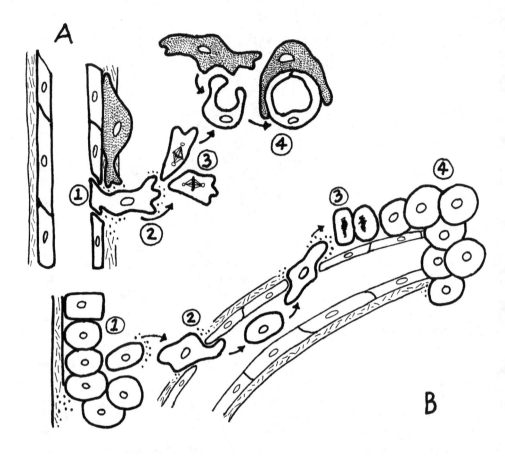

*Figure 1. **Angiogenesis (A) and tumor invasion (B).*** *Each process begins with an initiation event (1) in which cells break contacts with their neighbors and secrete proteases to digest the surrounding basement membrane, followed by cell migration (2) and proliferation (3). While angiogenic sprouts differentiate to form mature, lumenized vessels complete with surrounding pericytes (4), tumor cells continue sustained growth (4).*

degrading enzymes to digest the surrounding basement membrane. The endothelial cell then migrates away from the vessel into the interstitial space, forming the vascular sprout. The advancing vascular sprout degrades the surrounding type I collagen-rich stroma as it progresses. Endothelial cell proliferation follows this invasive angiogenic front. Finally, the vascular sprout differentiates to form a lumen-bearing vessel, recruits pericytes to its abluminal surface and completes its basement membrane. In tumors, this basement membrane is disorganized, discontinuous and leaky, often leading to ascites formation (2).

The process of angiogenesis requires invasion through surrounding tissue and subsequent cell proliferation, and is thus akin in many characteristics to the invasive behavior of metastasizing tumor (3) (Figure 1). Physiologic angiogenesis occurs during embryogenesis, morphogenesis, trophoblast implantation, tissue transplantation, wound healing and in the female reproductive cycle. Pathological angiogenesis occurs during tumor growth as well as in non-malignant conditions such as diabetic retinopathy, psoriasis, and rheumatoid arthritis (4). Turnover rates of capillary endothelium in the adult retina and regions of the brain are 0.01% whereas tumor-induced endothelial cell proliferation has been measured as high as 9.0%, similar to the maximal 13% rate observed in embryogenesis (5, 6). Under physiologic conditions, the process of blood vessel invasion is tightly controlled at the cellular and tissue levels by a multitude of finely tuned regulatory systems. Disruption of this regulation by tumors is essential for growth and metastasis of tumors and tumor-induced vasculature.

Tumor growth is divided into avascular and vascular stages. It has been well established that tumor vascularization is one of the rate-limiting steps for tumor growth and metastasis, and may occur as early as during dysplasia or carcinoma *in situ* (3, 7-9). A tumor mass larger than 0.125mm^2 has outgrown the capacity to acquire nutrients by simple diffusion (7). In such cases, the inner tumor mass becomes necrotic and hypoxic, a potent stimulus for the production of angiogenic factors, thus causing the angiogenic switch, the point at which tumors first become vascularized. Angiogenesis fosters tumor growth by providing a mechanism for the exchange of nutrients, oxygen, and waste products and by the release of autocrine and paracrine growth factors. These factors include vascular endothelial growth factor/vascular permeability factor (VEGF/VPF), fibroblast growth factors (FGFs), insulin-like growth factors (IGFs), platelet-derived growth factor (PDGF) and colony stimulating factor-1 (CSF-1) from intratumoral endothelium, inflammatory cells, stroma and tumor cells (10, 11).

Ovarian tumors secrete into the ascites VEGF and many other protein and lipid growth factors including interleukin 8 (IL-8) (12) and lysophosphatitic acid (LPA) (13). These growth factors can work both as autocrine growth factors for the cancer and as proangiogenic molecules. While ovarian tumor masses are very vascular, there are also considerable numbers of ovarian cancer cells in the ascites. The avascular nature of the ascites suggests that regulation of angiogenesis in ovarian tumor growth may occur early and by mechanisms not as prevalent in other tumors. As the increase in size of a tumor and its metastatic capacity are a function of its angiogenic state, it is vital to identify and characterize the molecular mechanisms regulating ovarian tumor angiogenesis.

2. PHYSIOLOGICAL AND PATHOLOGICAL OVARIAN ANGIOGENESIS

The female reproductive tract is the only site of cyclical physiological angiogenesis in the adult. Angiogenesis is an essential component of both the follicular and luteal phases of the ovarian cycle, tightly correlating with secretory endometrial maturation and ovulation. Cyclic ovarian angiogenesis is controlled by steroid hormones and polypeptide growth factors (14). The normal ovarian cycle is composed of several morphologically distinct angiogenic phases. The follicular phase begins with the development of a complex vascular network within the theca interna of the dominant follicle. These theca cells stain strongly for VEGF, implying that angiogenesis may be essential for follicular development (15). At ovulation, the basement membrane separating the theca and granulosa cell layers is proteolyzed, coinciding with a marked increase in angiogenesis centripetally from the theca toward the ruptured follicle. It has been demonstrated that ovarian angiogenesis is a requirement for early stages of folliculogenesis and luteal growth and that regression of angiogenesis coincides with follicular atresia and luteal regression (16). Following ovulation, there is a massive burst of angiogenesis that precedes actual corpus luteum formation. Individual sprouting vessels can be identified within 1-2 days after ovulation (17). These endothelial cells invade the corpus luteum and continue to grow through the first third of the ovarian cycle (17). Once ovulation has occurred, there is further angiogenic activity for the repair of the ovarian surface (18). During luteolysis the regression of newly formed vessels is accompanied by gradual foreshortening and rounding of endothelial cells and subsequent detachment from the corpus luteum (17). This physiological blood vessel regression does not appear to involve endothelial cell apoptosis (17). Angiogenesis in the growing ovarian corpus rubrum was found to be 4 to 20 times more intense than even the most angiogenic tumors (6), indicating a pre-programmed capacity for active angiogenesis that may become dysregulated in cancer.

Induction of angiogenesis is observed in numerous pathological non-malignant ovarian conditions including polycystic ovary syndrome, ovarian hyperstimulation syndrome, as well as benign and malignant neoplasms (14). All of these conditions are characterized by increased circulating and local levels of polypeptide growth factors such as VEGF and FGF-2, as is observed in physiological angiogenesis. There is an important distinction between pathological and physiological angiogenesis in that despite the marked similarities occurring in the mechanism of angiogenic initiation and progression, e.g. the involvement of VEGF and its receptor tyrosine kinases, profound differences should exist in the regulation of these events.

3. THE ROLE OF ENDOTHELIAL CELL-PERICYTE INTERACTIONS IN ANGIOGENESIS

The capillary is composed of two cell types, endothelial cells and pericytes. Interactions between these cells are critical for maintenance of microvascular integrity. Perturbations in endothelial cell-pericyte contact may contribute to decreased blood vessel integrity resulting in edema and pathological neovascularization. Specific loss of pericytes is observed in a number of diseases associated with pathological blood vessel growth including tumor growth, diabetic retinopathy, and retinopathy of prematurity (19, 20). Normally, pericytes surround the abluminal surface of the endothelium and the two cell types are surrounded by a discontinuous common basement membrane so that there are direct cell-cell contacts (Figure 2). Pericytes contain α-vascular smooth muscle actin and are believed to have contractile capacity, allowing them to influence microvascular tone (21). There are functional gap junctions between pericytes and endothelial cells (22, 23), but the importance of these connections in modulating endothelial cell-pericyte signaling remains unknown. Pericytes are known to inhibit endothelial cell migration and proliferation *in vitro* via a TGF-β mediated pathway (24, 25). While pericytes and endothelial cells individually produce the inactive, latent form of TGF-β, direct contact between the two cell types activates the cytokine to inhibit endothelial cell proliferation (26, 27). The ability of pericytes to inhibit endothelial cell proliferation and migration may explain why vascular beds having the lowest endothelial cell turnover rate have the highest numbers of pericytes.

Pericyte recruitment to the maturing neovessel appears to be dependent, at least in part, upon PDGF and VEGF secreted by neighboring stromal cells (28, 29). *In vivo* disruption of contacts between retinal pericytes and endothelial cells by treatment with PDGF-B, which presumably disrupts endogenous signaling between the two cell types, results in abnormal vascular remodeling and capillary regression (30). A reduction in pericyte number has been observed in mice genetically engineered to lack a functional PDGF-BB gene; however this reduction is variable in an organ-specific manner (29). Parallel to that finding is recent work that has demonstrated that pericyte association with tumor blood vessels varies with the type of tumor (6). Heterogeneity in pericyte coverage of blood vessels in tumors may be useful

358

as a diagnostic marker. Regulation of pericyte survival factors may be a novel direction for therapeutic development.

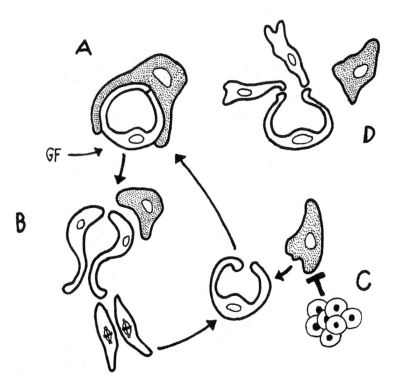

Figure 2. Endothelial cell-pericyte interactions during angiogenesis. In a quiescent capillary (A) the pericyte contacts directly the abluminal surface of the vessel, composed of a single endothelial cell. Upon stimulation by a growth factor (GF) such as VEGF or FGF-2, endothelial cells dissociate from pericytes (B), migrate away from the parent vessels and proliferate. As the angiogenic sprout differentiates to form a lumen, pericytes are recruited to return (C). However, tumor cells may produce factors that inhibit pericyte survival, migration, or association with endothelial cells, allowing the neovessel to continue its growth unchecked (D).

4. CONTROL OF TUMOR-INDUCED BLOOD VESSEL GROWTH BY PRO- AND ANTI-ANGIOGENIC FACTORS

The environment of fluid phase, or ascitic, ovarian tumors is strongly proangiogenic, despite ascites being avascular. This suggests that regulation of angiogenesis occurs on multiple levels, therefore implying multi-potential therapeutic targets. A multitude of soluble and extracellular matrix-associated polypeptide growth factors secreted by ovarian cancer cells act upon endothelial cells to initiate or extend blood vessel growth, and many such factors are present in ovarian cancer ascites (Table 1). However, under normal circumstances in the adult, endothelial cells are exceedingly quiescent. Recently, a cohort of endogenous anti-angiogenic factors has been discovered, providing support for the hypothesis that endothelial cell regulation is a dynamic balance between stimulation and inhibition. By its proangiogenic yet avascular nature, ovarian cancer ascites has the potential to help identify the mechanism(s) by which tumors defeat endogenous anti-angiogenic controls.

Table 1. Proangiogenic Factors

Cell Proliferation/Survival	Extracellular Matrix Proteolysis
$\alpha v \beta 3$ integrin	
FGF	MMP-2
VEGF	MMP-9
PDGF	MT1-MMP
IGF	

Cell Adhesion	Cell Motility	
Integrins	HGF	VEGF
Cadherins-catenins	EGF	FGF-2

4.1. Pro-Angiogenic Growth Factors
4.1.1. Vascular Endothelial Cell Growth Factor

VEGF is a potent endothelial cell mitogen, inducer of endothelial cell motility and stimulator of capillary tube formation (31). Originally purified from ovarian cancer ascites, VEGF is also referred to as vascular endothelial permeability factor (VPF) because of its ability to cause blood vessel leakage (32), presumably by disrupting endothelial cell-cell and cell-matrix contacts. VEGF is essential for blood vessel differentiation. Targeted disruption of the genes encoding VEGF or its receptors Flt-1 or Flk-1/KDR in mice results in embryonic lethality caused by incomplete blood vessel extension and differentiation (33). VEGF is a mitogen and a survival factor for the endothelium and promotes neovessel elongation (34). It is expressed by ovarian carcinoma and many other tumor cells, but not endothelial cells, suggesting a paracrine proangiogenic effect. Some ovarian tumor cells also express VEGF receptors (35), the first such demonstration of a non-endothelial cell type expressing Flt-1 and Flk-1/KDR. This expression indicates that an autocrine route of tumor cell proliferation may also occur in ovarian cancer. The local environment of the tumor, such as oxygen availability, may affect levels of VEGF produced by a tumor by regulation of VEGF transcription or translation (36). One ovarian cancer-produced growth factor, LPA, has been shown to induce gene expression and protein production of VEGF and interlukin-8 (IL-8) (13).

VEGF is involved in normal ovarian angiogenesis as well as in numerous pathological conditions in the ovary. VEGF immunoreactivity was localized to growing and mature luteal cells and was detected throughout the ovarian cycle until the onset of luteolysis (37). Luteolysis, which leads to the regression of the corpus luteum and its vasculature, has been associated with a rapid downregulation of VEGF mRNA (37). A number of studies have demonstrated altered gene expression and protein concentration of VEGF and its receptors in conditions such as benign and malignant neoplasia, follicular cyst formation, polycystic ovary syndrome and ovarian hyperstimulation syndrome (14). Graunulosa and theca cell layers of women with polycystic ovarian syndrome have been shown to contain elevated levels of VEGF mRNA and protein in the hyperthecotic stroma (38). In women with ovarian hyperstimulation syndrome, serum VEGF levels correlated with disease progression, specifically capillary leakage and leukocytosis (39). VEGF mRNA is also higher in the granulosa cells of hyperovulatory patients (40). Unresolved is the direct connection between the observed elevated VEGF mRNA and protein and how any increases in blood vessel density cause abnormal follicular growth and differentiation.

VEGF and its receptors have potential use as diagnostic and therapeutic targets in ovarian tumor malignancy. These proteins have been found in primary tumors and metastases, as well as in multiple ovarian cancer cell lines (35). Yeo and colleagues (41) suggest that due to the higher levels of VEGF protein found in malignant ovarian cancer effusions, measurement of VEGF levels in effusions may provide a useful biomarker for ovarian metastatic potential. Furthermore, Abu-Jawdeh and co-workers were able to differentiate malignant ovarian tumors from benign or borderline tumors based upon VEGF mRNA expression (42). Antibodies directed against VEGF are currently in phase I-II clinical trials sponsored by Genentech (San Francisco, CA) and the National Cancer Institute (NCI, Bethesda, MD). The anti-angiogenic compound SU5416 (Sugen, South San Francisco, CA) (43), which is purportedly a selective blocker of Flk-1/KDR receptor signaling, is in multiple phase I-III clinical trials (Cancer Trials Database, NCI/NIH; http://cancertrials.nci.nih.gov/), including a combination trial with carboplatin for ovarian cancer patients soon to open to accrual at the NCI. Preclinical studies are in progress to examine the effectiveness of the anti-

VEGF receptor antibody, DC101 (44), as well as therapies using soluble Flk-1/KDR extracellular domain constructs (45). These findings all suggest that VEGF and its receptors play significant, if not essential, roles in cellular processes that drive ovarian disease progression and are important prognostic and therapeutic targets.

4.1.2. Angiopoietins

The angiopoietins (Ang 1-4) are a family of proteins that associate with and either agonize or antagonize two endothelial cell-specific receptor tyrosine kinases, Tie-1 and Tie-2/tek (46). The angiopoietins are required in embryonic angiogenesis at a later stage than VEGF. Mice lacking Ang1 or Tie-2 suffer embryonic or early postnatal lethality due to abnormal vascular networks (47), suggesting they focus primarily on remodeling the embryonic capillary plexus. Ang1 appears to be important for endothelial sprouting via focal adhesion kinase (48) and in pericyte investment along the abluminal surface of the nascent vessel (37). Ang2 competes with Ang1 for binding to Tie-2 and therefore may act as a natural inhibitor; overexpression of Ang2 prevents blood vessel remodeling and also causes embryonic lethality (49). The ligand(s) for Tie-1 remain to be identified.

Angiopoietins interact with VEGF signaling to affect vascular remodeling during normal and pathological angiogenesis. Ang2 causes a loosening of cell-cell and cell-matrix interactions in the presence of VEGF (50). This allows endothelial cell migration and angiogenic sprout formation to occur, while also increasing leakage of plasma components into the extravascular space. In the absence of VEGF or other growth or survival signals, Ang2 expression results in apoptotic cell death (50). Overexpression of Ang1 results in blood vessels resistant to leakage and can overcome constitutive ectopic expression of VEGF (51).

Currently, little is known of the regulation of the angiopoietins in ovarian cancer. Higher levels of Ang2, Tie-1 and Tie-2 mRNA were detected in cutaneous angiosarcomas versus normal skin (52). Elevated levels of Ang1, Tie-2, VEGF and CD31 but not Tie-1 were detected in human non-small cell lung carcinomas (53). The critical balance between angiopoietins and VEGF may be perturbed during ovarian tumor growth; increased Ang2 and VEGF, along with a decrease in Ang1, may lead to vessel leakage and subsequent ascites accumulation.

4.1.3. Fibroblast Growth Factors

362

The fibroblast growth factor family currently contains 18 members similar to one another in primary sequence and some functional properties such as heparin binding (54). Acidic FGF /FGF-1 was discovered in a rat ovarian cancer cell line (55). FGF-2 (basic FGF) is a heparin-binding endothelial cell and pericyte mitogen and inducer of cell motility originally identified as a mouse 3T3 cell growth-stimulatory activity from pituitary and angiogenic corpus luteum (56, 57). FGF-2 is deposited into the subendothelial matrix, and may be released into the extracellular milieu during cell injury, death or non-lethal disruption of the plasma membrane (58).

FGF-2 is a potent *in vivo* mitogen and motogen for endothelial cells (59) and induces angiogenesis *in vivo* (60). FGF-2 is overexpressed during the proliferative phase of infantile hemangiomas and declines during the involution phase of the tumor (61). It has been shown to induce ovarian cancer cell migration, cell proliferation, and tumor vascularity. In a study of patients with advanced epithelial ovarian cancer, serum levels of FGF2 were elevated in 92.3% of all cases studied, and in 88.3% of ovarian ascites studied (62). FGF-2 mRNA is increased in several ovarian cancer cell lines (63) and ovarian cancer patients have high urinary FGF-2 levels, compared to other cancer types (64). Tumor-associated macrophages have been shown to produce FGF-2 to support new vessel growth in a paracrine fashion (65). Thus, there exists a complex paracrine angiogenic loop that occurs during ovarian cancer tumor growth and vascularization.

Several anti-FGF therapies are currently in development. Interferon-alpha administered in low daily doses has been shown to inhibit FGF-2 production *in vitro* and in xenografts (66). Blockade of FGF signaling using the compound SU6668, a tyrosine kinase inhibitor with activity against FGF receptor, VEGF receptors, and PDGF receptors, is in phase I trials. Inhibition of FGF2-induced endothelial cell migration and angiogenesis may be accomplished by anti-FGF2 and anti-FGF-receptor antibodies. Thrombospondin-1 (67) and the C-terminal 4N1K peptide (68) have been reported to block FGF-2 mediated angiogenesis.

4.1.4. Hepatocyte Growth Factor

Hepatocyte growth factor (HGF), also known as scatter factor, is a broad specificity polypeptide growth factor that has mitogenic, motogenic and morphogenic actions on a variety of epithelial and endothelial cell-types (69). It signals through its receptor, a product of the oncogene c-met. In normal tissues, HGF promotes wound healing, possibly by recruitment of fibroblasts to the site of injury. Interaction of HGF with c-met is considered to be a paracrine mediator of normal mesenchymal-epithelial interactions and has been implicated in the generation and spread of epithelial tumors including those of ovarian origin (70).

HGF is present in ovarian cancer ascites. It affects ovarian cancer by stimulating ovarian cancer cell migration and invasion (71), and inducing angiogenesis (69). Furthermore, while c-met is expressed in both normal ovarian surface epithelium and ovarian tumor cell lines, increased expression is found in a small proportion of ovarian cancers (70). *In vitro*, HGF can increase the dedifferentiation and invasiveness of human carcinoma cells when grown on collagen type I gels (72), underscoring that the microenvironment of the tumor cells affects metastasis. Dissection of the HGF signaling pathway demonstrates that HGF induces ovarian cancer migration and invasion via ras and phosphatidylinositol-3 kinase pathways (73). The presence of HGF in ovarian tumor ascites, its potent actions on ovarian cancer cells and its affects on host blood vessels suggest it to be a crucial factor in ovarian tumor progression. The HGF/c-met system is an underappreciated therapeutic target.

4.2. Anti-Angiogenic Factors

It is widely accepted that the conversion of avascular tumors to vascularized tumors, the angiogenic switch, is caused in part by a shift in the balance of local pro- and anti-angiogenic molecules (8). Several tumor suppressor genes affect this balance such that their loss may either remove an inhibitor or induce a stimulant. Normal expression of the tumor suppressor protein p53 increases transcription of the angiogenesis inhibitor thrombospondin-1 (74). The von Hippel-Lindau gene product and p16/Ink4 (75, 76) block angiogenesis by post-transcriptional inhibition of angiogenic stimulators, including VEGF. VEGF transcription is increased by activated H-ras (77), demonstrating that inhibition of angiogenesis can occur at transcriptional and post-transcriptional levels.

4.2.1. Endogenous Angiogenesis Inhibitors

A relatively new class of angiogenesis inhibitors is the collection of endogenous protein fragments (Table 2). In 1991, the N-terminal 16-kilodalton fragment of human prolactin was identified as an inhibitor of FGF-induced endothelial cell proliferation (78), and subsequently as an anti-angiogenic factor (79). Angiostatin, a fragment of plasminogen (80), and endostatin, a fragment of type XVIII collagen (81), were discovered based upon their anti-angiogenic activities. They appear to act specifically upon endothelial cells in the tumor vasculature, causing tumor vascular regression and tumor disappearance. Angiostatin appears to block angiogenesis by inducing endothelial cell apoptosis (82), while endostatin may prevent growth factor signaling through heparan sulfate proteoglycans (83). Angiostatin was more effective than endostatin in one study of ovarian tumor growth inhibition, and a combination of both drugs produced a super-additive inhibitory effect on tumor mass (84). Angiostatin is predicted to have a longer circulatory half-life than endostatin, due to endostatin's greater mass (M_r 20,000) and the binding of endostatin to the host vasculature, further reducing its availability to the tumor site (85). Angiostatin has been shown to potentiate the anti-tumor effect of ionizing radiation therapy (86, 87). Both of these proteins are currently in phase I solid tumor clinical trials. Vasostatin, a calreticulin fragment, has been demonstrated to be anti-angiogenic and to block tumor growth (88). Additionally, the naturally occurring Neovastat/AE-941 was discovered as an anti-angiogenic factor in a shark cartilage extract (89). Neovastat blocks the matrix metalloproteinases (MMPs) secreted by cancer cells and sprouting blood vessels that digest extracellular matrix and allow invasion (90).

4.2.2. Synthetic Angiogenesis Inhibitors

The other class of angiogenic inhibitors is composed of synthetic molecules. This growing class of compounds targets many different aspects of the angiogenic process (Table 2) and several currently are in clinical trial. Some of these agents, such as antibodies to the EGF receptor (C225), anti-VEGF and anti-VEGF receptor neutralize polypeptide growth factors or prevent target growth factor signaling. The tyrophostin family of tyrosine kinase inhibitors has yielded several drugs now on trial, including SU5416 (43), SU6668 (91), SU101 (92) and Iressa (93). These block KDR, KDR, FGF-R and PDGF-R, PDGF-R, and EGF-R respectively, with differing levels of specificity. Other drugs block matrix turnover, including Marimastat (British Biotech, Annapolis, MD) now in phase III clinical trials in ovarian cancer (94), AG3340 (95) (Agouron, La Jolla, CA), COL-3 (96) (Collagenex, Newton, PA) and BMS-275291 (96) (Bristol-Myers Squibb, Wallingford, CT). Drugs that directly act upon endothelial cells include thalidomide, squalamine, an inhibitor of the Na+/H+ exchanger NHE3 (97) (Magainin Pharmaceuticals, Plymouth Meeting, PA) and combretastatin (Bristol-Myers). Also currently under investigation is EMD121974 (Merck KcgaA, Darmstadt, Germany), a small molecule that disrupts cell adhesion by blocking endothelial cell surface integrins, and carboxyamido-triazole (CAI,

NCI), an inhibitor or non-excitable calcium influx that causes tumor mass reduction by targeting tumor cells and disrupting tumor vessels (98).

5. ADHESION AND PROTEOLYSIS DURING ANGIOGENESIS AND INVASION

Adhesive connections among cells and between cells and their surrounding matrix are crucial for the maintenance of normal tissue integrity. Cell adhesion molecules, integrins, and cadherins mediate signaling both from the extracellular environment into the cell, "outside>in" signaling, and from the nucleus to the cell surface, "inside>out" signaling. These connections are remodeled during angiogenesis to initiate changes in cell shape and polarity driven by stimulating growth factors and cytokines. Disruption of normal cell-cell and cell-matrix interactions in tumor cells may contribute to increased invasiveness and metastatic potential. Activated endothelial cells, like invasive tumor cells, secrete proteases to digest surrounding basement membrane and stromal matrix.

5.1. Cadherins-Catenins

Cadherins are a family of calcium-dependent cell surface adhesive proteins that include epithelial, neural, and vascular endothelial (E, N and VE) cadherins (104). They transmit signals from a cell-cell junction with a neighboring cell into the cytoplasm. Cadherins bind to the intracellular catenins, which associate with cytoskeletal elements such as α-actinin and signal into the nucleus (105, 106). VE-cadherin is specifically localized at endothelial cell-cell junctions (107). Ablation of VE-cadherin *in vivo* does not affect endothelial cell differentiation, but rather prevents formation of tube-like structures (108). Loss of cadherin expression or function or that of the other members of its signaling cascade generally leads to a reduction in the ability of tumor cells to adhere to each other and facilitates their detachment from the primary tumor and invasion of the surrounding tissue (109). Loss of E-cadherin expression has been correlated with a high invasive capacity and poor differentiation of several different types of epithelium-derived carcinomas such colorectal, breast, prostate and gastric carcinomas (110). E-cadherin can act as an invasion suppressor gene in epithelial tumor cells (111).

Regulation of E-cadherin expression in the ovarian surface epithelium (OSE) may be different than that seen in most other epithelial malignancies but also correlates with ovarian malignancy. E-cadherin is undetectable in normal OSE but is found frequently in transformed OSE and primary ovarian carcinomas (112). Ectopic expression of E-cadherin in immortalized but not malignant OSE was shown to initiate early pre-neoplastic changes by

Table 2. Endogenous and Synthetic Angiogenesis Inhibitors

Endogenous Inhibitors

Angiopoietin-2 (Ang2) (50)	16-kDa Prolactin fragment (79)
Angiostatin (80)	AE-941/Neovastat (89)
Endostatin (81)	Vasostatin (88)

Thrombospondin-1 and 4N1K fragment (68)
Tissue inhibitors of metalloproteinases (TIMPs) (99)

Synthetic Inhibitors

Target growth factor signaling
Anti-EGF-R (C225) (100)
Anti-VEGF and
 anti-VEGF-R (31)
SU-101 (92)
SU-5416 (43)
SU-6668 (91)

Target cell adhesion
αvβ3 peptide antagonists and
anti-αvβ3 antibody (101)

Target extracellular matrix proteolysis
AG-3340 (95)
BMS-275291 (96)
COL-3 (96)
Marimastat (94)

Target cell motility and proliferation
CAI (98)
Paclitaxel (102)
Squalamine (103)

committing OSE cells to a complex epithelial phenotype, potentially restricting their mesenchymal potential (113). While contrary to the conventional role for E-cadherin, these results suggest that ovarian carcinogenesis also may be advanced by inappropriate E-cadherin expression. Free floating malignant ascitic cells of ovarian cancer origin have been demonstrated to have a markedly decreased expression of E-cadherin, as compared to their solid tumor mass counterparts, a pattern consistent with common epithelial tumors of other origins (114). This suggests that varied expression of E-cadherin by ovarian tumor cells may be important in the invasive to metastatic continuum. It remains unclear how increased levels of a surface adhesion protein in ovarian epithelium may generate a more invasive cell type. Further analysis of changes in E-cadherin gene expression and its effect on downstream signaling molecules is an important future direction.

5.2. Integrins

Tumor cells also associate with the surrounding matrix via the integrin superfamily of cell surface adhesion molecules. Integrins bind diverse extracellular matrix molecules such as the collagens, fibrinogen, fibronectin, laminin, tenascin, thrombospondin, vitronectin and von Willebrand's factor via combinations of non-covalently linked α and β subunits (115). Signaling through integrins regulates invasion, metastasis, cell proliferation, apoptosis pathways, and cell shape (116-123). Normal integrin activity is also crucial for control of angiogenesis (101, 124). The integrin $\alpha v\beta3$ is expressed on the surface of migrating endothelial cells and reacts with a wide variety of extracellular matrix components, facilitating angiogenesis in essentially all tissues during development (101).

Integrin expression is perturbed in tumor angiogenesis and tumor cell invasion. The integrin $\alpha v\beta3$ has been specifically associated with tumor growth and tumor angiogenesis (124, 125). It has been detected in ovarian cancer cell lines and in human ovarian cancers (126). There is a gradient of expression of the $\alpha v\beta3$ integrin in ovarian tumor progression from low malignant potential to more invasive cancers (127). Disruption of $\alpha v\beta3$ signaling by the function blocking antibody LM609 results in blood vessel apoptosis in tumors (101), possibly by altering endothelial cell shape, a key regulator of endothelial cell survival (128). Currently, integrin signaling blockers, such as $\alpha v\beta3$ antagonizing peptides and anti- $\alpha v\beta3$ antibodies (Vitaxin), are being examined in phase II studies for their ability to induce vascular cell apoptosis and inhibit tumor angiogenesis, leading to tumor stasis or regression.

5.3. Proteases

5.3.1. Matrix Metalloproteinases and the Tissue Inhibitors of Metalloproteinases

Matrix metalloproteinases (MMPs) are a family of secreted or cell-surface associated zinc-dependent endopeptidases that selectively degrade basement membrane proteins during angiogenesis and tumor metastasis (129) (Figure 3). MMPs are secreted in latent form and are activated by partial proteolytic processing. The role of MMPs in angiogenic sprouting is critical, allowing endothelial cells access to the surrounding stroma (130). Endothelial cells produce MMP-1 (interstitial collagenase), MMP-2 and MMP-9 (gelatinases A and B), MMP-3 (stromelysin-1), MMP-14 {membrane type (MT)1-MMP} (131). Endothelial cell production of MMP-2 and MT1-MMP, key participants in invasive processes in many cell types, is induced when cells are cultured within a stromal type I collagen matrix, and blocking MMP activity with synthetic MMP inhibitors prevents tube formation (132). *In vivo*, synthetic MMP inhibitors prevent growth factor-induced angiogenesis in animal models (133, 134) and reduces tumor burden (134). And while mice deficient in MMP-2 display no defects in vasculogenesis and embryonic angiogenesis, tumor-induced angiogenesis is partially depressed (135). MMP-9 deficient mice have impaired long bone angiogenesis, although the contributions of endothelial cells to this defect is unknown (136).

MMPs are associated with metastatic tumor spread in a wide range of cancers (for examples see (137, 138)). Normal ovarian epithelial cells do not express MMPs (139). Epithelial ovarian carcinoma cells derived from primary ovarian tumors, metastatic lesions or ascites, produce elevated levels of gelatinolytic MMPs, specifically MMP-2 and -9 (140-142), as do the surrounding stromal cells (143). Cells recovered from primary tumors of mice bearing ovarian cancer xenografts express MMP-1, MMP-2 and MMP-3, while cells from peritoneal ascites express only MMP-1 and MMP-3 (144). Ovarian carcinoma cells have been shown to activate MMP-2 via a $\beta 1$ integrin-dependent post-translational modification of MT1-MMP (141, 145). This suggests that extracellular matrix-induced integrin aggregation can differentially regulate MMP activity. Several studies have linked the presence of MMPs, specifically MMP-2, to ovarian cancer progression. MMP-2 expression was determined to be low in benign cystadenoma and high in malignant primary and metastatic tumors (146, 147). MMP-2 expression in stromal cells correlated with increased malignancy in ovarian tumors, although the MMP-2 protein localizes to stromal cells and epithelial tumor cells (148). Also, MMP-2 protein has been localized at the invasive edge of high-grade ovarian carcinoma (149).

A correlation between MMP-2 and CA125 status in 10 ovarian cancer patients has been described (150). However, the potential use of MMP-2 levels as a prognostic or diagnostic indicator is uncertain. Analysis of MMP-2 levels in sera from 14 ovarian cancer patients were found to have no difference from control levels (147). These results indicate the necessity of further analysis before determining the clinical utility of MMP-2 measurements. Since MMPs play critical roles in tumor angiogenesis and metastasis, a multitude of synthetic therapeutic agents, MMP inhibitors or MMPIs, are being developed to block MMP function. The first generation

369

pan-MMP inhibitor batimastat (BB94) was used to treat mice bearing ovarian carcinoma xenografts, and decreased tumor burden at 14 days by 90% and increased survival five- to six-fold (151). Poor solubility of batimastat required intraperitoneal and intrapleural administration in phase I and phase I/II clinical trials on patients with malignant ascites and malignant pleural

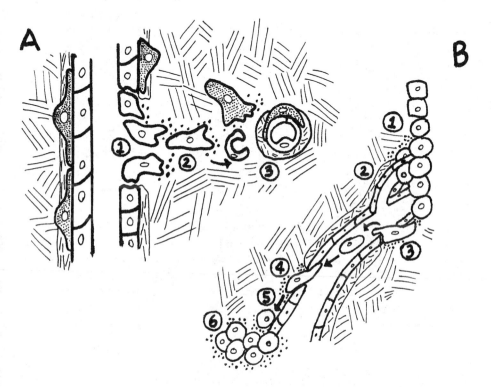

Figure 3. Matrix metalloproteinases in angiogenesis and tumor invasion. During angiogenesis (A) MMP activity is crucial during the initiation of the angiogenic sprout (1) as well as during endothelial cell migration through the interstitial space (2) and for basement membrane remodeling during vessel maturation. During tumor invasion, MMPs are believed to play roles in initiation of the tumor (1), tumor-induced angiogenesis (2), intravasation (3), extravasation (4), migration at the new site (5) and continued proliferation (6).

effusions (152, 153). Marimastat, a soluble analog of batimastat, was the first orally bioavailable MMPI to enter clinical trials. Phase I/II trials were conducted in patients with ovarian and other cancers (129). Efforts are underway to integrate marimastat and AG3340, a selective inhibitor of gelatinase A and B, collagenase-3, and stromelysin-1, as additions to cytotoxic chemotherapy or as a treatment after chemotherapy (129). Recent clinical trials of the MMPI BAY 12-9566, a butanoic acid analog, have been suspended (129).

A family of endogenous inhibitors, the tissue inhibitors of metalloproteinase (TIMPs), regulates MMP activity during angiogenesis and tumor cell invasion (99, 154). Currently, there are four known TIMPs (TIMP1-4), each of which has a distinct specificity for particular MMPs (155). TIMPs bind reversibly to the active site of MMPs, inhibiting their enzymatic activity. Thus, the extent of proteolytic activity produced by sprouting endothelial cells and invading tumor cells is determined by the balance of specific MMPs and TIMP concentrations (156).

TIMPs may inhibit angiogenesis by preventing MMP remodeling of the surrounding extracellular matrix. A combination of TIMP-1 and TIMP-2 inhibits Ang1-induced endothelial cell sprouting in fibrin gels (48). *In vitro*, TIMP-1 and TIMP-2 are capable of inhibiting endothelial cell tube formation (157) and TIMP-2 blocks FGF-2-stimulated endothelial cell proliferation, a function independent of its effects on MMP activity (158). Conversely, proangiogenic factors such as VEGF (159) and Ang1 (48) inhibit TIMP-2 but not TIMP-1 expression.

Since metastatic phenotype is associated with increased proteolysis, several groups have examined TIMP levels in cultured ovarian cancer cells and samples from ovarian cancer patients to determine if TIMP levels can be used as prognostic and diagnostic indicators. While normal OSE lack detectable TIMP expression, examination of several ovarian carcinoma cell lines demonstrated heterogeneous expression of TIMP-2 (160). Also, elevated levels of TIMP-2 protein have been documented in high-grade ovarian carcinoma (149). However, one study measuring TIMP levels in ovarian cancer tissues and normal ovary indicated no difference (161), and comparisons of TIMP-1 and TIMP-2 in the sera of women with advanced ovarian cancer versus normal controls revealed no changes (139). Therefore, additional studies regarding the usefulness of TIMP measurements in ovarian cancer are required.

5.3.2. Plasmin and Plasminogen Activation

The serine protease plasmin is converted from its zymogen form, plasminogen, via the plasminogen activators, urinary-type plasminogen activator (u-PA, urokinase) and tissue-type plasminogen activator (t-PA). Plasmin degrades several extracellular matrix proteins, primarily fibrin but also type IV collagen, fibronectin, laminin and vitronectin, and can activate MMPs. Plasmin activity is vital to matrix processing during angiogenesis

(162) and tumor metastasis (163). By its ability to remodel the extracellular milieu, plasmin is also capable of releasing extracellular matrix-associated growth factors such as VEGF and FGF-2.

u-PA is involved in matrix degradation during embryogenesis, wound healing, angiogenesis and metastasis (164). u-PA has been associated with ovarian cancer invasiveness. One study of 10 ovarian carcinoma cell lines demonstrated uPA production in all lines (165), while a comparison of normal OSE and ovarian carcinoma cells indicated a 17-38-fold decrease in uPA secretion in normal OSE (160). Elevated expression of u-PA in breast and ovarian tumor extracts and expression of the u-PA receptor in ovarian tumors is associated with increased invasion, a higher incidence of relapse, and short overall patient survival (166, 167).

u-PA activity is blocked by plasminogen activator inhibitors-1 and -2 (PAI-1 and PAI-2). PAI-1 is secreted by stromal cells surrounding the tumor and is sometimes elevated in metastases versus the primary tumor, while PAI-2 does not appear to be induced during metastatic progression (168). Currently, the usefulness of u-PA and PAI-1 levels in detecting ovarian cancer is uncertain. Several groups have concluded that plasma levels of PAI-1 correlated with cancer presence and higher stage of disease (169, 170). Abendstein and co-workers reported that u-PA and PAI-1 showed no significant relation to treatment response or overall patient survival (171), while Hoffmann and colleagues found that u-PA but not PAI-1 were correlated with increasing cell dedifferentiation (172). Perhaps because of the controversies regarding the potential prognostic significance of u-PA and PAI-1 as markers in cancer, fewer therapeutic drugs are in development than is the case with the MMPs.

6. CONCLUSION

Angiogenesis and metastatic invasion are complex processes that have significant similarities at the cellular and tissue level. Insights into how ovarian angiogenesis is initiated, maintained and eliminated during physiological and pathological ovarian angiogenesis may crossover towards understanding of how ovarian epithelial tumor cells invade surrounding tissue. State of the art screening technologies are expected to result in the identification and characterization of unique molecules and signaling pathways controlling the angiogenic/invasive processes. Novel therapeutics devised against these molecules may translate into reductions in mortality and morbidity due to ovarian cancer.

372

REFERENCES

1. Brown, M. R., Masiero, L., and Kohn, E. C. Tumor Angiogenesis and Metastasis. In: W. J. Hoskins, C. A. Perez, and R. C. Young (eds.), Principles and Practice of Gynecologic Oncology: Lippincott Williams and Wiklins, 2000.
2. Mesiano, S., Ferrara, N., and Jaffe, R. B. Role of vascular endothelial growth factor in ovarian cancer: ihibition of ascites formation by immunoneutralization. Am J Path 1998; 153: 1249-56.
3. Kohn, E. C. and Liotta, L. A. Molecular insights into cancer invasion: strategies for prevention and intervention. Cancer Res 1995; 55: 1856-1862.
4. Folkman, J. and Shing, Y. Angiogenesis, J Biol Chem 1992; 267: 10931-3.
5. D'Amore, P. A. and Thompson, R. W. Mechanisms of angiogenesis, Ann Rev Physiol 1987; 49: 453-64.
6. Eberhard, A., Kahlert, S., Goede, V., Hemmerlein, B., Plate, K. H., and Augustin, H. G. Heterogeneity of angiogenesis and blood vessel maturation in human tumors: implications for antiangiogenic tumor therapies Cancer Res 2000; 60: 1388-93.
7. Folkman, J. Tumor angiogenesis: Therapeutic implications. N Engl J Med. 1971; 5: 1182 - 1186.
8. Hanahan, D. and Folkman, J. Patterns and emerging mechanisms of the angiogenic switch during tumorigenesis. Cell 1996; 86: 353-364.
9. Liotta, L. A., Kleinerman, J., and Saidel, G. Quantitative relationships of intravascular tumor cells: tumor vessels and pulmonary metastases following tumor implantation. Cancer Res 1971; 34: 997-1003.
10. Folkman, J. and Klagsbrun, M. Angiogenic factors. Science 1987; 235: 442-447.
11. Folkman, J. Clinical applications of research on angiogenesis. New Eng J Med 1996; 333: 1757-1763.
12. Yoneda, J., Kuniyasu, H., Crispens, M. A., Price, J. E., Bucana, C. D., and Fidler, I. J. Expression of angiogenesis-related genes and progression of human ovarian carcinomas in nude mice. J Natl Cancer Inst 1988; 90: 447-454.
13. Fang, X., Gaudette, D., Furui, T., Mao, M., Estrella, V., Eder, A., Pustilnik, T., Sasagawa, T., Lapushin, R., Yu, S., Jaffe, R. B., Weiner, J. R., Erickson, J. R., and Mills, G. B. Lysophospholipid growth factors in the initiation, progression, metastases and management of ovarian cancer. Ann N Y Acad Sci 2000; 905: 188-208.
14. Abulafia, O. and Sherer, D. M. Angiogenesis of the ovary. Am J Obstet Gynecol 2000; 182: 240 - 246.
15. Gordon, J. D., Mesiano, S., Zaloudek, C. J., and Jaffe, R. B. Vascular endothelial growth factor localization in human ovary and fallopian tubes: possible role in reproductive function and ovarian cyst formation. J Clin Endocrin Metabol 1996; 81: 353-359.
16. Ferrara, N., Chen, H., Davis Smyth, T., Gerber, H. P., Nguyen, T. N., Peers, D., Chisholm, V., Hilan, K. J., and Schwall, R. H. Vascular endothelial growth factor is essential for corpus luteum angiogenesis. Nature Med 1998; 4: 336 - 340.
17. Augustin, H. G., Braun, K., Telemenakis, I., Modlich, U., and Kuhn, W. Ovarian angiogenesis: Phenotypic characterization of endothelial cells in a physiological model of blood vessel growth and regression. Am J Path. 147 1995; 339-351.
18. Neeman, M., Abramovitch, R., Schiffenbauer, Y. S., and Tempel, C. Regulation of angiogenesis by hypoxic stress: from solid tumors to the ovarian follicle. Int J Exp Pathol 1997; 78: 57-70.
19. Hirschi, K. K. and D'Amore, P. A. Pericytes in the microvasculature. Cardiovasc Res 1996; 32: 687-98.
20. Cogan, D. G. and Kuwabara, T. The mural cell in perspective. Arch Ophthalmol 1967; 78: 133-9.

21. Herman, I. M. and D'Amore, P. A. Microvascular pericytes contain muscle and nonmuscle actins. J Cell Biology 1985; 101: 43-52.
22. Larson, D. M., Carson, M. P., and Haudenschild, C. C. Junctional transfer of small molecules in cultured bovine brain microvascular endothelial cells and pericytes. Microvasc Res 1987; 34: 184-99.
23. Larson, D. M., Haudenschild, C. C., and Beyer, E. Gap junction messenger RNA expression by vascular wall cells. Circulation Research. 1990; 66: 1074-80.
24. Orlidge, A. and D'Amore, P. A. Inhibition of capillary endothelial cell growth by pericytes and smooth muscle cells. J Cell Biology. 1987; 105: 1455-62.
25. Sato, Y. and Rifkin, D. B. Inhibition of endothelial cell movement by pericytes and smooth muscles: activation of a latent transforming growth factor-beta 1-like molecule by plasmin during co-culture. J Cell Biol 1989; 109: 309-15.
26. Antonelli-Orlidge, A., Saunders, K. B., Smith, S. R., and D'Amore, P. A. An activated form of transforming growth factor beta is produced by cocultures of endothelial cells and pericytes. Proceedings of the National Academy of Sciences U.S.A. 1989; 86: 4544-8.
27. Sato, Y., Tsuboi, R., Lyons, R., Moses, H., and Rifkin, D. B. Characterization of the activation of latent TGF-beta by co-cultures of endothelial cells and pericytes or smooth muscle cells: a self-regulating system. J Cell Biol 1990; 111: 757-63.
28. Benjamin, L. E., Golijanin, D., Itin, A., Pode, D., and Keshet, E. Selective ablation of immature blood vessels in established human tumors follows vascular endothelial growth factor withdrawal. J Clin Invest 1999; 103: 159-165.
29. Lindahl, P., Johansson, B. R., Leveen, P., and Betsholtz, C. Pericyte loss and microaneurysm formation in PDGF-B deficient mice. Science 1997; 277: 242-5.
30. Benjamin, L. E., Hemo, I., and Keshet, E. A plasticity window for blood vessel remodeling is defined by pericyte coverage of the preformed endothelial network and is reguated by PDGF-B and VEGF. Development 1998; 125: 1591-8.
31. Ferrara, N. and Alitalo, K. Clinical applications of angiogenic growth factors and their inhibitors. Nature Med 1999; 5: 1359-64.
32. Senger, D. R., Galli, S. J., Dvorak, A. M., Perruzzi, C. A., Harvey, V. S., and Dvorak, H. F. Tumor cells secrete a vascular permeability factor that promotes accumulation of ascites fluid. Science 1983; 219: 983-985.
33. Carmeliet, P. Mechanisms of angiogenesis and arteriogenesis. Nature Med 2000; 6: 389-395.
34. Benjamin, L. E. and Keshet, E. Conditional switching of vascular endothelial growth factor (VEGF) expression in tumors: induction ofendothelial cell shedding and regression of hemangioblastoma-like vessels by VEGF withdrawal. Proceedings of the National Academy of Sciences U.S.A. 1997; 94:8761-8766.
35. Boocock, C. A., Charnock-Jones, S., Sharkey, A. M., McLaren, J., Barker, P. J., Wright, K. A., and al, e. Expression of vascular endothelial growth factor and its receptors flt and KDR in ovarian carcinoma. J Natl Cancer Inst. 1995; 87: 506-516.
36. Klagsbrun, M. and D'Amore, P. A. Vascular endothelial growth factor and its receptors. Cyt Grow Fact Rev 1996; 1: 259-270.
37. Goede, V., Schmidt, T., Kimmina, S., Kozian, D., and Augustin, H. G. Analysis of blood vessel maturation processes during cyclic ovarian angiogenesis, Lab Invest 1998; 78: 1385 - 1394.
38. Kamat, B. R., Brown, L. F., Manseau, E. J., Senger, D. R., and Dvorak, H. F. Expression of vascular permeability factor/ vascular endothelial growth factor by human granulosa and theca lutein cells. Am J Pathol 1995; 146: 157-65.
39. Abramov, T., Schenker, J. G., Lewin, A., Friedler, S., Nisman, B., and Barak, U. Plasma inflammatory cytokines correlate to the ovarian hyperstimulation syndrome. Hum Reprod 1996; 11:1381-6.

40. Doldi, N., Bassan, M., Messa, A., and Ferrari, A. Expression of vascular endothelial growth factor in human luteinizing granulosa cells and its correlation with the response to controlled ovarian hyperstimulation. Gynecol Endocrinol 1997; 11: 263-7.

41. Yeo, K. T., Wang, H. H., Hagy, J. A., Sioussat, T. M., Ledbetter, S. R., Hoogewerf, A. J., Zhou, Y., Masse, E. M., Senger, D. R., and Dvorak, H. F. Vascular permeability factor (vascular endothelial growth factor) in guinea pig and human tumor and inflammatory effusions. Cancer Res 1993; 53: 2912-8.

42. Abu-Jawdeh, G. M., Faix, J. D., Niloff, J., Tognazzi, K., Manseau, E., Dvorak, H. F. Strong expression of vascular permeability factor (vascular endothelial growth factor) and its receptors in ovarian borderline and malignant neoplasms. Lab Invest 1996; 74: 1105-1115.

43. Fong, T. A., Shawver, L. K., Sun, L., Tang, C., App, H., Powell, T. J., Kim, Y. H., Schreck, R., Wang, X., Risau, W., Ullrich, A., Hirth, K. P., and McMahon, G. SU5416 is a potent and selective inhibitor of the vascular endothelial growth factor receptor (Flk-1/KDR) that inhibits tyrosine kinase catalysis, tumor vascularization and growth of multiple tumor types. Cancer Res 1999; 59: 99-106.

44. Inoue, K., Slaton, J. W., Davis, D. W., Hicklin, D. J., McConkey, D. J., Karashima, T., Radinsky, R., and Dinney, C. P. Treatment of human metastatic transitional cell carcinoma of the bladder in a murine model with the anti-vascular endothelial growth factor receptor monoclonal antibody DC101 and paclitaxel. Clin Cancer Res 2000; 6: 2635-43.

45. Zhu, Z., Lu, D., Kotanides, H., Santiago, A., Jimenez, X., Simcox, T., Hicklin, D. J., Bohlen, P., and Witte, L. Inhibition of vascular endothelial growth factor induced mitogenesis of human endothelial cells by a chimeric anti-kinase insert domain-containing receptor antibody. Cancer Lett 1999; 136: 203-13.

46. Gale, N. W. and Yancopoulos, G. D. Growth factors acting via endothelial cell-specific receptor tyrosine kinases: VEGFs, angiopoietins, and ephrins in vascular development. Genes Dev 1999; 13: 1055-66.

47. Suri, C., Jones, P. F., Patan, S., Bartunkova, S., Maisonpierre, P. C., Davis, S., Sato, T. N., and Yancopoulos, G. D. Requisite role of angiopoietin-1, a ligand for the TIE2 receptor, during embryonic angiogenesis. Cell 1996; 87: 1171-1180.

48. Kim, I., Kim, H. W., Moon, S.-O., Chae, S. W., So, J.-N., Koh, K. N., Ahn, B. C., and Koh, G. Y. Angiopoietin-1 induces endothelial cell sprouting through the activation of focal adhesion kinase and plasmin secretion. Circ Res 2000; 86: 952-9.

49. Maisonpierre, P. C., Suri, C., Jones, P. F., Bartunkova, S., Wiegand, S. J., Radziejewski, C., Compton, D., McClain, J., Aldrich, T. H., Papadopoulos, N., Daly, T. J., Davis, S., Sato, T. N., and Yancopoulos, G. D. Angiopoietin-2, a natural antagonist for Tie2 that disrupts in vivo angiogenesis. Science 1997; 277: 55-60.

50. Hanahan, D. Signaling vascular morphogenesis and maintenance. Science 1997;277:48-50.

51. Thurston, G., Suri, C., Smith, K., McClain, J., Sato, T. N., Yancopoulos, G. D., and McDonald, D. M. Leakage-resistant blood vessels in mice transgenically overexpressing angiopoietin-1. Science 1999; 286:2511-4.

52. Brown, L. F., Dezube, B. J., Tognazzi, K., Dvorak, H. F., and Yancopoulos, G. D. Expression of Tie1, Tie2, and angiopoietins 1,2 and 4 in Kaposi's sarcoma and cutaneous angiosarcoma. Am J Pathol 2000; 156:2179-83.

53. Takahama, M., Tsutsumi, M., Tsujichi, T., Nezu, K., Kushibe, K., Taniguchi, S., Kotake, Y., and Konishi, Y. Enhanced expression of Tie2, its ligand angiopoietin-1, vascular endothelial growth factor, and CD31 in human non-small cell lung carcinomas. Clin Cancer Res 1999; 5:2506-10.

54. Gerwins, P., Skoldenberg, E., and Claesson-Welsh, L. Function of fibroblast growth factors and vascular endothelial growth factors and their receptors in angiogenesis. Crit Rev Oncol Hematol 2000; 34:185-94.

55. Clark, J. L., Jones, K. I., Gospodarowicz, D., and Sato, G. H. Growth response to hormones by a new rat ovary cell line. Nat New Biol 1972; 236: 180-1.

56. Armelin, H. A. Pituitary extracts and steroid hormones in the control of 3T3 cell growth. Proc Natl Acad Sci USA 1973; 70:2702-6.

57. Gospodarowicz, D. Purification of a fibroblast growth factor from bovine pituitary. J Biol Chem 1975; 250:2515-20.

58. Healy, A. M. and Herman, I. M. Density-dependent accumulation of basic fibroblast growth factor in the subendothelial matrix. Eur J Cell Bio 1992; 59 56-67.

59. Moscatelli, D., Presta, M., and Rifkin, D. B. Purification of a factor from human placenta that stimulates capillary endothelial cell protease production, DNA synthesis and migration. Proceedings of the National Academy of Science U.S.A.1986; 83:2091-5.

60. Basilico, C. and Moscatelli, D. The FGF family of growth factors and oncogenes. Advances in Cancer Research 1992; 59:115-65.

61. Takahashi, K., Mulliken, J. B., Koszkewich, H. P., Rogers, R. A., Folkman, J., and Ezekowitz, R. A. B. Cellular markers that distinguish the phases of hemangioma during infancy and childhood. J Clin Invest 1994; 93: 2357-64.

62. Barton, D. P., Cai, A., Wendt, K., Young, M., Gamero, A., and DeCesare, S. Angiogenic protein expression in advanced epithelial ovarian cancer. Clin Cancer Res 1997; 3:1579-86.

63. Crickard, K., Gross, J. L., Crickard, U., Yoonessi, M., Lele, S., Herblin, W. F., and Eidsvoog, K. Basic fibroblast growth factor and receptor expression in human ovarian cancer. Gynecol Oncol 1994; 55:277-84.

64. Nguyen, M., Watanabe, H., Budson, A. E., Richie, J. P., Hayes, D. F., and Folkman, J. Elevated levels of an angiogenic peptide, basic fibroblast growth factor, in the urine of patients with a wide spectrum of cancers. J Natl Cancer Inst 1994; 86:356 - 361.

65. Lewis, C. E., Leek, R., Harris, A., and McGee, J. O. Cytokine regulation of angiogenesis in breast cancer: the role of tumor-associated macrophages. J. Leukoc Biol 1995; 57:747-51.

66. Dinney, C. P., Bielenberg, D. R., Perrotte, P., Reich, R., Eve, B. Y., Bucana, C. D., and Fidler, I. J. Inhibition of basic fibroblast growth factor expression, angiogenesis, and growth of human bladder carcinoma in mice by systemic interferon-alpha administration. Cancer Res 1998; 58:808-14.

67. DiPietro, L. A., Nebgen, D. R., and Pelverini, P. J. Downregulation of endothelial cell thrombospondin 1 enhances in vitro angiogenesis. J Vasc Res 1994; 31:178-85.

68. Kanda, S., Shono, T., Tomasini-Johansson, B., Klint, P., and Saito, Y. Role of thrombospondin-1-derived peptide, 4N1K, in FGF-2-induced angiogenesis. Exp Cell Res 1999; 252:262-72.

69. Rosen, E. M. and Goldberg, I. D. Regulation of angiogenesis by scatter factor. Exs 1997; 79:193-208.

70. Corps, A. N., Sowter, H. M., and Smith, S. K. Hepatocyte growth factor stimulates motility, chemotaxis and mitogenesis in ovarian carcinoma cells expressing high levels of c-met. Int J Cancer 1997; 73:151-5.

71. Sowter, H. M., Corps, A. N., and Smith, S. K. Hepatocyte growth factor (HGF) in ovarian epithelial tumour fluids stimulates the migration of ovarian carcinoma cells. Int J Cancer 1999; 83:476-80.

72. Wong, A. S., Leung, P. C., and Auersperg, N. Hepatocyte growth factor promotes in vitro scattering and morphogenesis of human cervical carcinoma cells. Gynecol Oncol 2000; 78: 158-65.

73. Ueoka, Y., Kato, K., Kuriaki, Y., Horiuch, S., Terao, Y., Nishida, J., Ueno, H., and Wake, N. Hepatocyte growth factor modulates motility and invasiveness of ovarian carcinomas via Ras-mediated pathway. Br J Cancer 2000; 82 891-9.

74. Dameron, K. M., Volpert, O. V., ., Tainsky, M. A., and Bouck, N. Control of Angiogenesis in fibroblasts by p53 regulation of thrombospondin-1. Science 1994; 265:1582 - 1584.

75. Siemeister, G., Weindel, K., Mohrs, K., Barleon, B., Martiny-Baron, G., and Marme, D. Reversion of deregulated expression of vascular endothelial growth factor in human renal carcinoma cells by von Hippel-Lindau tumor suppressor protein. Cancer Res 1996; 56:2299-01.

76. Wizigmann-Voos, S., Breier, G., Risau, W., and Plate, K. H. Up-regulation of vascular endothelial growth factor and its receptors in von Hippel-Lindau disease-associated and sporadic hemangioblastomas. Cancer Res 1995; 55:1358-64.

77. Rak, J., Mitsuhashi, Y., Sheehan, C., Tamir, A., Viloria-Petit, A., Filmus, J., Mansour, S. J., Ahn, N. G., and Kerbel, R. S. Oncogenes and tumor angiogenesis: differential modes of vascular endothelial growth factor up-regulation in ras-transformed epithelial cells and fibroblasts. Cancer Res 2000; 60:490-8.

78. Ferrara, N., Clapp, C., and Weiner, R. The 16K fragment of prolactin specifically inhibits basal or fibroblast growth factor stimulated growth of capillary endothelial cells. Endocrinol 1991; 129:896-900.

79. Clapp, C., Martial, J. A., Guzman, R. C., Rentier-Delure, F., and Weiner, R. I. The 16-kilodalton N-terminal fragment of human prolactin is a potent inhibitor of angiogenesis. Endocrinol 1993; 133: 1292-9.

80. O'Reilly, M. S. and Holmgren, L. Angiostatin: a novel angiogenesis inhibitor that mediates the suppression of metastases by a Lewis lung carcinoma. Cell 1994; 79:315-328.

81. O'Reilly, M. S., Boehm, T., Shing, Y., Fuhai, N., Vasios, G., Lane, W. S., Flynn, E., Birkhead, J. R., Olsen, B. R., and Folkman, J. Endostatin: an endogenous inhibitor of angiogenesis and tumor growth. Cell 1997; 88:277-285.

82. Lucas, R., Holmgren, L., Garcia, I., Jimenez, B., Mandriota, S. J., Borlat, F., Sim, B. K., Wu, Z., Grau, G. E., Shing, Y., Soff, G. A., Bouck, N., and Pepper, M. S. Multiple forms of angiostatin induce apoptosis in endothelial cells. Blood 1998; 92:4730-41.

83. Hohenester, E., Sasaki, T., Olsen, B. R., and Timpl, R. Crystal structure of the angiogenesis inhibitor endostatin at 1.5 A resolution. EMBO 1998; 17:1656-64.

84. Yokoyama, Y., Dhanabal, M., Griffioen, A. W., Sukhatme, V. P., and Ramakrishnan, S. Synergy between angiostatin and endostatin: inhibition of ovarian cancer growth. Cancer Res 2000; 60:2190 - 2196.

85. Chang, Z., Choon, A., and Friedl, A. Endostatin binds to blood vessels in situ independent of heparan sulfate and does not compete for fibroblast growth factor-2 binding. Am J Path 1999; 155:71-6.

86. Gorski, D. H., Mauceri, H. J., Salloum, R. M., Gately, S., Hellman, S., Beckett, M. A., Sukhatme, V. P., Soff, G. A., Kufe, D. W., and Weichselbaum, R. R. Potentiation of the antitumor effect of ionizing radiation by brief concomitant exposures to angiostatin. Cancer Res 1998; 58:5686-9.

87. Mauceri, H. J., Hanna, N. N., Beckett, M. A., Gorski, D. H., Staba, M. J., Stellato, K. A., Bigelow, K., Heimann, R., Gately, S., Dhanabal, M., Soff, G. A., Sukhatme, V. P., Kufe, D. W., and Weichselbaum, R. R. Combined effects of angiostatin and ionizing radiation in antitumour therapy. Nature 1998; 394:287-91.

88. Pike, S. E., Yao, L., Jones, K. D., Cherney, B., Appella, E., Sakaguchi, K., Nakhasi, H., Teruya-Feldstein, J., Wirth, P., Gupta, G., and Tosato, G. Vasostatin, a calreticulin fragment, inhibits angiogenesis and supports tumor growth. J Exp Med 1998; 188:2349-56.

89. Dupont, E., Savard, P. E., Jourdain, C., Juneau, C., Thibodeau, A., Ross, N., Marenus, K., Maes, D. H., Pelletier, G., and Sauder, D. N. Antiangiogenic properties of a novel shark cartilage extract: potential role in the treatment of psoriasis. J Cutan Med Surg 1998; 2:146-52.

377

90. Wojtowicz-Praga, S. Clinical potential of matrix metalloprotease inhibitors. Drugs R D 1999; 1:117-29.

91. Laird, A. D., Vajkoczy, P., Shawver, L. K., Thurnher, A., Liang, C., Mohammadi, M., Schlessinger, J., Ullrich, A., Hubbard, S. R., Blake, R. A., Fong, T. A., Strawn, L. M., Sun, L., Tang, C., Hawtin, R., Tang, F., Shenoy, N., Hirth, K. P., McMahon, G., and Cherington, J. M. SU6668 is a potent antiangiogenic and antitumor agent that induces tumor regression of established tumors. Cancer Res 2000; 60:4152-60.

92. Strawn, L. M., Kabbinavar, F., Schwartz, D. P., Mann, E., Shawver, L. K., Slamon, D. J., and Cherington, J. M. Effects of SU101 in combination with cytotoxic agents on the growth of subcutaneous tumor xenografts. Clin Cancer Res 2000; 6:2931-4.

93. Ciardiello, F., Caputo, R., Bianco, R., Damiano, V., Pomatico, G., DePlacido, S., Bianco, A. R., and Tortora, G. Antitumor effect and potentiation of cytotoxic drugs activity in human cancer cells by ZD-1839 (Iressa), an epidermal growth factor receptor-selective tyrosine kinase inhibitor. Clin Cancer Res 2000; 6:2053-63.

94. Gore, M., A'Hern, R., Stankiewicz, M., and Slevin, M. Tumour marker levels during marimastat therapy. Lancet 1996; 348:263-264.

95. Shalinsky, D. R., Brekken, J., Zou, H., McDermott, C. D., Forsyth, P., Edwards, D., Margosiak, S., Bender, S., Truitt, G., Wood, A., Varki, N. M., and Appelt, K. Broad antitumor and antiangiogenic activities of AG3340, a potent and selective MMP inhibitor undergoing advanced oncology clinical trials. Ann N Y Acad Sci 1999; 878:236-70.

96. Heath, E. I. and Grochow, L. B. Clinical potential of matrix metalloprotease inhibitors in cancer therapy. Drugs 2000; 59:1043-55.

97. Akhter, S., Nath, S. K., Tse, C. M., Williams, J., Zasloff, M., and Donowitz, M. Squalamine, a novel cationic steroid, specifically inhibits the brush-border Na+/H+ exchanger isoform NHE3. Am J Physiol 1999; 276:C136-44.

98. Kohn, E. C., Alessandro, R., Spoonster, J., Wersto, R. P., and Liotta, L. A. Angiogenesis: role of calcium-mediated signal transduction. Proc. Natl. Acad. Sci. USA. 1995; 92:1307-1311.

99. Brew, K., Dinakarpandian, D., and Nagase, H. Tissue inhibitors of metalloproteinases: evolution, structure and function. Biochim Biophys Acta 2000; 1477:267-83.

100. Baselga, J., Pfister, D., Cooper, M. R., Cohen, R., Burtness, B., Bos, M., D'Andrea, G., Seidman, A., Norton, L., Gunnett, K., Falcey, J., Anderson, V., Waksal, H., and Mendelsohn, J. Phase I studies of anti-epidermal growth factor receptor chimeric antibody C225 alone and in combination with cisplatin, J Clin Oncol 2000; 18:904-14.

101. Brooks, P. C., Clark, R. A. F., and Cheresh, D. A. Requirement of vascular integrin avb3 for angiogenesis. Science 1994; 264:569-571.

102. Klauber, N., Parangi, S., Flynn, E., Hamel, E., and D'Amato, R. J. Inhibition of angiogenesis and breast cancer in mice by the microtubule inhibitors 2-methoxyestradiol and taxol. Cancer Res 1997; 57:81-6.

103. Sills, A. K., Williams, J. I., Tyler, B. M., Epstein, D. S., Sipos, E. P., Davis, J. D., McLane, M. P., Pitchford, S., Cheshire, K., Gannon, F. H., Kinney, W. A., Chao, T. L., Donowitz, M., Laterra, J., Zasloff, M., and Brem, H. Squalamine inhibits angiogenesis and solid tumor growth in vivo and perturbs embryonic vasculature. Cancer Res 1998; 58:2784 - 2792.

104. Ohene-Abuakwa, Y. and Pignatelli, M. Adhesion molecules in cancer biology. Adv Exp Med Biol 2000; 465:115-26.

105. Aberle, H., Schwartz, H., and Kemler, R. Cadherin-catenin complex: protein interactions and their implications for cadherin function. J Cell Biochem 1996; 61:514-23.

106. Jou, T. S., Stewart, D. B., Stappert, J., Nelseon, W. J., and Marrs, J. A. Genetic and biochemical dissection of protein linkages in the cadherin-catenin complex. Proc. Natl. Acad.Sci. U.S.A. 1995; 92:5067-5071.

378

107. Caveda, L., Martin-Padura, I., Navarro, P., Breviario, F., Corada, M., Gulino, D., Lampugnani, M. G., and Dejana, E. Inhibition of cultured cell growth by vascular endothelial cadherin (cadherin-5/VE-cadherin). J Clin Invest 1996; 98:886-92.

108. Vittet, D., Buchou, T., Schweitzer, A., Dejana, E., and Huber, P. Targeted null-mutation in the vascular endothelial-cadherin gene impairs the organization of vascular-like structures in embryoid bodies. Proceedings of the National Academy of Sciences U.S.A. 1997; 94:6273-8.

109. Hoffman, A. G., Burghardt, R. C., Tilley, R., and Auersperg, N. An in vitro model of ovarian epithelial carcinogenesis: changes in cell-cell comunication and adhesion occurring during neoplastic progression. Int J Cancer 1993; 54:828-838.

110. Ahmad, A. and Hart, I. R. Mechanisms of metastasis, Crit Rev Oncol/Hematol 1997; 26:163-73.

111. Vleminckx, K., Vakaet, L., Mareel, M., Fiers, W., and van Roy, F. Genetic manipulation of E-cadherin expression by epithelial tumor cells reveals an invasion suppressor role. Cell 1991; 66:107-119.

112. Sudfeldt, K., Piontkewitz, Y., Ivarsson, K., Nilsson, O., Hellberg, P., Brannstrom, M., Janson, P. O., Enerback, S., and Hedin, L. E-cadherin expression in human epithelial ovarian cancer and normal ovary. Int J Cancer 1997; 74:275-80.

113. Auersperg, N., Pan, J., Grove, B. D., Peterson, T., Fisher, J., Maines-Bandiera, S., Somasiri, A., and Roskelley, C. D. E-cadherin induces mesenchymal-to-epithelial transition in human ovarian surface epithelium, Proc Natl Acad Sci USA. 1999; 96:6249-54.

114. Veatch, A. L., Carson, L. F., and Ramakrishman, S. Differential expression of the cell-cell adhesion molecule E-cadherin in ascites and solid human ovarian tumor cells. Int J Cancer 1994; 58: 393-9.

115. Gille, J. and Swerlick, R. A. Integrins: role in cell adhesion and communication., Ann N Y Acad Sci 1996; 797:93-107.

116. Varner, A. J. and Cheresh, D. A. Integrins and Cancer. Curr Opin Cel Biol 1996; 8:724-730.

117. Ruoslahti, E. and Reed, J. Anchorage independence, integrins and apoptosis. Cell 1994; 77:477-478, 1994.

118. Meredith, J. E. and Schwartz, M. Integrins, adhesion, and apoptosis. Trend Cell Biol 1997; 7:146-150.

119. Chicurel, M. E., Singer, R. H., Meyer, C. J., and Ingber, D. E. Integrin binding and mechanical tension induce movement of mRNA and ribosomes to focal adhesions. Nature 1998; 392:730-733.

120. Schwartz, M. A., Schaller, M. D., and Ginsberg, M. H. integrins: emerging paradigms of signal transduction. Ann Rev Cell Dev Biol 1995; 11:549-599.

121. Yamada, K. M. and Miyamoto, S. Integrin transmembrane signaling and cytoskeletal control. Curr Opin Cel Biol 1995; 7:681-689.

122. Giancotti, F. G. Integrin signaling: specificity and control of cell survival and cell cycle progression. Curr Opin Cel Biol 1997; 9:691-700.

123. Hynes, R. O. and Bader, B. L. Targeted mutations in integrins and their ligands: their implications for vascular biology. Thromb Haemost 1997; 78: 83-7.

124. Brooks, P. C., Stromblad, S., Klemke, R., Visscher, D., Sarkar, F. H., and Cheresh, D. A. Anti-integrin alpha v beta 3 blocks human breast cancer growth and angiogenesis in human skin. J Clin Invest 1995; 96:1815-1822.

125. Varner, J. A., Brooks, P. C., and Cheresh, D. A. The integrin avb3: angiogenesis and apoptosis. Cell Adhes Comm 1995;3:367-374.

126. Cannistra, S. A., Ottensmeier, C., Niloff, J., Orta, B., and DiCarlo, J. Expression and function of beta 1 and alpha v beta 3 integrins in ovarian cancer. Gynecol Oncol 1995; 58:216-225.

127. Liapis, H., Adler, L. M., Wick, M. R., and Rader, J. S. Expression of alpha(v)beta3 integrin is less frequent in ovarian epithelial tumors of low malignant potential in contrast to ovarian carcinomas. Human Path 1997; 28: 443-449.

128. Ingber, D. Extracellular matrix and cell shape: potential control points for inhibition of angiogenesis. J Cell Biochem 1991; 47:236-41.

129. Nelson, A. R., Fingleton, B., Rothenberg, M. L., and Matrisian, L. M. Matrix metalloproteinases: biologic activity and clinical implications. J Clin Oncol 2000, 18:1135-49.

130. DeClerck, Y. A. Interactions between tumour cells and stromal cells and proteolytic modification of the extracellular matrix by metalloproteinases in cancer. Eur J Cancer 2000; 36:1258-68.

131. Haas, T. L. and Madri, J. A. Extracellular matrix-driven matrix metalloproteinase production in endothelial cells: implications for angiogenesis. Trends Cardiovasc Med 1999; 9: 70-7.

132. Haas, T. L., Davis, S. J., and Madri, J. A. Three dimensional type I collagen lattices induce coordinate expression of matrix metalloproteinases MT1-MMP and MMP-2 in microvascular endothelial cells. J Biol Chem 1998; 273: 3604-10.

133. Galardy, R., Grobelney, D., Foellmer, H. G., and Fernandez, L. A. Inhibition of angiogenesis by the matrix metalloprotease inhibitor N-{2R-2-(hydroxamidocarbonymethyl)-4 methylpentanoyl)]-L-tryptophan methylamide. Cancer Res 1994; 54:4715-4718.

134. Wojtowicz-Praga, S. M., Dickson, R. B., and Hawkins, M. J. Matrix metalloproteinase inhibitors. Invest New Drugs 1997; 15: 61-75.

135. Itoh, T., Tanioka, M., Yoshida, H., Yoshida, T., Nishimoto, H., and Itohara, S. Reduced angiogenesis and tumor progression in gelatinase A-deficient mice. Cancer Res 1998; 58:1048-51.

136. Vu, T. H., Shipley, J. M., Bergers, G., Berger, J. E., Helms, J. A., Hanahan, D., Shapiro, S. D., Senior, R. M., and Werb, Z. MMP-9/gelatinase B is a key regulator of growth plate angiogenesis and apoptosis of hypertrophic chondrocytes. Cell 1998; 93:411-422.

137. Liotta, L. A. and Stetler-Stevenson, W. G. Tumor invasion and metastasis: an imbalance of positive and negative regulation. Cancer Res 1991; 51: 5054-5059.

138. Coussens, L. M. and Werb, Z. Matrix metalloproteinases and the development of cancer. Chem Biol 1996; 3:895-904.

139. Stack, M. S., Ellerbroek, S. M., and Fishman, D. A. The role of protolytic enzymes in the pathology of epithelial ovarian carcinoma. Int. J Oncol 1998; 12:569-76.

140. Kohn, E. C., Francis, A., Liotta, L. A., and Schiffmann, E. Heterogeneity of the motility responses in malignant tumor cells: a biological basis for the diversity and homing of metastatic cells. Int J Cancer 1990; 46:287.

141. Fishman, D., Bafetti, L. M., Banionis, S., Kearns, A. S., Chilukuri, K., and Stack, M. S. Production of extracellular matrix-degrading proteinases by primary cultures of human epithelial ovarian carcinoma cells. Cancer 1997; 80:1457-1463.

142. Young, T. N., Rodriguez, G. C., Rinehart, A. R., Bast, R. C., Pizzo, S. V., and Stack, M. S. Characterization of gelatinases linked to extracellular matrix invasion in ovarian adenocarcinoma: purification of matrix metalloproteinase 2. Gynecol Oncol 1996; 62: 89-99.

143. Naylor, M. S., Stamp, G. W., Davies, B., and Balkwill, F. R. Expression and activity of MMPs and their regulators in ovarian cancer. Int J Cancer 1994; 58: 50 - 56.

380

144. Liebman, J. M., Burbelo, P. D., Yamada, Y., Fridman, R., and Kleinman, H. K. Altered expression of basement membrane components and collagenases in ascitic xenografts of OVCAR-3 ovarian cancer cells. Int J Cancer 1993; 55:102-9.
145. Ellerbroek, S. M., Fishman, D. A., Kearns, A. S., Bafetti, L. M., and Stack, M. S. Ovarian carcinoma regulation of matrix metaloproteinase-2 and membrane type 1 matrix metaloproteinase through beta 1 integrin, Cancer Res 1999; 59:1635 - 1641.
146. Campo, E., Merino, M. J., Tavassoli, F. A., Charonis, A. S., Stetler-Stevenson, W. G., and Liotta, L. A. Evaluation of basement membrane components and the 72 KDa Type IV collagenase in serous tumors of the ovary. The American Journal of Surgical Pathology 1992; 16: 500 - 507.
147. DeNictolis, M., Garbisa, S., Lucarini, G., Goteri, G., Masiero, L., Ciavattini, A., Garzetti, G. G., Stetler-Stevenson, W. G., Fabris, G., Biagini, G., and Prat, J. 72 kilodalton type IV collagenase, type IV collagen and Ki-67 antigen in serous tumors of the ovary: a clinicopathologic, immunohistochemical and serological study. Int J Gynecol Path 1996 15: 1996.
148. Autio-Harmainen, H., Karttunen, T., Hurskainen, T., Hoyhtya, M., Kauppila, A., and Tryggvason, K. Expression of 72 kDA type IV collagenase (gelatinase A) in benign and malignant ovarian tumors. Lab Invest 1993; 69: 312-21.
149. Afzal, S., Lalani, E., Foulkes, W. D., Boyce, B., Tickle, S., Cardillo, M. R., Baker, T., Pignatelli, M., and Stamp, G. W. Matrix metalloproteinase-2 and tissue inhibitor of maetalloproteinase-2 expression and syntehtic matrix metalloproteinase-2 inhibitor binding in ovarian carcinomas and tumor cell lines. Lab Invest 1996; 74: 406 - 421.
150. Garzetti, G. G., Ciavattin, A., Lucarini, G., Goteri, G., Romanini, C., and Biagini, G. Increased serum 72 kDa metalloproteinase in serous ovarian tumors: comparison with CA125. Anticancer Res 1996; 16.
151. Davies, B., Brown, P. D., N, E., J, C. M., and Blakwill, F. R. A synthetic matrix metalloproteinase inhibitor decreases tumor burden and prolongs survival of mice bearing human ovarian carcinoma xenografts. Cancer Res 1993; 194:2087 - 2091.
152. Beattie, G. J. and Smyth, J. F. Phase I study of intraperitoneal metalloproteinase inhibitor BB94 in patients with malignant ascites. Clin Cancer Res 1998; 4.
153. Parsons, S. L., Watson, S. A., and Steele, R. J. Phase I/II trial of batimastat, a matrix metalloproteinase inhibitor, in patients with malignant ascites. European Journal of Surgical Cancer 1997;23: 526-31.
154. Nagase, H. and Woessner, J. F. Matrix metalloproteinases. J Biol Chem 1999; 274:21491-21494.
155. Gomez, D. E., Alonso, D. F., Yoshiji, H., and Thorgeirsson, U. P. Tissue inhibitors of metalloproteinases: structure, regulation and biological functions. Eur J Cell Biol 1997; 74:111-122.
156. Corcoran, M. L., Kleiner, D. E., and Stetler-Stevenson, W. G. Regulation of matrix metalloproteinases during extracellular matrix turnover. Adv Exp Med Biol 1995; 385:151-9.
157. Schnaper, H. W., Grant, D. S., Stetler-Stevenson, W. G., Fridman, R., D'Orazi, G., Murphy, A. N., Bird, R. E., Hoythya, M., Fuerst, T. R., and French, D. L. Type IV collagenase(s) and TIMPs modulate endothelial cell morphogenesis in vitro. Journal of Cell Physiology 1993; 156:235-46.
158. Murphy, A. N., Unsworth, E. J., and Stetler-Stevenson, W. G. Tissue inhibitor of metalloproteinases-2 inhibits bFGF-induced human microvascular endothelial cell proliferation. J Cell Physiol 1993; 157: 351-358.
159. Lamoreaux, W. J., Fitzgerald, M. E., Reiner, A., Hasty, K. A., and Charles, S. T. Vascular endothelial growth factor increases release of gelatinase A and decreases release of tissue

inhibitor of metalloproteinases by microvascular endothelial cells in vitro. Microvasc Res 1998; 55:29-42.

160. Moser, T. L., Young, T. N., and Rodriguez, G. C. Secretion of extracellular matrix-degrading proteinases is increased in epithelial ovarian carcinoma. Int J Cancer 1994; 56:552-559.

161. Takemura, M., Azuma, C., Kimura, T., Kanai, T., Saji, F., and Tanizawa, O. Type-IV collagenase and tissue inhibitor of metalloproteinase in ovarian cancer tissues. Int J Gynaecol Obstet 1994; 46:303-9.

162. Mignatti, P. and Rifkin, D. B. Plasminogen activators and matrix metalloproteinases in angiogenesis. Enzyme Protein 1996; 49:117-37.

163. Andreasen, P. A., Kjoller, L., Christensen, L., and Duffy, M. J. The urokinase-type plasminogen activator system in cancer metastasis: a review. Int J Cancer 1997; 72:1-22..

164. Conese, M. and Blasi, F. The urokinase/urokinase-receptor system and cancer invasion. Baillieres Clin Haemat 1995; 8:365-389.

165. Karlan, B. Y., Amin, W., Band, V., Zurawski, V. R., and Littlefield, B. A. Plasminogen activator secretion by established lines of human ovarian carcinoma cells in vitro. Gynecol Oncol 1988; 31:103-12.

166. Schmitt, M., Wilhelm, O., Janicke, F., Magdolen, V., Reuning, U., Ohi, H., Moniwa, N., Kobayashi, H., Weidle, U., and Graeff, H. Urokinase-type plasminogen activator (uPA) and its receptor (CD87): a new target in tumor invasion and metastasis. J Obstet Gynaecol 1995; 21:151-165.

167. Pedersen, H., Brunner, N., Francis, D., Osterlind, K., Ronne, E., Hansen, H. H., Dano, K., and Grondahl-Hansen, J. Prognostic impact of urokinase, urokinase receptor, and type 1 plasminogen activator inhibitor in squamous and large cell lung cancer tissue. Cancer Res 1994; 54:4671-4675.

168. Pujade-Lauraine, H., Lu, H., Mirshahi, S., Soria, J., Soria, C., Bernadou, A., Kruithof, E. K. O., Lijnen, H. R., and Burtin, P. The plasminogen activation system in ovarian tumors. Int J Cancer 1993; 55:27-31.

169. Ho, C. H., Yuan, C. C., and Liu, S. M. Diagnostic and prognostic values of plasma levels of fibrinolytic markers in ovarian cancer. Gynecol Oncol 1999; 75: 397-400.

170. Kuhn, W., Schmalfeldt, B., Reuning, U., Pache, L., Berger, U., Ulm, K., Harbeck, N., Spathe, K., Dettmar, P., Hofler, H., Janicke, F., Schmitt, M., and Graeff, H. Prognostic significance of urokinase (uPA) and its inhibitor PAI-1 for survival in advanced ovarian carcinoma stage FIGO IIIc. Br J Cancer 1999; 79:1746-51.

171. Abendstein, B., Daxenbichler, G., Windbichler, G., Zeimet, A. G., Geurts, A., Sweep, F., and Marth, C. Predictive value of uPA, PAI-1, HER-2, and VEGF in the serum of ovarian cancer patients. Anticancer Res 2000; 20: 569-72.

172. Hoffmann, G., Pollow, K., Weikel, W., Strittmatter, H. J., Bach, J., Schaffrath, M., Knapstein, P., Melchert, F., and Pollow, B. Urokinase and plasminogen activator-inhibitor (PAI-1) status in primary ovarian carcinomas and ovarian metastases compared to benign ovarian tumors as a funcion of histopathological parameters. Clin Chem Lab Med 1999; 37: 47-54.

Index

α2 antiplasmin 333
α2 macroglobulin 333
Activin 294-297
Activin receptor 295,299
Amino terminal fragment 335
Angiogenesis 355,360
Angiopoietin 361
Angiostatin 363,364
Antennapedia complex 233,234

Bax 138,139
BRCA 6-8,30,33,35-48,138,140,172,186
Bithorax complex 232,233
Borderline malignant potential tumors 105
Brenner tumor 195
Breast/ovarian cancer 35,172
Bystander effect 135, 136

c-kit 286
CA125 8,11,15,63-76,79-81,83,85,100-102,107-8,120,121,138,162,164,166,168,241,276,287,343,368
Call-Exner bodies 187,196
Carboplatin 107,110
Cathepsin B 343
CD44 306-311,318,322
Chocolate cyst 189
Choriocarcinoma 201,202
Cisplatin 107,109,110-112,138
Collagen 166,168,187,197,306,312,314,317,318,336,339,354,362,367,370
Colony stimulating factor (CSF) 285,287,288,337,338
Colony stimulating factor receptor 285,288-290
Comparative genomic hybridization 62
Corpus albicans 188
Corpus luteum 188
Creatine kinase 82
Crystals of Reinke 197
Cyclophosphamide 107,109,111,112,145
Cytoreductive surgery 104
Cytosine deaminase 134

Doppler imaging, color 120,122,123
Doxorubicin 111
Dysgerminoma 198,199,201

E-cadherin 162,164,166,168,173,174,270,306,320-322,364,367
Endometriod carcinoma 191,193
Endothelial differentiation gene (Edg) 259-263,265-266,270,277
Endometrial sinus tumor 199,201
Endostatin 363,364
Epidemiology 3,5,30,119
Epidermal growth factor (EGF) 15,147,169,338
Epidermal growth factor receptor (EGFR) 15,81,139,170,247,248,251,252-254,269,337,364
Epithelio-mesenchymal conversion 166,167
ErbB 16,17,113,137,139,140,142,143,247,252-254,261,269,338
Expression array analysis 62,81
Extracellular matrix (ECM) 168,305,306,312,314,317,319,321,331-333,335,336,339,353,358
Extracellular response kinase (ERK) 262-267,269-274

Familial ovarian cancer 31,33,36,38,40,172
Fibroblast growth factor 362,370
Fibroma 197
Fibrosarcoma 197
Focal adhesion kinase 273,319,339
Follicles 187
Follicle stimulating hormone (FSH) 294,297,298

Ganciclovir 135,136
Gelsolin 260
Gemcitabine 111
Gene therapy 133,142,145,146
Germ cell tumor 189,223
Glucocorticoids 288m289
Granulosa cells 162,187,294,297
Granulosa cell tumor 195,196,201,297,299

Hand-foot-genital syndrome 236
Hepatocyte growth factor 362
HER-2/*neu* 9,84,141,170,261
hTERT 215,216,220-222
Homeobox genes 231
Hox genes 233-243

Hyaluronan 307-311,318,319

Immunopotentiation 133,134
Immunotherapy, active 142,143
Immunotherapy, passive 142
Inclusion cyst 164
Inhibin 294,298,299
Inhibin receptor 298,299
Integrin 163,306,312,315-320,322,339,364,367,368

Kallikrein 82

Laminin 169,314-318,333,367,370
Laparoscopy 104,108,186
Laparotomy 108
Leutinizing hormone (LH) 294
Leydig cells 197
Lynch syndrome 172
Lysophosphatidic acid (LPA) 12-14,80,81,86,101,259-277,338,355
Lysophosphatidylcholine 260,273,274,360

Matrix metalloproteinase (MMP) 12,14,269,332,333,335-339,341-343,364,367-370
Mesothelial cells 305,310,317,318,339
Mesothelioma 191
Microarray analysis 285
Microsatellite instability 37
Mixed epithelial tumor 189
MLH gene 37,38,41,46
Mucinous tumor 191,192
Multidrug resistance 144,145
Mutation compensation 133,137

N-cadherin 163,166,173

Ovarian dysplasia 19
Ovarian intraepithelial neoplasia 19
Ovarian "Pap" test 4,19,85
Ovarian surface epithelium 161,163-176

p53 10,62,138,140,141,147
Paclitaxel 107,110,138,141
Pericytes 357

Peutz-Jeghers syndrome 198
Phosphatidylinositol 3-kinase 262,263
Plasmin 332,334,340,343,370
Plasminogen activator inhibitor (PAI) 332,337,339-341,371
Platelet activating factor 260,273
Platelet derived growth factor (PDGF) 357
Polyembryoma 201
Positive predictive value 4,63,120
Psammoma bodies 188,191
Premalignant lesion 18,38
Prostasin 82
PTEN 138

Rho 261,262
Ribozyme 137,138

Schiller-Duval bodies 200
Second-look surgery 108,110,112,223
Serous tumor 190
Smad 295,296,299
Small cell carcinoma 189
Sphingosylphosphorylcholine 260,262,273,274

Telomere 213,214
Telomerase 15,215-224
Teratoma 189,202,203
Thecoma 197
Thrompospondin 364
Thymidine kinase 134,135,136
Tissue inhibitor of metalloproteinases (TIMP) 334,337-339,370,371
Tissue-type plasminogen activator 332,335,370
Topotecan 110
Transabdominal ultrasound 64,121
Transforming growth factor (TGF) β 295,296,299,357
Transvaginal ultrasound 8,64,68,73-75,85,120,121,124
Tumor suppressor genes 134,138
Tunica albuginea 164

Urinary-type plasminogen activator (uPA, urokinase) 12, 14-15,269,289,332,333,335,337-341,343,370,371
Urinary-type plasminogen activator receptor (uPAR) 332,335,340,341

Vascular endothelial growth factor 269,338,355-361,364,370

Vinrelbine 110

Wilms tumor 222

Yolk sac tumor 199,201